Palliative Care: An Integrated Approach

Palliative Care: An Integrated Approach

Jenny Buckley, RGN, RNT, MA (Nursing), Diploma in Palliative Care
Head of Education
St Wilfrid's Hospice
Chichester, UK

WILEY-BLACKWELL

A John Wiley & Sons, Ltd., Publication

This edition first published 2008

© 2008 John Wiley & Sons, Ltd

Wiley-Blackwell is an imprint of John Wiley and Sons, formed by the merger of Wiley's global Scientific, Technical and Medical business with Blackwell Publishing

Registered office
John Wiley & Sons Ltd, The Atrium, Southern Gate, Chichester, West Sussex, PO19 8SQ, United Kingdom

Editorial office
John Wiley & Sons Ltd, The Atrium, Southern Gate, Chichester, West Sussex, PO19 8SQ, United Kingdom

For details of our global editorial offices, for customer services and for information about how to apply for permission to reuse the copyright material in this book please see our website at www.wiley.com/wiley-blackwell.

Library of Congress Cataloging-in-Publication Data is available

ISBN: 9780470058855

A catalogue record for this book is available from the British Library.

Set in 10/12 pt Palatino by SNP Best-set Typesetter Ltd., Hong Kong
Printed in Singapore by Markono Print Media Pte Ltd

1   2008

Contents

Foreword

The rapidly evolving field of palliative care has received increasing recognition and interest in response to the growth in the populations living with chronic, debilitating and life-threatening illnesses, and a focus by health-care professionals, across disciplines, on developing and implementing effective approaches to address physical, psychological, social and spiritual pain that contribute to suffering, undermining the quality of life and preventing a death with comfort and dignity. In recent years there has been an increasing number of books written about palliative care and, although some have contributed to the body of knowledge of palliative care, none has taken such a thorough and comprehensive integrative holistic approach to palliative care across settings (hospital, home, community). Although written from the context of palliative care in the UK, the home of the hospice movement, the book has universal application. It provides clear insight into many of the complex issues that arise in the delivery of palliative care and provides an invaluable resource to all disciplines involved in palliative care in hospital, hospice and community settings. The author of the book, drawing from an extensive career in providing critical as well as palliative care, has effectively combined the theory and practice of palliative care into one book and has linked patient stories with practical advice, thereby delineating clinical practice in a way that reflects the daily concerns of clinicians. A central aim of the book is to reaffirm that palliative care is within the scope of all health-care professionals in any setting. An integrative approach is taken where the orthodox approach to treatment and care is discussed alongside a complementary approach and the art and science of palliative care are made explicit. The concept of holism, namely the patient being able to use their own inner resources, i.e. empowerment, is clearly evident throughout. This book points out that we cannot sit beside patients and support them in using their own resources until we know how they are feeling. Asking the questions often takes great courage but, as the author of the book states, 'until we do, we follow our own agenda, not that of the patient'. This book will give the clinician the confidence to follow the patient's agenda.

The scientific foundation of palliative care is advancing rapidly and the author effectively integrates both research and recognised theorists and experts in the field on palliative care in a way that moves the clinician to evidence-based application and practice. Existing data and evidence, drawn from clinical and research settings, are provided in a manner that is practical, informative and useful for clinicians. Key psychoneuroimmunology research is reviewed with reference to practice, as are the critical concepts of resilience, hope and decision-making for both patients and the health-care professionals. Palliative care is addressed, not only from the provision of care to the patient and family, but from the importance of self-awareness, self-care and reflective practice for the clinician providing the care. Extensive information on cultural considerations, impact on second, third and fourth generations, and implications for vulnerable groups are found throughout the book. A cadre of assessment screening tools and guidelines necessary to provide quality, evidence-based care to individuals with life-limiting illness and their families is presented. Important implications for practice are discussed at the end of each chapter and case studies and short reflections on practice, and insightful poems springing from practice, are used to move the reader's thinking forward. Excellent resources and suggestions with implications for practice permeate each chapter, along with an extensive reference list at the end of the book.

The book flows logically from a comprehensive review of the important historical and cultural perspectives on the evolution of palliative care, to a comprehensive discussion of communication skills, and the psychosocial and spiritual approaches to care that focus on the importance of helping the patient determine the pace at which information is shared and the person's desired level of autonomy, to an integrated approach to pain and symptom management, to living with progressive disease and death, and finally to the bereavement period. Each chapter, however, is designed to stand on its own, and as such provides clinicians with indepth information, practical clinically relevant tables and boxes, and other helpful tools and guides on a specific topic area.

This book is an invaluable read and a resource for all health-care professionals who want to take an evidence-based, holistic, integrative and insightful approach to providing comprehensive palliative care to adults, children and their families.

Dr Kaye Herth
Dean, College of Allied Health and Nursing
Minnesota State University
Mankato, USA

Contributors' biographies

Jenny Buckley, RGN, RNT, MA(Nursing), Diploma in Palliative Care

Jenny Buckley is Head of Education at St Wilfrid's Hospice in Chichester. Her career in nursing spans four decades! Her early clinical years were spent in critical care and acute medicine. Her most memorable jobs by far were as a staff nurse on the liver unit at King's College Hospital and later as a ward sister on the liver unit at the Royal Free Hospital. She became a nurse tutor before having a career break to have her three children. She returned to work as a staff nurse on the inpatient unit at St Wilfrid's Hospice, then as a clinical nurse specialist and now as Head of Education. Her MA research was on hope and the dying person.

Kay de Vries, PhD, MSc, PGCEA, BSc(Hons), RGN, RM

Kay de Vries currently holds a joint post with the Faculty of Health and Medical Sciences, Division of Health and Social Care, University of Surrey, Guildford and the Princess Alice Hospice, Esher, Surrey. Her role at the University involves teaching on specialist subjects (end-of-life care for older people and people with dementia and other palliative care subjects), research methodology and supervision of BSc, MSc and PhD students, plus involvement in a number of research projects. Her role at the Hospice involves management of the education department, plus teaching on specialist subjects within the hospice and the wider community, e.g. hospitals, nursing and residential homes and other hospices.

Amanda Free, BBS, DCH, DRCOG, Dip Pall Med

Amanda Free is a GP with a Special Interest (GPSI) and Macmillan GP Facilitator in Palliative Care, Surrey PCT, GP Principal, Integrated Care Partnership, Epsom and a GP Associate, GSF Core Team. Having trained at St George's and completed her VTS she has worked as a partner in general practice in Epsom ever since. Her main interest is in providing holistic and personal care to her patients. In 2003 she completed her Diploma in Palliative Medicine and became a Macmillan GP Facilitator in Cancer and Palliative Care in Surrey. In 2006 the post was expanded to include a GPSI role and an honorary contract with Princess Alice Hospice. The aim of this post is to ensure that patients at the end of life in the community receive appropriate care, and that all agencies are working together to achieve this. Since 2004 she has worked with Keri Thomas as a GP Associate on the Gold Standards Framework (GSF) team, with a lead role in the care of patients with non-cancer-related illness.

Kaye Herth, PhD, RN, FAAN

Kaye Herth is Dean, College of Allied Health and Nursing, Minnesota State University, Mankato, USA. She earned a diploma in nursing from St Luke's Hospital School of Nursing, Racine, WI, a Bachelor of Science degree in nursing from Northern Illinois University, DeKalb, IL, Master of Science degree in nursing at the University of Minnesota, and a PhD degree in nursing from Texas Woman's University, Denton, TX. She has extensive clinical, teaching and administrative experience at several universities, and in hospitals, hospices and community health settings. Her research has focused on hope, humour and grief in those individuals with a chronic or terminal illness and the impact on their family/significant others, as well as homeless families and children. Her instruments to measure hope have been translated into 12 foreign languages and are used throughout the world. She has over 62 publications in reviewed professional journals and over 200 presentations at regional, national and international professional conferences. She has co-authored a book on hope and hopelessness and published chapters in eight major nursing and healthcare texts addressing hope, humour and grief. Kaye serves on the editorial boards of four professional journals and as a manuscript reviewer for seven professional journals. She was included in the biographical directory entitled *Two Thousand Outstanding Scientists of the 20th Century*. She has received numerous honours and awards for her scholarship, leadership and professorship, including her selection as a Fellow in the American Academy of Nursing and as a Sigma Theta Tau International Nursing Honor Society Distinguished Lecturer.

Marie Price, CQSW, Dip SW, Dip Couns, Cert Couples counselling

Throughout her career Marie has been interested in the impact of loss, bereavement and change on individuals, families, groups and organisations. As a social worker, her work was mainly with children; through this she became acutely aware of how the situations experienced impacted on their lives into adulthood, affecting their ability to make relationships and to live their lives in a meaningful, productive way. This included children coming into care and the implications, through to children who were being adopted, and to the loss for the birth parents, the adoptive parents who may not have been able to have their own children and again the children themselves. Her career then concentrated on working in hospices where the ultimate/permanent loss was anticipated – the loss through death. During this time she became aware of how all the losses accumulated through life were often there to be worked through and that included losses and situations that no one else may be aware of – the hidden losses that may not be spoken of for a variety of reasons, such as shame, guilt or a wish to protect those close to them. In addition to qualifying as a social worker Marie is a counsellor and currently works for the University of Chichester and Chichester Counselling Services as a tutor/lecturer, as well as having a private practice for clients and supervision.

Keri Thomas MB, BS, MRCGP, DRCOG, MSc (Pall Med)

Keri Thomas is National Clinical Lead of the Gold Standards Framework Centre, based in Walsall PCT, aiming to enable top quality care for all people nearing the end of life. As a GP for 22 years, and the originator of the Gold Standards Framework (GSF) for community palliative care in 2001, she continues to lead the GSF Programme in both primary care and care homes. GSF is extensively used across the country, with about two thirds of all GP practices, a large number of care homes using the specifically adapted GSF for Care Homes Programme, and several international partner projects developing. She is Hon. Senior Lecturer at University of Birmingham and Chair of the newly developed charity Omega, the National Association for End of Life Care, focusing on enabling, training and supporting the generalist workforce to provide quality end of life care. She has written and lectured extensively in the UK and abroad on community palliative care and end of life care. She was formally National Clinical Lead for Palliative Care (Generalist) in the Department of Health's End of Life Care Programme, and has been involved in consultation for various national strategic groups, including the Prime Minister's Strategy Group, several Parliamentary consultations, and the emerging National NHS End of Life Care Strategy in England. Her greatest achievement, however, is as wife and mother of five children.

Acknowledgements

My thanks to Jim McCarthy, who invited me to write this book, and to Emma Hatfield, Emma Lonie, Magenta Lampson and all at Wiley-Blackwell for their expertise and support.

Thanks also to the Board of Trustees and Senior Management Team at St Wilfrid's Hospice for granting me sabbatical leave to kick start this project. In particular, thank you to my colleagues Bridget Halward and Lynne Morgan for their moral support and encouragement, and to Nicola Gardner who came to my rescue, yet again, this time with her word processing skills.

Thank you to Bev Applin, Dr Kaye Herth, Dr Suzy Jordache, Michele Kent, Brenda Waters and Sally Reynolds for reviewing this text and their subsequent helpful comments. I am indebted to my many colleagues who have been students at St Wilfrid's over the years; their stories and knowledge shared enrich this book. My gratitude also to my lovely family for their support on the many book-designated Sundays. I am also extremely grateful to Darrel, George, Mike and all at the Dunhill library at St Richard's Hospital for their patience with me and their help in locating appropriate literature. Grateful thanks to the following people for their contributions in the following chapters:

- Kay de Vries in Chapters 3 and 9.
- Kaye Herth in Chapter 6
- Marie Price in Chapter 9
- Amanda Free in Chapter 14
- Keri Thomas in Chapter 14.

Last but by no means least a heartfelt thank you to Gloria Smith, Jenny Guy, Pink June and their team without whose unstinting support over many years this book would not have happened.

Dedications

This book is dedicated to Steve, Tom, Aimée and Katie who give meaning to every moment of my life and to our dear friend Seraphina.

Also to my Aunt Edith Fincham who features in Chapter 9 of this book, Howard, Niki, Jane and David featured in the poem in Chapter 3, and Eva Marie and Nicky, subjects of poems in Chapter 4. All too old to die young.

Chapter 1
Historical and cultural perspectives on the evolution of palliative care

KEY POINTS

- **Introduction**: palliative care is one of the success stories in the health service. In a death-denying society, as a result of work in the hospice movement, good-quality palliative care is now high on the government's agenda.
- **Death in society**: as health care has improved, death has been marginalised. Today society grapples with Victorian Romanticism, which portrays death of a loved one as unbearable, and twentieth-century denial, which sees death as a failure (Aries 1983). Death is a normal part of living.
- **Dame Cicely Saunders and the origins of contemporary palliative care**: Dame Cicely became a doctor with the intention of making a difference to the quality of dying for cancer patients. Her remarkable story has led to the modern-day organisation and approach to the care of people who are dying.
- **An international perspective**: international networking and some of the initiatives that exist to keep palliative care high on the international agenda are explored.
- **Definitions**: these shape our attitude and approach to the work that we do. Current definitions are presented and some discussion is raised about their implications. Definitions should implicate the patient's role. When they do not, are they disempowering? A health-promoting approach is encouraged.
- **End-of-life care**: the End-of-Life Programme examines current initiatives concerned with providing equity, continuity and choice to patients who receive palliative care. The tools used for this are the Gold Standards Framework, Preferred Place of Care initiative and Liverpool Care Pathway.
- **Culture**: in a multicultural society information about, and access to, palliative services among many minority ethnic groups cause some concern. Aspects of research in this area are highlighted. The tensions that can exist in professional roles as a result of dominant philosophical approaches are discussed.
- **Service user involvement**: recent legislation has set the scene for service users to be involved at all stages in shaping services. It is hoped that this will lead to less need for patient groups taking an adversarial role. Local initiatives in involving service users are important.

INTRODUCTION

This first chapter aims to provide a historical and cultural perspective on the evolution of palliative care; it then goes on to describe and discuss definitions and frameworks for the delivery of contemporary palliative care. The twentieth century heralded enormous advances in medical science and the introduction of the National Health Service. The health of the nation's people was being valued as never before. Diagnosis, cure and health promotion dominated in this new health-care system. Death was marginalised. Intellectually we all know that we are going to die, but emotionally perhaps we deny this. Possibly this is why health-care professionals have, over the years, failed to give good end-of-life care. Dying is not a dress rehearsal.

In the middle of the twentieth century Dame Cicely Saunders and other committed colleagues, both in this country and around the world, challenged a death-denying health-care system. The hospice movement was born. Palliative care is considered to be one of the great success stories in health care over the past 40 years. The challenge now is to continue to transfer and embed what has developed in the hospice sector into the mainstream NHS (Ellershaw and Murphy 2005).

The document *Building on the Best: Choice responsiveness and equity in the NHS* (Department of Health or DH 2003a) highlighted that patients and carers want choice over care at the end of their lives. In another recently published government report, *Our Health, Our Care, Our Say: A new direction for community services* (DH 2006), there was recognition that more investment is needed in end-of-life care and a statement to endorse an earlier call that is relevant to increased expenditure. The government is on board; the scene is set; provision of a high-quality palliative care service is the remit of every health-care professional working in all areas of health care.

DEATH IN SOCIETY

Historical perspective

Advances in public health, e.g. understanding infection control, the importance of clean water and the introduction of immunisations for all, have meant that, since the second half of the twentieth century, the death of children and young adults is rare. It is over 60 years now since the end of World War II. In this country we have a society that is less 'used' to death than ever before. In line with many parts of Europe, North America and Australia, death now is less often sudden and unexpected, and more often associated with chronic disease of long duration (Clark 2004).

Political initiatives over the past 20 years have encouraged people to take greater charge of their own health, e.g. *Promoting Better Health* (DH 1987) and *The Health of The Nation* (DH 1991a). Against this backdrop and a continuing focus on health promotion, coupled with the media's almost obsessive preoccupation with the 'body beautiful', it probably makes it emotionally more difficult now, than ever before, to accept ill health and dying. Conversely the efficiency of the media can make us witness to the atrocities of violent death in our own society and around the world, sometimes on the scale of genocide. Deaths from famine, natural disasters and manmade disasters are also brought to our attention all too regularly. It is impossible to make a blanket statement on what effect this dichotomy may have on each person's attitude to mortality.

Sociologists have been commenting on the depersonalisation of death for some years. They identify a process in which the care of those who are dying and of death has been taken out of the hands of family and friends, and put into the hands of health-care professionals and funeral directors. With this process, the customary mourning practices have disappeared (Gorer 1955; Aries 1983; Walter 1994; Clark 2005b). Gorer (1955) pinpoints the beginning of the end of mourning customs to World War I, when the magnitude of the number of deaths and the need to keep the war effort going hindered mourning.

Spiritual care

Historically the spiritual care of those who are dying was of paramount importance and this was often portrayed in literature by the clergy, who had a predominant role at the deathbed. The events of World War I diminished the role of spirituality in dying, according to Walter (1994). In a Christian religious context, absolution from sin before death represents spirituality. Who would not absolve a soldier dying in terrible circumstances for his country? There was a sense of the clergy feeling humbled and inadequate. Doctors and public health workers have supplanted priests at the bedside of those who are dying (Walter 1994). Although we know that a person's spirituality does not necessarily exist in a religious context, it has been represented by clergy in the formal structure of society.

Today society grapples with the influence of Victorian Romanticism which portrayed the death of a loved one as unbearable and twentieth-century denial that sees death as a failure (Aries 1983). Gorer's (1955) statements about a society that reports death daily and proliferates media and journal articles about death, also being a society that finds it difficult to talk about their own personal grieving seem as relevant now as they did then.

DAME CICELY SAUNDERS AND THE ORIGINS OF CONTEMPORARY PALLIATIVE CARE

Historically contemporary palliative care services are embodied within the hospice movement, which was launched by the opening of St Christopher's Hospice (a registered charity) in Sydenham, south London on 24 July 1967. This was the first teaching and research hospice of its kind in the world. The founder of the hospice movement was Dame Cicely Saunders. Dame Cicely, first a nurse and then a social worker, trained in medicine with the sole intention of challenging the dominant model that valued cure at the expense of being responsive to the individual experiences of those who are dying.

In the 1950s, around the world about a dozen homes had been set up as charities to care for dying people. It was while working as a volunteer in one such home, St Luke's Hospital in Bayswater, that Dame Cicely witnessed pain being controlled much more effectively than in general hospice wards, and 'much more besides'. At this time she worked as an almoner at St Thomas' Hospital. She spoke to the surgeon for whom she worked about this. He told her that there was much more to learn about pain and that she would only be frustrated in any efforts to make a difference unless she was a doctor. It was then that she decided to enter medical school and he helped her with this (Clark 2006).

A patient, David Tasma, who died of cancer in London's Archway Hospital in 1947, has been credited as being the inspiration for Dame Cicely's work with dying people (Clark 2006). He was a young man who had been in the Warsaw Ghetto. Cicely, as an almoner, was drawn to him and their relationship intensified 'into a fragile loving friendship' (Clark 2006). The two discussed the idea of creating more 'home like' places where people could die. David had said to her, 'I want only what is in your mind and in your heart'. Clark (2006) describes this combination of emotion and intellect as being the guiding theme in her subsequent work. David Tasma left Dame Cicely £500 in his will, saying that 'I'll be the window in your home'. In her Templeton Prize speech, given in 1981, Dame Cicely said:

> Here was a commission from a dying man who felt he had made no impact on the world, a commission to give meaning to his life by creating a home dedicated to openness and to the balance of mind and heart, of skill and friendship.
>
> Saunders in Clark (2006, p 158)

It was a momentous achievement that 19 years later St Christopher's was opened. Dame Cicely has described it as building the home around the window (Clark 2006, p xvi).

For the first 18 years of its existence Dame Cicely was the medical director at St Christopher's. During this time she developed a home care service and a specialist education unit. She continued to research pain control and the effectiveness of the hospice. She was well known for her international lecture tours and she regularly published – some 220 works in total. She also taught in the education unit. She left no stone unturned. On a study day I ran recently a delegate described how Dame Cicely had visited her primary school in south London to explain the work of the hospice. She remembers it as having death explained clearly to her and fear being removed.

Notably her writings are almost always firmly grounded in practice. In her paper on the treatment of intractable pain, she writes of keeping analysed detailed records of 900 patients who had died (Saunders 2006a). She regularly tape-recorded interviews with her patients in order that she could reflect on their descriptions of physical pain and their experiences of facing death. Many of her earlier articles, in particular, are based on case histories.

Other palliative pioneers

Dame Cicely is not the only person responsible for palliative care becoming part of mainstream medical and health care. Many have made valuable contributions, but notably Eric Wilkes, Robert Twycross, Neil MacDonald, Derek Doyle, Elisabeth Kübler-Ross, Balfour Mount and Colin Murray Parkes and, I'm sure, many others working on both sides of the Atlantic. Significant landmarks that can be attributed to their efforts are the General Medical Council according palliative medicine a specialist status in 1987 and the inception of the National Council for Specialist Hospice and Palliative Care Services shortly afterwards, which, from 2004, has been known as the National Council for Palliative Care (NCPC). It is important now to stop seeing hospices as buildings and to see them rather as representing a philosophy of care.

Future challenges

One challenge for the future is to continue to develop a palliative approach in all health-care settings – in hospitals, care homes and at home. In *Building on the Best: Choice, responsiveness and equity in the NHS* (DH 2003a) it is highlighted that patients and carers want choice over end-of-life care. The End-of-Life Programme (NHS Confederation 2005) is committed to taking forward training programmes, so that all adult patients nearing the end of life will have access to high-quality palliative care. One aim of the programme is that people will have a choice about where they die. This initiative is being managed by strategic health authorities (SHAs).

The second future challenge is concerned with the considerable body of knowledge and research that has built up over the years. Historically this is embedded in cancer care because this is where it all began. We need to continue to examine and, where appropriate, transfer knowledge and evidence accrued in cancer care to the care of people with all other life-threatening illnesses. It is also important to keep developing the evidence base for all aspects of care. How far things have come since Dame Cicely first met David Tasma in 1947.

The National Council for Palliative Care

It is appropriate here to look at the aims of the NCPC and what the provision of specialist palliative care services in the UK is at this time. The NCPC aims to:

- identify and develop policy proposals that enable improved palliative care and wider access to this
- influence the policies of the governments in England, Wales and Northern Ireland to this end
- identify good clinical practice management and disseminate.

The strategy is (NCPC 2005a):

- to promote improvement in the quality and availability of palliative care to patients with cancer, their families and carers
- to promote the extension of palliative care to patients with other life-threatening conditions, their families and carers.

The current provision of specialist palliative care services, as of January 2006 in England, Wales and Northern Ireland, was (NCPC 2005b):

- 193 specialist inpatient units providing 2774 beds, of which 20% were NHS beds
- 295 home care services; at present this figure will include both primary advisory services delivered by hospices or NHS-based community palliative care teams and more sustained care delivered in patients' homes
- 314 hospital-based services
- 234 day-care services
- 314 bereavement support services.

AN INTERNATIONAL PERSPECTIVE

From the inception of the idea of St Christopher's, international links were made. In 1967 an American colleague wrote to Dame Cicely from New York:

> I think you should realise that you have two obligations. One is to continue your work which you are doing in the development of your own centre at St Christopher's and the other is to teach the world what you have learned.

Clark (2005a, p 11)

In the period 1959–67 her published letters include correspondence with colleagues in many different parts of the USA, Switzerland, Sri Lanka, the Netherlands, France and South Africa. As Medical Director at St Christopher's she visited North America regularly and made strong professional bonds with Balfour Mount at the palliative services at the Royal Victoria Hospital in Montreal. She was a regular visitor to the international conferences that he has hosted every 2 years from 1976. She also visited many other countries, including Yugoslavia, Belgium, Australia, Israel and South Africa (Clark 2005a). There are many examples of international collaboration in the palliative care arena. The *Oxford Textbook of Palliative Medicine* is now in its third edition (Doyle et al. 2005) and it contains contributions from all members of the multidisciplinary team around the world.

World Health Organization

The United Nations Specialised Agency for Health, i.e. the World Health Organization (see www.who.int/cancer/palliative/pain ladder/en/index.html), has a remit for palliative care. The WHO is governed by 192 member states throughout the world assembly. In collaboration with the International Organization for the Relief of Pain, the WHO has established the three-step pain relief ladder that is generally adopted by all specialist palliative care units and based on the early work of Dame Cicely and her colleagues.

Some 52 million people die in the world each year with approximately one in ten of these deaths being from cancer. Millions more suffer from other life-threatening illnesses such as AIDS. Often the need is greatest where resources are poor. Barriers to caring for those who are dying include lack of financial resources, non-availability of vital medicines, no opportunity for training or support, and long-standing conflicts and natural disasters. In spite of these obstacles, it is now estimated that palliative care services exist, or are being developed, in 100 countries (Help the Hospices 2006).

The *Hospice Information Bulletin* is a magazine produced jointly by St Christopher's and Help the Hospices. Through this publication 6000 people in over 100 countries in the world are contacted (Help the Hospices 2006). Help the Hospices, in partnership with palliative care associations around the world, has produced a report called *Suffering at the End of Life – The state of the world* and it was published by the Help the Hospices (2005). This report highlights current issues by using facts and figures, case studies and photographs. Below are some extracts from it.

Facts and figures

> There are currently more than 13 million children under 15 years of age who have lost one or both parents to AIDS. Most live in sub-Saharan Africa. By 2020, the number is expected to increase to more than 25 million. AIDS brings psychosocial distress and material hardship to children. They may be pressed into service to care for ill and dying parents, required to drop out of school to help with farm or household work, or experience declining access to food and health services. Many are at risk of exclusion, abuse, discrimination and stigma.
>
> Help the Hospices (2005, p 11)

Table 1.1 summarises the findings of 64 studies and shows the symptoms experienced by patients with specific diseases (Solano et al. 2006).

Table 1.1 Prevalence of symptoms in advanced diseases, based on a systematic review of 64 studies

Symptoms	Cancer	AIDS	Heart disease	COPD	Renal disease
Pain	35–96	63–80	41–77	34–77	47–50
Depression	3–77	10–82	9–36	37–71	5–60
Anxiety	13–79	8–34	49	51–75	39–70
Confusion	6–93	30–65	18–32	18–33	?
Fatigue	32–90	54–85	69–82	68–80	73–87
Breathlessness	10–70	11–62	60–88	90–95	11–62
Insomnia	9–69	74	36–48	55–65	31–71
Nausea	6–68	43–49	17–48	?	30–43
Constipation	23–65	34–35	38–42	27–44	29–70
Diarrhoea	3–29	30–90	12	?	21
Anorexia	30–92	51	21–41	35–67	25–64

From Solano et al. (2006). Reproduced with the permission and help of the authors.
AIDS, acquired immune deficiency syndrome; COPD, chronic obstructive pulmonary disease.

Hospice or palliative care has been identified as a relatively cheap and effective means of meeting the needs of those nearing the end of their lives, thereby ensuring that they do not suffer unnecessarily.

The case of Uganda shows that palliative care is not just for wealthy industrialised nations. Uganda was the first African country to make palliative care for people with AIDS and cancer part of its national health plan (2000–2005). A clear national policy has been established, with appropriate education for health professionals at all levels. Affordable morphine has been made easily available in the country.

Help The Hospices (2005, p 19)

The role of governments

The role of governments in developing and promoting palliative care is crucial. Hospice and palliative care associations from around the world drew up a Declaration on Hospice and Palliative Care in March 2005, which asked governments to take 15 actions, including the following:

- Include hospice and palliative care as part of all governmental health policy, as recommended by the WHO.
- Make access to hospice and palliative care a human right.
- Make resources available for hospice and palliative care programmes and services.
- Make necessary drugs available, including affordable morphine to the poorest.

www.wwpca.net

The global community must act now to meet the enormous challenge of providing palliative care for all who need it. To ensure that suffering at the end of life is not inevitable, let each and every one of us play our part. We all stand to benefit.

Help The Hospices (2005, p 26)

DEFINITIONS

Definitions are important although we often pay them little regard. Definitions may well help to shape our attitude and approach to the work that we do. For an equable and coordinated approach to care, we all need to have a common understanding of the what, why, how, when and where of palliative care.

Health

Illich's definition of health embraces the concept of a 'healthy death'. He stated that 'health designates the ability to adapt to changing environments, to growing up and ageing, to healing when damaged, to suffering and to the peaceful expectation of death. It also embraces the future and therefore includes anguish and the inner resources to live with it' (Illich 1975). Viewing health as a process of adaptation, rather than simply an absence of disease, can create a useful approach to palliative care. The emphasis is on supporting people in their adaptation and helping them to remain in control of their illness experience for as long as possible (Buckley 2002a).

Palliative care

Perhaps the most widely quoted definition of palliative care is the one published by the National Institute for Health and Clinical Excellence (NICE), which leans heavily on NCHSPC (1995). It is as follows:

> Palliative care is the active holistic care of patients with advanced progressive illness. Management of pain and other symptoms and the provision of psychological, social and spiritual support is paramount. The goal of palliative care is the best possible quality of life for patients and their families.
>
> NICE (2004b, p 20)

This definition has quickly become recognised as appropriate for the care of patients with any life-threatening/long-term condition.

The definition, as quoted here, can carry an implicit suggestion of disempowerment. There is no real suggestion of the contributions that the ill person and their friends and relatives might make to their illness management. However, within the NICE manual (2004b), there is such a suggestion. It states, for example, that 'patients, families and other carers should play the central role in making decisions about the care they receive' (NICE 2004b, p 21) and 'user empowerment must therefore underpin good supportive and palliative care' (NICE 2004b, p 21). This definition is also given in NCPC (2005b). However, as in the NICE guidelines, this document goes on to describe a more active role for patients.

Holism

The increasing use of the word holism is also of some concern. It is a word that is becoming embedded in nursing theory, e.g. in philosophies of care, curricula and writing. An analysis of the literature suggests that its emergence as an ideal is dogged by lack of clear definitions (Smart 2005). In many instances it simply seems to mean consideration of the whole, i.e. psychological, social and spiritual, as well as physical. Within the discipline of complementary therapies, the heart of holism is seen as supporting people in utilising their own inner resources; thus patients are experts on themselves (Daniel 2001b). A definition should have purpose and clarity; including the word holism has the potential to hamper that.

By adopting a definition that contains the words holism, psychological, social, spiritual and physical, particularly with a poorly defined sense of what holism means, we are in danger of being intrusive and controlling for some of our patients. Holism and its tool, individualised palliative care, has granted us permission to peel away the layers of the onion that is patient care, but perhaps we do not always need to do so because the knowledge that we gain may not be necessary for the care of a patient and may have costs to them as a person (Smart 2005).

This is not to devalue the philosophy of an approach that encompasses understanding patients' perceptions and feelings, and supporting their coping styles. Nor does it devalue the notion of supporting the physical, psychological, social and spiritual needs. It is simple to recognise that not everyone wants or needs this full-on approach.

An alternative definition presented here is:

> The aim of palliative care is to support the patient, their family and friends in adapting to embracing a peaceful expectation of death. To this end expert assessment skills are paramount. Control of pain and difficult symptoms are a priority. Expert support should be offered where needed and wanted in all areas, physical, psychological, social and spiritual. The goal of palliative care is achievement of the best quality of life for patients, their family and friends and the creation of precious memories in the dying trajectory.

Terminal care

It has been suggested that the use of the word 'palliative' has replaced the word 'terminal' and that this may be indicative of a death-denying society (Praill 2000). Perhaps it is more indicative of the evolution of a palliative service rather than a substitution of words. 'Terminal care' is a term used within palliative care. It refers to a period when, despite the best efforts of patients, carers, friends, relatives and the multidisciplinary team, symptoms become more difficult to manage. Typically it is heralded by loss of energy, no interest in eating, and some psychological withdrawal from family and friends. The onset and duration of this period are as unique as every human being. Indeed, some people do not have a 'terminal phase' either as a result of an acute occurrence or because they simply do not experience it. It is an important period to recognise. Sometimes a palliative approach, e.g. small appetising meals, managed exercise and organising anticipated enjoyable activities, can become a burden to the patient. They may not want to dampen the enthusiasm of friends, relatives and professionals in their attempts to care. Relatives and friends may need additional support at this time. When a loved one no longer wants to eat, for example, they may need help to understand this. Preparing food translates into nurturing and eating is often a mutually enjoyable event. Relinquishing this may feel like withdrawing love and friendship at some level.

Generalist and specialist palliative care

Good quality palliative care is the remit of every health-care professional. The NCPC (2005b) sees two distinct categories of health-care and social-care professionals providing palliative care: generalist and specialist palliative care teams. They provide day-to-day care for patients, relatives and friends in the community hospitals, care homes and indeed all care settings. Generalists do not nurse dying people exclusively – they are only part of their caseload. Specialist palliative care teams will usually have had extra training and will be caring for people with life-limiting disease only. Traditionally, these teams have been hospice and hospital based.

Generalists should be able to assess and meet the physical, psychological, social, spiritual and informational needs of patients and families in their care. Importantly they should be aware of their own limits in knowledge, skills and competency in palliative care, and know when to seek advice from a specialist palliative care team (NCPC 2005b).

Specialist palliative care is provided by a specialist multidisciplinary care team. Such a service should include the following:

- Assessments of, advice for and care of patients, families and friends in all care settings, including hospitals and care homes.
- Specialist inpatient facilities in hospital or hospice.
- Intensive coordinated home support for patients with complex needs who wish to stay at home. This may be a specialist service providing advice alongside the GP and district nurse or perhaps a hospice-at-home service, i.e. specialist nursing, medical advice and access to all other members of the care team in the patient's home.
- Day-care facilities offering a range of opportunities for assessment and review of all needs. They can provide support and friendship groups, and also complementary and creative therapies.
- Advice and support to all people involved in patient care.
- Bereavement support care.
- Education and training in palliative care.

The specialist teams should include palliative medical consultants, palliative care nurses, physiotherapists, occupational therapists, dietitians, pharmacists, social workers, and those able to give psychological and spiritual support (NCPC 2005b). Integral to most specialist palliative care services is a complementary therapy service and, in many, a well-defined creative therapies service. There is overwhelming anecdotal evidence, and a growing more formal evidence base, that these therapies help to enhance quality of life for the dying person.

Supportive care

The term 'supportive care' is recent but is now firmly established on the health-care agenda, largely as a result of the NICE (2004b) manual *Improving Supportive and Palliative Care for Adults with Cancer,* and its accompanying publication *Supportive and Palliative Care: The research evidence* (NICE 2004a). Supportive care in the past has been piecemeal and patchy and still is. It is hoped that the 20 key recommendations from the NICE manual (2004b) can start to rectify this, not just for cancer patients, their relatives and friends, but for all facing progressive disease.

The definition of supportive care quoted here is from the NICE manual (2004b) and has been adopted by the NCPC (2005b):

Supportive care helps the patient and their family to cope with cancer and the treatment of it from pre diagnosis, through the process of diagnostics and treatment, to cure, continuing illness or death and bereavement. It helps the patient to maximise the benefits of treatment to life and correlate as well as possible with the effects of the disease. It is given equal priority alongside diagnosis and treatment. Supportive care should be fully integrated with diagnosis and treatment. It encompasses:

- Self help and support
- User involvement
- Information giving
- Psychological support
- Symptom control
- Rehabilitation
- Complementary therapies
- Spiritual support
- End of life bereavement care.

Three exciting nationally coordinated initiatives – the Gold Standards Framework, the Preferred Place of Care document and the Liverpool Care Pathway – are an important part of a supportive and palliative care approach in the UK. The NHS End-of-Life Care Programme has been established to promote the spread of these three frameworks into the cancer and non-cancer populations.

END-OF-LIFE CARE NATIONAL PROGRAMME

The Gold Standards Framework

The Gold Standards Framework (GSF) has grown from a local initiative by Dr Keri Thomas, a GP Macmillan Facilitator in Huddersfield. The original project involved 12 GP practices in Huddersfield. In 2006 the GSF was being used by over 2000 primary care teams in the UK covering a quarter of the population (Thomas 2005).

The GSF is an evidence-base programme of assessment and care, developed for the use of primary health-care teams. It provides a home pack for patients to facilitate sharing of information. Assessment tools, e.g. pain assessment and other symptom assessments, have also been developed for use with it. The aim of the GSF is to improve and optimise the quality of life for patients, their families and friends in the last year of life. It aspires to providing equal opportunity, good quality, end-of-life care regardless of location and diagnosis. By using the GSF, practices should be able to improve communication and teamwork. Each practice nominates a key nurse and GP for each patient whom they place on a practice-based palliative care register. Each practice should have a monthly meeting to review patients on this register. Improvement of the seven Cs is frequently quoted as being the main goals:

- Communication
- Control of symptoms
- Continuity of care
- Coordination

- Care support
- Care of those who are dying
- Continued learning.

The GSF practices should also hold 6-monthly significant events meetings and attend central meetings to share experiences and develop protocols. It is from these meetings that the 'toolkit' previously referred to, containing a variety of assessment tools, and guidelines for practice have been developed (Thomas 2003).

A central NHS GSF team provides continued support for SHAs, primary care trusts (PCTs) and cancer networks.

Using GSF in the community can improve communication advance care planning and monitoring of patients enabling more patients to die where they choose. It has also been shown to reduce un-needed hospital admissions.

There is evidence of strong central government support for the GSF. It was mentioned in the House of Commons Select Committee Report in July 2004, the Labour and Conservative Party Manifestos in April 2005 and is embedded in the National Service Frameworks, e.g. for chronic heart disease and chronic renal disease (Thomas 2005).

The Preferred Place of Care/Preferred Priorities of Care

The NHS Cancer Plan (DH 2000b) stated that cancer patients should be able to live and die in a place of their own choosing where this is possible. Nationally 56% of us would prefer to die at home, but only 20% of us actually do (NCPC 2003).

The Preferred Place of Care/Preferred Priorities of Care (PPC) is the initiative of the Lancashire and Cumbria Cancer Network. The aim is to put the patient at the centre of care planning, in the hope that autonomy and control will be fostered: 'Many patients feel these factors are taken away in the terminal stages of their illness' (Storey 2003). Some sections of the PPC documentation are designed to be completed by carers and some by health professionals. The document is divided into four parts, as follows:

Section 1

Family profile – explains details relating to dependence and identifies who key carers will be.

Section 2

Records discussions of the patients' and families' understanding of the diagnosis and possible outcomes.

It is here that the practitioner proceeds to discuss what consideration has been given to where and by whom, they would like to be cared for when their condition deteriorates.

Section 3

Provides a comprehensive assessment of health and social services available to the patients and any services currently being accessed.

Section 4

This is a variance sheet allowing space for patients and professionals to document changes.

Storey (2003)

It is impressed upon patients that they can change their mind at any time. An accompanying NHS leaflet also explains that choices may not always be honoured for various reasons, e.g. a change of physical condition, a carer becoming ill or tired, and a lack of resources to meet a particular need (Department of Health 2004b).

By collecting documents after the death of a patient, it is hoped to gather data on what actually happens. Why do people who wish to die at home die in hospital? Is it lack of resources or poor communication between professionals? Or is it not listening to patients and relatives? These data will be invaluable and will help determine whether it is a reality to offer home as a choice of place to die. Do we have enough resources in the right places?

The Liverpool Care Pathway

The stimulus for the development of care pathways in this country was the government's White Paper – *A First Class Service – Quality in the New NHS* (DH 1998). Embodied within this paper were initiatives that created the expectation that quality of delivered care must be benchmarked, audited and inspected to ensure compliance. This paper was the launch of clinical governance, the NICE and the Commission for Health Improvement (CHI). A care pathway is an agreed plan of care ideally constructed by a multidisciplinary team. It provides a central organising tool for all clinical care and is designed to replace all other documentation and become a multiprofessional document. 'The care pathway includes expert opinion, guidelines, protocols, evidence-based practice and research and development where possible' (Ellershaw and Murphy 2005, p 132). The Liverpool Care Pathway (LCP) was developed as a joint initiative between the Marie Curie Hospice in Liverpool and the Royal Liverpool Hospital. It was developed 10 years ago as a tool to enhance education programmes for the care of those who are dying (Ellershaw and Wilkinson 2003). It is designed for use in the last days of life.

The fundamentals incorporated in the LCP are not complex. The diagnosis for those who are dying includes easily demonstrable criteria, e.g. the patient is bed bound, semi-comatose, only taking sips of fluid, can no longer swallow tablets. The multiprofessional team must agree that two or more of these criteria have been met to stimulate the implementation of the LCP. In a well-run area this should avoid conflicting messages being given to relatives and friends about whether or not the patient is dying.

One of the first actions that the LCP recommends is to review all medications, discontinue non-essential medicines and prescribe medication for potential symptoms as needed, e.g. pain, nausea. These are very simple and easy steps to follow. As someone who frequently listens to multidisciplinary team members practising generalist palliative care, issues of continuing with all medications and being unable to get prompt consultations re difficult symptoms when they arise, are factors that still cause a good deal of distress to patients, relatives, friends and professional carers.

The LCP was developed for use in hospitals but is increasingly being used in the community as a natural extension of the GSF.

In the NICE supportive care manual (NICE 2004b, p 11), key recommendation 14 states:

> In all locations, the particular needs of patients who are dying from cancer should be identified and addressed. The Liverpool Care Pathway for the Dying provides one mechanism for achieving this.

So, similar to the GSF, there is evidence that the LCP is being adopted by mainstream NHS organisations. It is estimated that over 25% of hospices in the UK are now using the LCP. Evaluation has shown that, in the generic health-care setting in Liverpool, over 50% of patients on the LCP are non-cancer patients (Ellershaw and Murphy 2005). This trend has also been demonstrated in other hospitals (Murtagh et al. 2004; Mirando 2005).

As with the GSF there is a national team to support the LCP, based at the Marie Curie Palliative Care Institute in Liverpool. An audit and research team supports four continuing associated programmes. They are: non-cancer, benchmarking, education and international. An annual national conference focuses on research and new developments.

'It is well recognised within our society and within the healthcare system that hospice care is synonymous with quality care of the dying' (Ellershaw and Wilkinson 2003, p xi). In a society where over 56% of people die in hospital (NCPC 2003), it is exciting to think that the LCP could be at the fingertips of all health-care professionals wherever they are. It provides the framework for a good quality of dying.

CULTURE

Multicultural Britain

In the mid-1990s there was concern that uptake of hospice and other specialist palliative care services among black and minority ethnic (BME) patients was low. Research identified several factors that constituted this perceived low uptake. There was a lack of accurate data on ethnicity of people using services. At this time, in many units cancer was still the focus for palliative care. Deaths from cancer occur mainly in the population of people aged 55 years and over. There was a smaller proportion of BME groups in this age range and many may emigrate back to their country of origin in later life, which could help to account for low uptake. Added to this, cancer is not the main cause of illness among the black and Asian communities. It was also found that there is little or no information available to BME patients or their carers about palliative services (Hill and Penso 1995).

The research, called Opening Doors (Hill and Penso 1995), targeted three specific sites for an indepth analysis – Brent, Newham and Birmingham. It concluded by making 11 recommendations. This summary by Baroness Cumberlege from the report highlights some of the main areas for concern and action:

> One of the most important aspects of the report is the evidence it shows of an understanding of the particular needs of the black and ethnic minority communities for hospice and specialist palliative care. However, awareness on its own is not enough. Although much progress has been made, access to, and knowledge of these services by people for ethnic minority communities is still not as good as it should be. The report shows that better liaison between agencies involved and more information on current needs are necessary. Training in cultural awareness, interpreting services and targeting information in appropriate languages are some of the ways services can be made friendlier to their users.
>
> Hill and Penso (1995, p 4)

A follow-up study commissioned by the then National Council for Hospice and Specialist Palliative Care Services (Firth 2001) made further recommendations: it suggested more availability of culturally sensitive tools, e.g. pain assessment charts, more sensitivity to different cultural practices, e.g. large family gatherings and mourning rituals. It also suggested regular meetings of health-care professionals, community leaders and patient groups, and the subject of more culturally sensitive recruitment of nurses was raised. This study makes 11 recommendations for practice and 5 for further research, including looking at beliefs and attitudes to illness and death, care and the role of carers, attitudes to disclosure, autonomy and informed consent, attitudes and responses to pain, and referral patterns (Firth 2001).

Neuberger (2003) highlights that her experiences in terminal care demonstrate that, on occasion, services can be totally culturally appropriate. However, in conditions once considered terminal and now viewed as chronic, e.g. some cancers, HIV, heart disease, she views cultural sensitivity as often lacking. Despite several national attempts to encourage better end-of-life care incorporating psychological, social and spiritual considerations, 'services are still patchy and depending too much on individual enthusiasts' (Neuberger 2003, p 208).

Interprofessional culture

Offering a service to patients that recognises them as unique human beings presents a challenge. It requires a good deal of individual motivation and excellent communication within the team, which must include patients and their families/friends. As human beings, we operate on an intellectual and emotional level. Sometimes we make intellectual decisions that conflict with our emotions, e.g. a mother giving a baby up for adoption may be making an intellectual decision that carries emotional suffering. Similar things happen in health care, often with very little professional awareness of it. However, the suffering as a result of 'faulty' decision-making is not that of the professionals but that of the patient, family and friends. This is vividly demonstrated by continuation of aggressive futile treatments.

Doctors

Western doctors traditionally work within a strong philosophical framework based on curing. When making decisions about active treatment in the face of futility, experience supports ignoring hard evidence. The doctor may operate at an emotional level and continues futile treatments. The consequences for patients, relatives and friends are far reaching. Essentially, because of invasive painful procedures, they are robbed of their last moments together. This cannot be reversed. Anguished moments replace potentially precious ones.

Nurses

Nurses work in a philosophical framework of caring. They often 'come into their own' when a patient cannot be cured. I heard a doctor gently talking to an elderly woman who had an aggressive chest infection. He sensitively explained that antibiotic therapy could be optional. She understood. She replied that she had a daughter and three grandchildren who loved her and she loved them and life. He prescribed the antibiotics. The conversation with the patient was stimulated by nurses advising him not to prescribe. The nursing staff were critical of him in spite of knowing that he had spoken to the patient. In their opinion, she had suffered enough. Their philosophical framework of care in this instance was misguided and created unnecessary tension. It begs the question of how it may have impinged on their relationship with the patient.

Therapists

Maintaining independence when disease is progressing can be synonymous with maintaining hope (Buckley and Herth 2004). Physiotherapists, occupational therapists and speech and language therapists have a vital role to play in this important aspect of care. Although they know their value at this critical time, they often find themselves with feelings of sadness and failure when patients can no longer remain independent and their role becomes redundant.

These are complex issues. Developing a stronger sense of personal and professional awareness is crucial to our decision-making and this is addressed in Chapter 4. Having a good knowledge of what patients understand and feel about a situation is also a vital component of decision-making; this is discussed in Chapter 3.

We can do a good day's work caring for our patients physically and organisationally. However, supporting patients emotionally and spiritually requires added energy and motivation. Those who are dying do not have a strong voice in the main, so the personal motivation of their carers becomes an even more vital factor. Health professionals need to feel supported to be able to keep caring for those who are dying. Staff support systems and self-care are vital and are discussed in Chapter 4.

SERVICE USER INVOLVEMENT

A new system of patient and public involvement in health care has been implemented in recent years. Community health councils have been replaced by patient and public involvement forums (PPIFs). These forums have many responsibilities, including monitoring and reviewing services and seeking patient views. Every PCT and NHS trust has a patient advice and liaison service (PALS), with members who monitor trends and highlight gaps in services. A national independent public body, the Commission of Patient and Public Involvement in Health, provides a voice for patients and the public; it advises on systems of patient and public involvement and on major issues that arise. In addition, local authorities with responsibilities for the Social Services have an overview and scrutiny committee to take on the role of scrutinising health services, including the NHS (DH 2003b). A strong philosophy behind the new framework is that patients and the public will be included in shaping services, e.g. assessing need and writing policies. It is hoped that this will shape a more user-friendly service and the new patient organisations will be less involved in adversarial roles, as was often the case for community health councils.

Historical perspective

One could say that palliative care as we know it today has been shaped around patient involvement, e.g. the giving of regular morphine was a result of an extensive study by Dame Cicely Saunders (2006a), during which she analysed 900 records and tape-recorded patients' stories of pain and response to pain relief. A doctor remarked to her at a symposium in 1963 'I always thought that regular giving was the answer'. 'Patients' voices have provided the answer' (Saunders 2006a, p 6), was Dame Cecily's reply.

Contemporary initiatives

At St Christopher's, two patient groups have been set up: one for ward-based patients and one for home-based patients. The Beacon project in Brighton, which provides a service for people with HIV and AIDS, has a user forum so that service users are involved at all stages of the service provided there (Munroe and Oliviere, 2003). These are just two examples of practice.

It may be perceived that user involvement in palliative care presents a particular challenge because of limited life expectancy, and some specialist palliative care teams are resistant to forming user groups. Munroe and Oliviere (2003) warn against this type of stereotyping. It should not be assumed that, as patients pass from active to palliative care, they are not well enough to take part in user activity. This has the potential to create a divide between patients and staff, particularly if patients are coming from areas where they have had active user involvement. In Chichester, patients are involved in planning and delivering study days for health-care professionals. These are in their infancy but so far have proved to be valuable learning experiences.

Palliative care service users are already involved in a wide range of activities: self-help groups, education groups, user consultation forums. The challenge for the future is to extend these activities and evaluate the effectiveness in terms of impact on both service and patients involved.

CONCLUSION

This chapter has given an overview of the history of and cultural perspectives on the evolution of the modern palliative care movement. The challenge is now to continue to develop frameworks and approaches that will extend a good-quality palliative service to people dying of any illness, in any setting, in any country of the world.

MAIN IMPLICATIONS FOR PRACTICE

- It is important to understand what the philosophical approach to palliative care is in your place of work. If the approach in practice does not match the philosophy or, indeed, if palliative care is not included in your philosophy or mission statement, raise these points at an appropriate forum, e.g. ward meetings.
- A palliative approach should, where possible, aim to help people use their own inner resources and avoid disempowerment.
- Be mindful that sometimes rehabilitative aspects of care and, indeed, life-sustaining activities (e.g. eating) can become burdensome in the terminal stage of someone's illness.
- All health-care professionals practising generalist palliative care should know how to contact their local specialist teams for advice.
- Services should be culturally sensitive and all health-care organisations should design policies and educational approaches that will help to establish this as a routine part of care. This important aspect should not depend on the enthusiasm of individuals.
- Interprofessional culture is important when making individual and group decisions. Understanding of our own profession's philosophical approach and that of our colleagues is a fundamental step in understanding our decision-making.
- User involvement is as important in palliative care as in active care. It should not be assumed that, because people are receiving palliative care, they will not feel well enough for user involvement. Assumptions are disempowering for patients, friends and relatives, and may lead to social isolation.

SUGGESTED FURTHER READING

Ellershaw J, Wilkinson S (2003) *Care of the Dying: A pathway to excellence.* Oxford: Oxford University Press.

Monroe B, Oliviere D (2003) *Patient Participation in Palliative Care. A voice for the voiceless.* Oxford: Oxford University Press.

Thomas K (2003) *Caring for the Dying at Home.* Oxford: Radcliffe Medical Press.

Websites

www.helpthehospices.org.uk
www.ncpc.org.uk
For information on the Preferred Place of Care initiative contact www.cancerlancashire.org.uk.
www.goldstandardsframework.nhs.uk
www.endoflifecare.nhs.uk
www.who.int

Chapter 2
Facing progressive disease and death

KEY POINTS

- **Psychosocial care**: offering psychosocial care is an integral part of palliative care. All health-care professionals have some responsibility for this. Research suggests that psychiatric morbidity may go undetected as a result of limited access to specialist mental health services.
- **Partnership – maintaining the balance**: support needs to be fine tuned to each person. The aim is to avoid being intrusive and disempowering, but also not to push people to be autonomous against their wishes. As a person becomes more ill in some cases they can fluctuate between wanting an active and wanting a passive role from day to day, hour to hour.
- **Approaches to care**: two popular perspectives for underpinning and informing a psychosocial approach to palliative care are briefly critiqued. These are the stage theories of grief and the narrative model of care.
- **Giving the bad news**: aspects of giving bad news are discussed in terms of providing information at a pace dictated by the patient. The aim of doing this is to maximise the potentiality for a healthy adaptation to facing progressive disease and dying. A more detailed account of giving bad news is included in Chapter 3.
- **Denial/avoidance**: denial is a much-used word in palliative care. As a coping mechanism, denial has value. Misuse of the word can be counter-productive to quality care. Sometimes the word 'avoidance' would be more appropriate. Sometimes denial is socially constructed. Assessment of denial is included in Chapter 3.
- **Anger**: dying patients may get angry at many things. It may not be a response to their predicament. Conscientious assessment is vital. Angry people need our time and care.
- **Anxiety**: the physical manifestation of anxiety can divert from the underlying psychological cause. Anxiety states can be relatively simple to help with but may go undiagnosed. Recognition of anxiety symptoms needs to be higher profile.
- **Depression**: this may go undiagnosed in palliative care. Better access to specialist mental health practitioners is needed. In the interim, senior nurses and doctors need to learn how to assess for depression.
- **Social pain**: potential family and financial problems are highlighted. However, more concepts of social care are discussed in Chapter 8.

This chapter identifies broad principles for caring for people who face progressive disease and death. It is not a comprehensive overview of every emotional response or theoretical framework. Rather it draws on experience and highlights aspects of psychological care that can be problematic in the clinical area, because they are either not identified or are misunderstood. In looking at approaches to care, the importance of helping the patient to dictate the pace at which information is shared and the level of autonomy that they want is highlighted. This way the potential for a more 'healthy' adaptation to facing progressive disease and death is exploited.

PSYCHOSOCIAL CARE

The psychosocial care of patients facing progressive disease and death has been defined by the National Council for Hospice and Specialist Palliative Care Services (1997, page 6) as:

> Psychological approaches concerned with enabling patients and those close to them to express thoughts, feelings and concerns relating to their illness, assessing individual needs and resources, and ensuring that psychological and emotional support is available. A range of formal and planned interventions may be used to relieve psychological distress, e.g. anxiety, anger, low mood and intrusive thoughts. For some people this will also include the recognition and treatment of specific psychiatric disorder such as depressive illness.

Within the same document, the council identifies the different levels of skills that are needed to help make this definition a reality:

- Level 1: skills that are general communication skills desirable for all professionals
- Level 2: excellent interpersonal and communication skills – advanced communication skills
- Level 3: skills that are required by a specialist in psychosocial care.

Communication is a vital component for good quality palliative care. That said, a series of research studies in the UK and European countries indicates that a high proportion of people after a diagnosis of cancer remain dissatisfied with their interactions with professionals (Wilkinson et al. 1999b). As a result of this research there has been a government-backed national initiative to improve the communication skills of senior doctors and nurses in oncology and palliative care. The advanced communication skills programme is being rolled out by the Cancer Action Team with the intention of bringing professionals up to level 2 of the Council recommendations. This is discussed in more detail in Chapter 3.

The provision of level 3 skills within specialist palliative care is, however, patchy. An analysis of 97 returned questionnaires from hospices enquiring about psychosocial care revealed that 83% employed a chaplain and all had access to one; 75% employed a social worker and a further 6% had access to one; 43% employed one or more counsellors, although 25% indicated that they did not have access to one; only 9% employed a full- or part-time psychiatrist and 7% employed a psychologist.

The authors concluded that psychiatric morbidity may go undetected and untreated as a result (Lloyd-Williams et al. 1999a). This issue is raised again later in Chapter 13 when discussing depression as a prevalent symptom.

PARTNERSHIP – MAINTAINING THE BALANCE

The aim of the health professional in palliative care is to support patients and their families and friends without being inappropriately intrusive or disempowering. Many patients find the help that they need from within themselves, their family and friends, and may need minimal input from professionals.

In the Canadian Needs Studies (Vachon et al. 1991, 1995), patients with cancer were asked to list their biggest problems since receiving their diagnosis. The first and second biggest problems mentioned were most commonly difficulty in accepting the diagnosis. However, about two-thirds in one group and three-quarters in another said that they had resolved this problem. They relied on themselves, their family, their doctor and their spouses/partners for help in learning to live with their diagnosis. It seemed that their primary coping method was to confront the situation in a practical way, e.g. accepting treatment, making a will and making plans for their family after their death.

A study of 40 patients from a unique, culturally diverse, Jewish/Middle Eastern population showed that an overwhelming majority of participants could communicate their fears to close friends and family, and they received their support from them. Six of the 40 stated that their doctor and/or oncology/palliative department had helped. God and their religion were cited as support by some of the religious patients (Blinderman and Cherny 2005).

There are patients who need more help than others from professionals as they make an adjustment to facing death; however, the research quoted here implicates that they may be in the minority. In research by Rothenbacher et al. (1997), although a majority of cancer patients wanted an active role in making decisions about their care, 28% said that they desired a passive role. Sheldon (1997) states that patients should not be forced to be autonomous if that is not their wish.

It becomes more complex as people are closer to death. Often their level of physical and emotional energy fluctuates from day to day and so therefore does their ability to engage in social discourse and decision-making. Health professionals in the palliative situation must learn to reassess the situation automatically each time that they are with the patient in order to gauge the level of help and emotional support that they give.

When people are dependent physically, they become vulnerable and it is easy for well-meaning professionals to threaten, or remove, their autonomy. For example, I once nursed a woman who was dying and her only visitors were some friends and a neighbour. She had three adult daughters living in various parts of the world. She was adamant that she did not want them contacted. As she became weaker the ward sister and neighbour decided that they would contact the daughters anyhow. They felt sure that this was the 'right' thing to do. Two of the daughters came to the ward and the mother refused to see them. The other telephoned and the mother refused to talk with her. This intrusive action caused considerable emotional distress to this dying woman and her daughters. Not everyone will resolve emotional and spiritual issues in the dying period. And just because we think that it is an ideal to strive for, or something that we might want ourselves, we must be mindful not to impose this ideal inappropriately.

Brewin (1996) put forward the notion of friendly professional interest as an approach to psychosocial and spiritual care. He says:

> Professional friendship is not quite the same as ordinary friendship, but much that applies still holds true. A friend is warm and welcoming at each meeting. A friend pays compliments. A friend has at least some idea of how the patient feels: some idea of what she has been going through; understands how her moods might vary (maybe hope one day, despair the next). A friend listens; knows the value of praise; asks how she can help. A friend is just as ready to talk seriously (if that is what the patient wants), as to joke or gossip. A really supportive professional doesn't go over the top emotionally, but is always concerned; doesn't stay too long; knows when to be silent: doesn't ask too many questions.
>
> Brewin (1996, p 76)

Brewin recommends this approach for doctors and this is endorsed by Randall and Downie (2006). I think that it encapsulates what health-care professionals are aiming to achieve when they take a palliative approach.

APPROACHES TO CARE

The dominant models of grief and bereavement theory in the latter part of the twentieth century are termed the 'stage theories of grief'. A superficial analysis of these models is that people have to pass through a series of stages described in psychological and cognitive terms before they can 'recover' from grief or, in the case of facing one's own death, reach acceptance. It may be that the authors of these models have not done enough to dispel the myth that they represent a linear process. In the context of the original books, e.g. Kübler-Ross (1970), Parkes (1972) and Worden (1983), it is quite clear that all these three see the phases/stages that they describe as being intermingled and capricious.

Kübler-Ross's (1970) seminal work is based on the stories of over 200 dying patients whom she listened to, recorded and content analysed. The stages that she describes – denial and isolation, anger, bargaining, depression and acceptance – have been applied to bereaved individuals as well as those who are dying. More recently she wrote that they have been much misunderstood over the last three decades. She says:

> . . . they are tools to help us frame and identify feelings. But they are not stops on some linear time line of grief. Not everyone goes through all of them or goes in a prescribed order.
>
> Kübler-Ross and Kessler (2005, p 7)

In inexperienced hands, if the stage theories are misunderstood as linear processes, they mitigate against good communication, particularly if the health professional fails to assess but works on assumptions. For example, a dying person who is angry may not be in the 'angry stage' but have a legitimate concrete reason for their anger, e.g. the wrong meal has been delivered, again.

Walter (1994) brings a sociological perspective to grief and bereavement and challenges the dominant model that he perceives has prompted the concept of 'letting go' and 'moving on' when someone has died. He highlights the value of a biographical model in which the dead person is talked about by the bereaved person. This way the bond with the dead is continued and they can still have influence within the family. 'My Aunt Edith died when she was 13. I was born 10 years later. Each household in the family displayed her photograph. Guess what? She always helped her mum, worked hard at school, practised at the piano, did her homework and had impeccable manners.' Aunt Edith was our role model (I have two sisters) and an example of the value of the biographical model. Incidentally, I am now 56 and I still regard her as my Aunt Edith.

In tune with Walter (1994) is the growth of the use of the narrative role for caring. This idea is underpinned by the approach that we can best understand our patients and how they cope by listening to their individual stories, and this is something that has always been at the heart of good care. However, using narrative as a form of communication between patient and professional has, in some places, become part of the documentation of care replacing the nursing process, e.g. Johns (2004). It seems logical that patient care is more sensitive to individual need if the patient's voice is predominant in our notes. This concept is explored more in later chapters.

In palliative care some supporters of the narrative model see it as a valued replacement of the staged models. They feel that labels, similar to denial, can impact negatively on patient care because these labels provide a framework that may preclude people from listening attentively to unique stories (Telford et al. 2006).

It could be argued that the professional's integrity and self-awareness are the key. A well-motivated professional with sound education in palliative care should be able to listen to unique stories and respond to stages such as denial intelligently and flexibly with no negative impact on the patient.

Finally, a well rounded life should have a beginning, a middle and an end. Not just for reasons of symmetry but because I may be mortal, the social system of which I am part is immortal and my arrival into and departure from that social system are important events that must be prepared for.

Too many things militate against a fitting approach to death. Despite all evidence to the contrary we insist on assuming we are immortal and assuring each other that all of us are on a space walk, immune from the laws of celestial gravity. 'Don't worry' says the doctor, 'it's only a little ulcer'; 'come now', says the nurse, 'you mustn't talk like that, you're going to be alright.'

But the relinquishment of life is possible, particularly if, through illness, our body has lost its appetite for living. Those who have the privilege of caring for the person who is about to die know that the final phase of life can be a time of peaceful acceptance, a time of calm which contrasts with the tensions and frustrations of the battle for survival.

Parkes – extracts from the foreword that he wrote for Kübler-Ross (1970)

GIVING THE BAD NEWS

The way that the diagnosis of a life-threatening illness is given to someone becomes an important point of their narrative. I have not kept a record but, in my career as a palliative care nurse, I estimate that almost all the patients with whom I have had a relationship at some point recount the story of hearing the bad news. If it is done well it leaves the person feeling valued and respected at one of the most significant events in their life. Conversely, if the person is told in a seemingly uncaring way, it has the opposite effect.

Listen to these two accounts:

Mrs B being told she has motor neurone disease:

'. . . I had been told to bring someone with me if I wanted, so I took the whole family (husband and two adult children). It is just as well I did because when he told me – and I did want to know – it was such a shock I fainted. Dr X was so nice to all of us. He was concerned I was so upset. I could see the hurt in his eyes.'

Mrs B told me this story in such a way that we both laughed about her fainting at such an important time.

Mrs F being told that her cancer was more aggressive than first thought:

' ". . . you are to have a mastectomy, chemotherapy and radiotherapy." I said "Why?" He just shrugged and said, "I don't want to see you here again in a year's time." "But two weeks ago you said I would be fine and I just needed some radiotherapy." I was crying by this time, he just shrugged his shoulders again and said "go away and think about it and let me know what you decide." With that, he showed me out. I was still crying.'

Buckley (1998)

Most of us have an unconscious assumption that we will die when we are old and that (irrationally) death happens to other people. Although we know from the media that people die regularly in appalling circumstances, for the majority of the world's population, it all seems remote. Being constantly acutely aware of all the dangers would make daily living untenable. Stedeford (1994) states that we need to be defended against the constant possibility of death in order to survive. She calls this existential denial and says that, without it, it would be difficult to cross the road, travel abroad and make plans for the future. As life goes on and people whom we know die we start to assimilate the threat for ourselves. The giver of bad news is unlikely to know in advance at what level of assimilation of their own death the ill person has reached.

The consensus in the literature is that an essential element of giving bad news is to find out just what the ill person already knows and feels about what is happening (Buckman 1993a; Kübler-Ross 1993; Faulkner and Maguire 1994; Wilkinson and Mula 2004). As well as giving the clinicians something to build on, it also gives insight into any psychological adjustment that has already been made. Experts also agree that the level of information and detail given about the diagnosis and prognosis must be guided by both verbal and non-verbal clues from the patient.

Here is an account of Mr T recalling how his wife was told that her cancer had metastasised:

> You might as well go off and have a good holiday. We can't change things. By summer it will be too late to go away . . . It left us with nothing, J was devastated. At least the previous doctors had said they would be able to offer help to make J feel better.

> Buckley (1998)

Buckman (2005) suggests that a clear signal is needed before proceeding, e.g. 'Are you the kind of person who likes to know full details of what is going wrong – or would you prefer just to hear about the treatment plan?'. A strategy for giving bad news is outlined more fully in Chapter 3, accompanied by discussion of the evidence base for truth telling.

Vachon (2005) highlights the particular importance of equating information about prognosis to the patient's need. The practitioner should realise that, just as there is a right to know, there is a corresponding right not to know. When a patient chooses not to know about the prognosis it is important that the key health professional involved is prepared to 'walk with the patient along the path they have chosen' (Vachon 2005, p 965) and be open to talking with the patient should he or she change his or her mind.

Narratives suggest that, when patients feel out of control, strong feelings of fear, anxiety and hopelessness can dominate (Buckley 1998). It is imperative that patients be given some control over the pace and nature of the information that they are given. That way it is logical to conclude that the patient will be assisted in making a more healthy adaptation to the predicament.

Giving bad news – some examples of potential cultural considerations

In a multicultural society it is important to be mindful of the customs and practice of different cultural groups without stereotyping. The use of a sound approach to communicating as outlined in Chapter 3 helps to avoid this.

Traditionally in Chinese, Arabic and Muslim families, there is a history of the family not wanting the patient to know the diagnosis. There is a preference that the health professional speak first to the relatives and that they manage giving the information to the patient.

In Arabic countries, many people thought that the word cancer was synonymous with death. There may be a fear that, if the patient knows that they have cancer, they will 'give up' and not accept treatment. Some Muslim families may forbid the word 'cancer' and use euphemisms such as 'serious infection' instead.

In some traditional Asian cultures, cancer, for example, holds a stigma and this can have far-reaching consequences, particularly for women, e.g. a young wife who becomes ill may be sent back to her own family. The Asian TV and radio programmes have very active health education to try to address such issues. Also, there may often be quite strict ideas about how information should be shared. The health professional may find that, rather than talk to the patient and spouse initially, they may be asked to participate in a family conference from which the patient is absent.

The Jewish faith is very life affirming and when orthodox Jewish patients say that they want to know the truth, it is wise to tread very gently because they may not really be ready for it (Macdonald 2004).

In African–Caribbean communities, death is viewed as a great loss no matter what the age of the patient. There may be efforts to protect young people from the truth. There is no stigma attached to disease but it is important that the language used does not indicate that a disease is infectious – if it is not. This fear may lead to the patient being less supported (Macdonald 2004).

In the British culture, perhaps one of the big issues for someone being diagnosed with a chronic illness is being a burden – either emotionally or financially – on their family. Many people perceive their life as being very busy and that finances are tight.

Having said all this, there is evidence that cultural background does not necessarily affect a patient's desire to know the diagnosis (Fielding and Hunt 1996; Seo et al. 2000). My colleague is Malaysian by birth. She has lived in the UK for many years. She has been a palliative care nurse in the UK for many years. Her mother became terminally ill in Malaysia. She went home. The predominant culture in her family at home was not to tell her mother or talk to her about it. Her mother did want to talk to her and they shared many precious moments reviewing the life of her mother, sharing and, to some extent, reassuring her about her fears. It was a special time. However, my colleague's siblings found this hard and it took a while after her mother had died to resolve these issues with them.

Many people from different ethnic backgrounds originally are now second, third or fourth generation in the UK. As our philosophy in health care in this country states: each person is unique, we must always assess and never assume what people's customs and practices are. The later generations of immigrant parents have been brought up in the UK and are British. Sometimes their home traditions may be very different to a 'traditional' UK experience, sometimes not. Within all family groups there will almost certainly be a different perception by each generation of what the 'cultural norm' is.

For the health-care professional there may be a tension between their belief that they should speak directly with the patient about their diagnosis and the relatives' insistence that they should speak to them. This is always going to be difficult. It happens within all cultures that health-care professionals may be invited to collude with the relatives. Sometimes, working within the traditions of the culture will be the right response and sometimes not. Ideally the health-care professional should be able to ask the patient what their preference is and follow that.

It is vital that skilled interpreters are used if language is a problem. When an interpreter is not available, an appropriate high commission or embassy may be able to advise. A member of the family may interpret but care will need to be taken that no bias about that individual's thoughts and feelings distort the information given. Culturally sensitive recruiting of health-care staff will help to produce a more user-friendly environment in many circumstances.

DENIAL/AVOIDANCE

Denial has been most extensively described as a coping mechanism by Kübler-Ross (1970) in her seminal work *On Death and Dying*, in which she interviewed over 200 patients. She describes her book as telling the stories of her patients, in which they describe their agonies, expectations and frustrations.

Denial acts as a buffer against shocking news. It has been described as the most primitive defence mechanism. It gives patients time to collect themselves and perhaps mobilise other less radical defence mechanisms. Kübler-Ross (1970) is at pains to highlight that, although denial or partial denial was used by almost all of the 200+ patients whom she interviewed, it is not simply an initial response. It occurs during the illness trajectory at different times.

> Man cannot look at the sun all the time neither can they face death all the time.
>
> Unknown author (Kübler-Ross 1970)

So while some people may be able to consider their own death, at other times they 'put that consideration away', and get on with living. Denial is not an all-or-none phenomenon. A patient may talk realistically about illness in the morning but by the evening deny that he has it (Dein 2005).

Later on in their illness a patient may use 'isolation' more than denial. This is when people talk about their health and illness concurrently. Then, in a conversation acknowledging their impending death a person may also refer to a future that is clearly (to the listener) not possible. Niki, at 18, was dying of colon cancer. She had been very 'accepting' and realistic throughout her illness. She had worked out how good could come of her death, i.e. her large extended family would now be screened for early signs of colon cancer in the future. She had also planned her funeral. One day, within days of her death, she began talking about getting married. She said that she had a fiancé, she described in detail plans for the wedding. After marrying they would live in London. She would do her nurse's training and nurse terminally ill children. Later they would have a family of their own.

Kübler-Ross (1970) sees this expression of a hope for the future as nurturing, at a time when reality cannot be faced. The eyes need a rest from the sun. I think I understand this from a personal perspective. We were in the process of adopting our daughter. She had lived with us for 3 months. We loved her totally. We were told, because of changes in the adoption law, that we may not be able to keep her. The next 3 months were very difficult. I could not contemplate parting from her. Never. I hatched an escape plan. We would leave the country together (she had no passport). I spent hours pondering the logistics; the size of the bag I would make her cradle in, the potential problem of her popping her head out of the bag at customs, etc., etc. She is 18 now. This is one of the family stories that always gets a roar of laugher. It seems absurd now. At the time that impossibly implausible plan helped me to survive a wildly difficult time.

Not many theorists address this particular aspect. In its oscillation it is not dissimilar to the dual process model of bereavement described by Stroebe and Schut

(1999). In this dual process, people oscillate between being focused on restoration, e.g. coping with everyday life and looking to a future without the dead person, and less focused, e.g. crying, grieving and perhaps dreaming and imagining that the dead person may return.

Kübler-Ross (1970) advises us not to embellish or encourage the unreality of the 'lost future hope' and not to challenge it either. Gently, by non-verbal means, we must support the person telling of what is their hoped-for story of life.

Denial is a term that is embedded in the language of health care. However, it is a word that can represent ambiguity and be misinterpreted, and as such become counterproductive to patient care. A 'true denial' is a subconscious process. It revives and reinterprets a portion of painful reality, avoiding what it threatens to be and holding fast to what has been (Wool 1988).

Avoidance

This is when a person is well aware of the truth of the situation, but chooses not to talk about it. Thus avoidance is a chosen defence mechanism.

Mutual pretence awareness (Vachon 2003)

Patients, relatives and professionals can become involved with mutual pretence awareness. This is when all concerned know that the patient is going to die but no one is talking about it. This may or may not be comfortable for the patient.

Denial as a social process (Vachon 2003)

Denial can be encouraged with the collusion of others and thereby serve as a protective mechanism for family and friends. Professionals can be consciously or subconsciously invited to collude. There is the potential for this becoming a very lonely space for the patient.

Assessment of 'denial'

It is important to talk with the patient to assess if denial indeed exists. It is possible that the patient has not been told the diagnosis! It is possible that they are not being 'allowed' to talk about what is happening to them by their family, friends and professionals. Consciously or subconsciously it may be a relief to others that the patient seems to be using denial as a defence and leads to subtle reinforcement of the denial by them. It is important that the professional stays open minded and be alert for cues from the patient indicating that denial is no longer present and they want to talk, perhaps ask questions. To minimise defensive behaviour, the health professional needs to be self-aware and practise self-care. These aspects are considered in Chapter 4.

To assess for denial invite patients to tell the story of their illness. Ask them to explain how they felt at each significant event. Check to see if they feel that they have been fully informed (Maguire 2000). Give them an opportunity to ask questions. From this it should be apparent what the nature of the denial is, i.e. conscious or subconscious. Is it a choice? Is it socially constructed in some way? A more detailed strategy for communicating with someone about denial is presented in Chapter 3.

Challenging denial

If this is to happen, ideally it should be done by someone with a good deal of experience in delivering psychological care. Research shows that employment of psychologists or psychiatrists in palliative care units is something of a rarity (Lloyd-Williams et al. 1999a). The more difficult psychological issues are often dealt with by the social worker, chaplain or senior members of the medical and nursing teams. Challenging denial should be clearly motivated by concern for the patient. It is not sufficient to challenge denial because the professional feels that it is a desirable goal for the patient and family to accept what is happening. This sort of intervention is an assumption of responsibility by the health professional that does not belong (Vachon 2003).

Patients in denial may apparently not be open to new treatments. Inclusion in drug trials, for example, requires patients to sign a consent form which indicates that treatment has been discussed. One solution in this circumstance is to present the patient with a hypothesis:

> Supposing you were in a very difficult situation and there really was no alternative, are you the sort of person who would like to consider some very new or experimental treatment? The patient may say 'Well, yes, I suppose if I had to' and then a discussion about the treatment could be gently led by the healthcare professional. They may however say 'No, I am not going to be a guinea pig'. It would probably then be best to leave it there.
>
> Macdonald (2004, p 68)

In a study of terminally ill patients with very advanced disease, Connor (1992) concluded that, in the main, denial at this late stage also served a protective function. Predominantly, however, the patient or loved ones were practising mutual pretence in attempts to avoid hurt. In these sorts of circumstances, gentle challenging can usually be helpful and result in the creation of precious quality time for all concerned, and pretence can be pushed aside (Connor 1992).

Holmberg (2006) is a professor at the Department of Teacher Education, Malmö, Sweden. She presents a case history of the communication between her and her dying 36-year-old son. She writes:

> When the son, through gentle guidance from the palliative care team finally realised that he was dying, he stopped denying and took control over his last days. The communication between him and his mother again was open, close and warm and the mother and son could share their grief.
>
> Holmberg (2006, p 15)

In challenging denial it is important to be gentle so that fragile defences are not disrupted, but to be firm enough that any awareness can be explored and developed.

Maguire (2000, p 299)

Bargaining

Bargaining is a coping strategy described in Kübler-Ross's (1970) original work. She describes it as being less used than denial but equally helpful. It is really an attempt to postpone death. The person may ask several people about the prognosis and implicitly encourage them to lengthen it. These are often the patients who make a supreme effort to attend a family function, and sometimes this energy seems to keep them alive. This has been likened to Frankl's (1946) observations to fellow inmates in a Nazi concentration camp. He gives one example of an inmate who was convinced that the camp would be liberated on a certain date. His energy as a result of this hope fuelled not only him but also his immediate friends in the camp. When the date came and they were not liberated, he died in his sleep that night. I remember nursing a woman who had three daughters. She was determined to attend the wedding of her third daughter and, in spite of her advanced state of cancer, she did. She returned to the hospice that night exhausted but happy. The first thing that she said as she came through the door was: 'I have had a marvellous time, and guess what? I am to be a grandmother. I must see that baby.' The baby was due in 8 months. I simply put my arm around her shoulders and did not commit myself verbally at all. Later in Chapter 3 bargaining is referred to when looking at communicating about prognosis.

ANGER

Sometimes people experience anger as a result of their frustration with their predicament. It is important to acknowledge anger and try to assess the reasons for it. It can be very rewarding to sit with someone and say: 'Please tell me why you are so angry.' When it works well a list can be produced. There may be some things on the list for which the professional may be able to offer some practical support; others cannot be fixed. Acknowledging this may help. It may be that someone's anger has nothing to do with the diagnosis, so avoid the trap of labelling someone 'in the anger stage' by careful assessment. Never assume.

Anger about the diagnosis and prognosis

Anger can help people to feel more in control at a time when they feel helpless. Vachon (2005) regards it as an honest reaction closer to the truth than repression, and therefore may be healing. Sometimes anger can be focused on the 'Why me?' question. 'I don't know why you, I'm sorry this has happened to you' is a good starting point. It may be that the person has good reason to be angry, e.g. delayed diagnosis. If this is established as a fact, empathising and acknowledging this is important. Sometimes the patient may find it helpful to write about the anger in a journal or letter. Sometimes a chance to talk to a person with whom they are angry may help. Listening to the patient's story is important. When a person has talked through anger and there is nothing that can be done, it might be helpful to suggest that going on being angry is exhausting and life could be made more enjoyable if it was left behind (Stedeford 1985).

Anger can be free floating. Certain people, or indeed everyone, can be a target with no particular rationale. Relatives and friends can find this particularly difficult. Sometimes offering the angry patient some 'time out', e.g. respite in the local hospice, can help diffuse a fraught home life. Relatives and friends get a rest and time away from home sometimes helps to diffuse the anger. However, a person whose anger continues to disrupt home or ward life may well benefit from a referral to mental health staff, e.g. social worker, clinical psychologist or psychiatrist. Some people may attempt to suppress their anger and this can lead to depression. Kübler-Ross (1970) advises that we should find a way of letting the angry person know that we care and have time for them. Avoiding an angry person may fuel their anger. We all need to find our unique way of showing the angry person that we care.

ANXIETY

Patients who are suffering unduly from anxiety will exhibit many different symptoms. Physically these can include restlessness, tension, insomnia, shortness of breath, numbness, apprehension and gastrointestinal upsets, to mention just a few. The physical symptoms may be difficult to relate to anxiety and they may dominate, obscuring the psychological reason for it. Furthermore, certain medications, e.g. steroids, can magnify the physical symptoms, so it is very important to be alert to the signs of anxiety. Many palliative care patients will be anxious.

Some people's manifestations of an anxiety state are more straightforward and the psychological symptoms dominate. People will be worrying excessively about one or several issues and have difficulty controlling these feelings on most days. With anxiety disorders, once diagnosed, there is much that can be done in terms of minimising the effect of this occurrence. Among these interventions are good sound communication skills, and a range of psychological interventions including counselling, group work, stress management skills, relaxation and visualisation; there is a growing body of evidence for the effectiveness of these. They are discussed more fully in Chapters 7 and 11. Thus, taking a reflective approach to a patient's behaviour and reporting potentially anxiety-related symptoms early can go a great way towards optimising a patient's quality of life.

DEPRESSION

Research indicates that as many as one in three cancer patients will suffer from episodes of depression or anxiety at some stage in their illness (Ibbotson et al. 1994; Fulton 1998). It is also probable that 30–33% of relatives also become anxious or depressed (Pitceathly and Maguire 2000). It is generally accepted that depression frequently remains undiagnosed in palliative care (Lloyd-Williams et al.

2003). Barraclough (1994) estimates that depression will be a significant symptom for a quarter of all patients admitted to a palliative care unit. That said, recognition of anxiety and depression should be high on the list for all health-care professionals in generalist or specialist palliative care. This section therefore concentrates on being alert to the manifestations of depression and making an assessment, and there is a need to improve on this.

Reasons put forward for the under-diagnosis of depression in palliative care include some health-care professionals seeing depression as a reasonable response to facing death. Treatment may be seen as interfering with a normal response (Massie 1989). It may also be that professionals fail to distinguish between what is 'appropriate sadness' and what is depression. It is not unusual for a dying person to be tearful, sad, and experience feelings of fear and anxiety. However, these expressions of fear and sadness should not be unremitting. To improve the diagnosis and treatment of depression in palliative care we need to give it the same attention that we do physical symptoms, e.g. pain. The dearth of specialist mental health practitioners has already been highlighted.

The *Diagnostic and Statistical Manual of Mental Disorders*, fourth revision (DSM-IV; American Psychiatric Association 1994) criteria for major depressive disorder is widely used for diagnosing depression in the physically healthy population. Using this system to qualify for a diagnosis of depression, the physically healthy should exhibit one of the core symptoms and four other symptoms from the criteria. The two core criteria are depressed mood most of the day and anhedonia – a marked loss of pleasure or interest in activities. The other criteria are weight loss or gain, insomnia or hypersomnia, psychomotor agitation or retardation, fatigue, feelings of worthlessness or excessive or inappropriate guilt, diminished ability to concentrate or indecisiveness and recurrent thoughts of death or suicide, or planning a suicide attempt (Wilson et al. 2000).

The core criterion, loss of interest and diminished pleasure, needs some discussion when applied to palliative care. In advanced disease, functional decline will limit motivation to engage in social activities. It is not uncommon for dying people to re-focus their energy on priorities of a deeper significance and disengage from areas of interest that probably have secondary importance. However, when there is a marked loss of interest or pleasure in all activities, including interaction with relatives or friends, there is a consensus that this is a valid criterion for assessment for depression (Lynch 1995; Passick and Breitbart 1996).

The Hospital Anxiety and Depression Scale (HADS) represents the most widely used tool for assessing depression in palliative care (Lloyd-Williams et al. 2003). This 14-item scale, devised by Zigmond and Snaith (1983), excludes symptoms that may have an emotional and physical component, e.g. loss of appetite, changes in sleep pattern. The scale is in fact based on anhedonia. The HADS has now been translated into all European languages, Arabic, Japanese, Chinese and Urdu.

The 10-item Edinburgh Postnatal Depression Scale (EPDS) was compared with a present state examination for depression according to the *International Classification of Diseases*, 10th edn (ICD-10; WHO 1992) criteria in 100 patients with metastatic cancer receiving palliative care. In this study a cut-off threshold of 13 gave an optimum sensitivity of 81% and specificity of 79%. This scale has also been used in other palliative care settings with favourable results. Although designed for use in postnatal depression, it may well be a useful screening tool for patients receiving palliative care (Lloyd-Williams et al. 2003). Screening tools have a role to play in assessing for depression. However, they should be accompanied by sensitive questions about the patient's own perception of their mood together with questions that explore their feelings, e.g. of helplessness, hopelessness, inappropriate guilt and thoughts of self-harm or suicide. Lloyd-Williams et al. (2003) suggest that, when considering whether a patient is depressed, a useful guide may be that, if the person blames the illness for how he is feeling, he is probably experiencing sadness at the illness. If the person blames himself for the illness he may well be depressed.

As care of family and friends is an integral part of palliative care, it is important for health-care professionals to be alert to the potential for them being depressed. Advising a family member to consult their GP about a possible minor or major depression can make the difference between the success and failure of a planned home death.

In the absence of readily available psychiatric input, health-care professionals, usually doctors and/or nurses, will be left to assess for depression. They should bear in mind, when doing so, that research indicates that patients may underestimate their own distress (Lloyd-Williams et al. 2003) and relatives and friends, if asked, will describe psychological distress that is closer to how they feel than what the patient is feeling (Faller et al. 1995).

Strategies for supporting depressed patients mirror the principles of sound palliative care to some extent. They include good rapport and support. Relief of poorly controlled symptoms that may be contributing to depression is important. Supportive psychotherapy may help to reduce feelings of isolation for the patient. Also there are many antidepressants available with acceptable side-effect profiles and patients identified as depressed, even in the last 4–6 weeks of life, may still benefit from treatment (Lloyd-Williams et al. 2003).

SOCIAL PAIN

The potential for social pain is probably greater in today's materialistic society than ever before. Loss of employment can herald loss of status and self-esteem as well as loss of income. Loss of income these days can equate with loss of home and anguish about debts. People need early clear help and support to navigate their way through the benefits regulations. Even so they may have to manage on reduced income when expenditure may be going up, e.g. being at home may increase energy bills. Roles and relationships within the family will inevitably change as people are dying and these can be the source of great pain. These issues are given more attention in Chapter 8, which looks at living with dying (see also Chapter 13).

CONCLUSION

This chapter has aimed to give pointers on how to take a health-promoting approach to palliative care in broad terms. To this end it is important to provide a level of support that is adapted to the individual and flexible to changing needs. Finding the balance between not being intrusive and avoiding encouraging autonomy when it is not wanted can be a challenge. Potentially distressing aspects of facing progressive disease and death, e.g. denial, anger, anxiety and depression, are highlighted and explored further in Chapters 3 and 13. The strategies for communication in Chapter 3 provide some of the tools necessary to assess patients' understanding of the situation and give them choices about the level of psychological support that they receive.

MAIN IMPLICATIONS FOR PRACTICE

- Assessing the level of psychosocial and spiritual support needed by each patient is important. Although it is important to provide appropriate support it is equally important to recognise and value the patient's personal and social coping mechanisms.
- Patients should not be pushed to be autonomous if this is not their choice.
- The level of support needed by someone facing death will often oscillate. Professionals need to adjust to this and aim to respond accordingly.
- At each new juncture in the disease trajectory information should be given at the rate and depth signalled by the patient.
- When giving bad news it is important to be mindful of cultural nuances without stereotyping.
- The term 'denial' is open to different interpretations. A patient may truly have an intrapsychic denial; however, he or she may simply not want to talk or the denial can be *socially constructed* by others in a subconscious effort as a protection. This could leave the dying person isolated and fearful. It is important to assess this and be aware that oscillation between denial and acceptance is common as people get closer to dying.
- Where there is limited access to mental health services, senior nurses and doctors would do well to learn how to assess for depression and recognise anxiety states. Referral on to appropriate services is desirable.
- Services should be fine tuned to offering help and advice about social aspects of care, e.g. financial difficulties and housing problems.

SUGGESTED FURTHER READING

Downie RS, Randall F (2006) *The Philosophy of Palliative Care*. Oxford: Oxford University Press.

Kübler- Ross E (1970) *On Death and Dying*. London: Tavistock Publications. Reprinted 1989, 1991, 1992, 1995, London: Routledge.

Kübler-Ross E, Kessler D (2005) *On Grief and Grieving: Finding the meaning of grief through the five stages of loss*. London: Simon & Schuster.

Lloyd Williams M (2003) *Psychosocial Issues In Palliative Care*. Oxford: Oxford University Press.

Macdonald E (2004) *Difficult Conversations in Medicine*. Oxford: Oxford University Press.

Chapter 3
Communication skills

KEY POINTS

- **The impact of good communication**: good communication among patients, health professionals, relatives and friends is the cornerstone to high-quality care. Patients value face-to-face contact with health professionals. It is most successful when underpinned by a mutual understanding about what the patient knows and feels about their illness.
- **The impetus to teach communication skills**: in nursing this resulted from a steep rise in complaints about nurses in 1979. All complaints contained an element of poor communication. Following that research studies demonstrated that nurses were using aberrant communication skills on many occasions, including avoidance of answering questions and ignoring them. These behaviours have become known as blocking behaviours or avoiding and distancing. They are socially learnt, subconscious in the main and can become habitual.
- **Facilitative styles**: facilitative styles of communication require the health professional to respond to the cues of the patient's relatives and friends, provide information where necessary so that they can reflect on their own story and with support find their own way forward. Facilitating styles are non-verbal and verbal. They can be taught. Avoiding and distancing behaviours can be sophisticated. A review of these is included and you are invited to reflect on your own practice in their light.
- **What Howard taught me about nursing dying people**: learning from patients.
- **Helpful strategies**: some strategies for dealing with common issues, e.g. giving bad news, exploring denial and answering difficult questions, are outlined.
- **Communicating with people with dementia**: the principles of communicating with people with dementia are discussed. People with dementia will be more commonplace in the years to come.

THE IMPACT OF GOOD COMMUNICATION

Good communication is the key to the delivery of effective supportive palliative care services (National Institute for Health and Clinical Effectiveness or NICE 2004a). From a survey carried out by the National Cancer Alliance that involved talking with 75 patients we know that patients value being treated with human dignity and respect and having good communication with health professionals. They also want to be given clear information about their illness and receive psychological support when they need it (*The NHS Cancer Plan* – DH 2000b). Research over the past 50 years demonstrates the benefits of good communication. Some of the major works are briefly highlighted here.

As early as 1964 Revans found that, in wards where morale was good, the atmosphere was more conducive to good communication and patient stay was shorter than in wards where the reverse was true.

Experimental studies by Hayward (1975 – a study involving 68 patients), and one by Boore (1978) using physiological measures of stress for 80 patients, demonstrated that, by giving preoperative and pre-investigative information that included experiential as well as procedural details, patients reported lower anxiety levels than in control groups. Participants in the experimental groups were also more likely to comply with related clinical activities, e.g. postoperative exercises. In both studies attention was paid to ensuring that patients had understood the information given, usually by getting them to repeat it back to the researcher.

A more recent meta-analysis of 21 randomised controlled studies demonstrated that there is a correlation between effective doctor–patient communication and improved patient health outcomes (Stewart 1995). There is a consensus that effective communication can influence the rate of recovery and psychological functioning and, in line with the early research, that it can result in more effective pain relief and compliance with treatment (Razavi et al. 2000).

Good communication has an interpersonal perspective that is about health professionals and patients engaging emotionally. Both Hunt (1991) and Lanceley (1995) have researched the social interaction of conversation with cancer patients and conclude that it is collaboratively produced between patients and professionals. The conversations were of a friendly informal nature but were also frequently emotional. In a study of 29 patients, a good communicator was synonymous with a good nurse and described as having a kind caring attitude (Bailey and Wilkinson 1998). In a study of 16 dying patients 14 said that good relationships with professionals helped them to stay hopeful; 'noticing if I was down' and 'being interested in me' were two aspects of care that were valued (Buckley and Herth 2004). Patients value face-to-face communication with health-care professionals; for it to be most successful, it needs to be underpinned by a mutual understanding of what patients know and feel about their illnesses.

THE IMPETUS TO TEACH COMMUNICATION SKILLS

The impetus to teach communication skills in nursing came from a critical incident. In 1979 the NHS Ombudsman contacted the Royal College of Nursing (RCN) and

General Nursing Council. There was a rising level of complaints against nurses. These increasing numbers of complaints all had an element of inadequate communication. Subsequently research, looking at nurse–patient conversations in different settings, by Faulkner (1979) and Macleod-Clark (1981), who analysed 56 hours of conversation, found that verbal communication related, in the main, to physical care. Perhaps more worrying were many instances of nurses blocking and avoiding disease-oriented questions, information-seeking questions and expressions of anxiety, e.g.

> N: You are not wearing any make-up at the moment, no hair clips?
> P: No.
> N: And the doctor showed you the green consent form?
> P: Yes, I signed it. I shall get out from here soon, shan't I, darling? Because they do send in a home nursing help when I get home, don't they?
> N: I'll leave you in peace for a few minutes.

Other later studies supported these findings of Faulkner and Macleod-Clark. Maguire (1985) highlighted many examples of nurses ignoring signs of distress in cancer patients and considered that there was little acknowledgement of each patient's coping style or recognition of the patient's need to be nurtured or affirmed through communication. Wilkinson (1991) found a high trend for blocking behaviours used by nurses working with cancer patients. As part of her conclusions she felt that a nurse's communication style was affected by her own attitude to death and the dominant facilitation style of the ward sister.

Recently when teaching some medical students, they said that it was difficult if the consultants left them alone with a patient in outpatients. Invariably the patient would ask: 'What is wrong with me?' They said that they would reply by saying something like: 'Well, it's difficult to tell', and then try to change the subject. I said why not just say: '. . . I'm not allowed to say as I am still a student. However, do ask the consultant when she or he comes back or would you like me to ask on your behalf?' There was silence for a while and then one said, 'We are already fobbing the patients off . . . why do we do this?'

Addington-Hall et al. (1995) surveyed friends and relatives of 237 patients who had died as a result of a cerebrovascular accident. They highlighted that two-fifths of the sample felt that they had needed more information, and concluded that psychological support and communication among health-care professionals, patients, families and friends needed improvement.

Fourteen years after the initial approach via the Ombudsman to the nursing organisations re poor communication, the government acted again. In 1993 the Audit Commission again expressed concern about poor levels of communication (25% of patients interviewed felt a lack of individual care and attention and 20% felt that nurses could try harder to help them understand the information that they are given). This resulted in the Commission publishing a booklet called *Making Time for Patients: A handbook for ward sisters* (Audit Commission 1993). In it are many fundamental strategies for improving communication and continuity of care.

Communication is complex and, most professionals would probably agree, one of the most difficult things to get right in clinical practice. It is a positive, and one imagines a reasonably accurate, premise that no one sets out to develop faulty communication skills. Aberrant skills of avoiding and distancing are almost certainly learnt subconsciously, although, in early research (Macleod-Clark 1981), some nurses on reflection recognised that they were doing it. In many situations, however, the health-care professional may not have this insight. The behaviour becomes automatic, and it may be that this habitual behaviour hampers the skills of a professional with the emotional integrity very ably to support the dying person. Furthermore, it has been demonstrated that a poor ability to communicate increases stress, reduces job satisfaction and leads to emotional burnout of health-care professionals (Wilkinson 1994; Fallowfield 1995; Ramirez et al. 1995).

If aberrant skills are learnt subconsciously it follows that communication skills will not reliably improve with experience alone, as highlighted by Cantwell and Ramirez (1997). However, there is evidence that communication skills can be taught (Maguire 1990; Faulkner 1992; Langewitz et al. 1998; Wilkinson et al. 1999b; Razavi et al. 2000; Fallowfield et al. 2001), and maintained over time (Maguire et al. 1996; Wilkinson et al. 1999b).

As a result of this evidence and a clear need for action to improve communication skills, a commitment was made by the government in *The NHS Cancer Plan* (DH 2000b) that teaching advanced communication skills would be part of continuing professional development throughout the cancer networks. This commitment was reinforced in the NICE (2004b) guidelines on supportive and palliative care. Advanced communication skills courses are now being rolled out nationally through the cancer networks. One aim is to embed these courses in institutes for higher education. It is from this programme that much of the material in this chapter is drawn.

FACILITATIVE STYLES

Both our verbal and non-verbal behaviour are important in helping to facilitate good communication.

Non-verbal communication

Social psychologists will tell us that what we say with our bodies can be up to five times more powerful than our speech (Argyle 1978). This can be demonstrated easily. Think of a very sincere comment to make to a friend and then say it while rolling your eyes and taking up an aggressive body posture. Some of the main elements of non-verbal communication are posture, eye contact, facial expressions, gestures and the use of touch.

When talking with someone a closed body posture, e.g. folded arms and crossed legs, can be seen as inhibiting easy conversation. An open posture is more classically identified with someone who wants to listen. Often people in intense conversation mirror each other's posture, changing from time to time – one leads, the other follows. An anxious person may have a tense and alert musculature. A depressed person may have a rather closed and *drooping* posture.

Verbal facilitating skills

To be able to provide individualised care and support, it is important that the professional understands what the patient knows and feels about each key event as it happens. How they are coping, and who or what resources they have, are also essential areas to discuss. In addition, it is useful to establish what past experiences they may have had of a similar event and how they managed then (Wilkinson and Mula 2004).

Skilful use of key verbal behaviours during conversation holds the key to encouraging patients to share their thoughts and feelings, and raise appropriate questions. Listening to patients is an active skill and requires great concentration if the patient's cues are to be picked up. On paper the value of good verbal skills, e.g. the use of open questions, reflection, clarification and empathic statements, is difficult to portray. Watching role-play or a video of role-play, where it is used well, demonstrates vividly what useful tools they are. These are the skills highlighted and practised on the 3-day communication skills programme that is currently being rolled out nationally via the cancer networks (Cancer Action Team NHS 2007). I did this course after 35 years of nursing, during which I have also taught communication skills. I now find that, by using these skills more expertly in assessment, I can elicit more pertinent information in a shorter space of time, and often feel closer to the patient.

It can be challenging to pick up on all the cues that a patient gives. It is not unusual to walk away from a conversation and, on reflection, feel that you have missed opportunities to encourage patients to express fears. You can go back. You can return to the patient that day, or some days later even, and explain that you felt that you did not pick up on what they were saying and ask if they would like to talk more about the area that you feel you missed.

Avoiding and distancing: traps for young and old players

As discussed earlier it is common for professionals to avoid difficult issues with patients. These strategies are almost certainly socially learnt and can become habitual. Here are some examples of some more sophisticated avoiding and distancing strategies. Sometimes as professionals we use these strategies and still feel that we have done a good job. You can choose to reflect on your own practice by regarding this as a questionnaire.

The following strategies have been described by Faulkner and Maguire (1994), Heaven and Maguire (2003) and Wilkinson and Mula (2004). The following questionnaire is based on their work.

Neutral conversation

Starting a conversation by talking about neutral safe topics, e.g. the weather, the ward, the patient's home, is sometimes recommended as building a relationship. To some extent this may be true, but if things do not move on beyond neutral, then this may be regarded as blocking. The patient may be taking cues from the professional and keeping it neutral and *safe*. Then you have to ask who is *protecting* whom? Faulkner and Maguire (1994) found that most conversations between nurse and patients followed this neutral pattern.

> Do you use neutral conversation predominately with patients?
>
> ☐ Never   ☐ Sometimes   ☐ Often   ☐ Habitually

Normalising

This is a form of reassurance that has good intentions, i.e. making the patient feel better. The patient faced with death may, for example, have a young family and say something like 'I can't leave my children'. The professional may reply by saying kindly, 'It is natural to feel the way you do; all mothers would'. This will almost certainly effectively block any more expression of emotional pain. At a later stage it may be helpful to know that others have faced these issues and had similar feelings. Timing here is important.

> Do you normalise patients' fears and anxieties prematurely?
>
> ☐ Never   ☐ Sometimes   ☐ Often   ☐ Habitually

Selective attention to cues

A patient may be facing a situation that raises a whole range of issues. These may cover practical as well as psychosocial, body image and sexual issues. For the less reflective or inexperienced professional, a trap is to select an area that they feel expert in, e.g. the practical management of a stoma. This opposes use of non-verbal and verbal facilitating skills in supporting the patient to express all fears and anxieties, then summarising them and making a plan of care. The net result here is that the patient gets information and reassurance only in the area in which the professional feels comfortable.

> Do you select issues that you feel safe with, as opposed to others that you are less confident about, and use this as your guide in reassuring patients?
>
> ☐ Never   ☐ Sometimes   ☐ Often   ☐ Habitually

Giving false reassurance

Patients may be expressing fears and anxieties. Before rushing in with what may be very articulate and well-informed reassurance, it is important to elicit just what the concerns are and then address them specifically, e.g. a patient may say that they think they may be dying. After gently establishing that the person does want to address this area now, ask what specific fears and anxieties they have about this. This opposes working on assumptions of what you think the fears are. And this is what you are doing unless you ask a question such as 'Can you bear to tell me exactly what is worrying you about dying?'.

How often do you use false reassurance?

☐ Never ☐ Sometimes ☐ Often ☐ Habitually

Passing the buck

This is when a patient may express a concern and, instead of encouraging more disclosure and expression of anxieties, the professional immediately suggests referral to a third party, e.g. a breast care nurse. The referral may be entirely appropriate but it need not preclude the patient expressing how they are feeling at that moment. Listening to the patient can help them to feel more supported and will result in a more comprehensive referral to the third party.

How often do you pass the buck?

☐ Never ☐ Sometimes ☐ Often ☐ Habitually

Switching focus

This is when the professional may stay with the content that is being expressed by the patient but manages to steer the conversation to what might feel like safer territory for themselves. Here are three examples of switching focus.

Switching time

Patient: When the surgeon told me it had spread I was totally devastated . . .

Professional: Are you feeling better now?

Here the time frame has been moved and a leading question has been asked. This will almost certainly block the patient from expressing emotion about the past event.

Do you switch time frames?

☐ Never   ☐ Sometimes   ☐ Often   ☐ Habitually

Switching topic

Patient: I'm so frightened that the treatment isn't going to work . . . I know it's experimental . . . and I felt so ill last time I had chemo.

Professional: You felt ill. Tell me more about that.

Here the professional is picking up on content with which she feels safe. The more emotionally laden content re fear and doubts about treatment has been ignored. The chances are that the patient will not be able to steer the conversation back to fears about the treatment.

Do you switch topic?

☐ Never   ☐ Sometimes   ☐ Often   ☐ Habitually

Switching person

Patient: I think I am coming to the end of things . . . it all seems so hopeless now . . . .

Professional: How is your wife coping?

Here, confronted by a person feeling hopeless facing fears of death, the professional looks for an easier option by talking about a third person.

Do you switch person?

☐ Never   ☐ Sometimes   ☐ Often   ☐ Habitually

Personal note

If I had filled in this questionnaire early in my career I would have been ticking habitually for many of these behaviours. This is not because I am an uncaring person. I had less emotional integrity than I have now, the behaviours were socially learnt and I had no insight that I was using them. I still use some of these strategies on occasions. The difference now is that I reflect more and know when I have used them. This gives me the opportunity perhaps to go back to a situation that has not gone well.

WHAT HOWARD TAUGHT ME ABOUT NURSING DYING PEOPLE

Four factors are known to impact on communication behaviour: fears, e.g. of unleashing strong emotions, of doing more harm than good; or beliefs that, for example, emotional problems are inevitable and there is no point talking about them unless you have answers. The third factor is inadequate skills and the fourth lack of, or perceived lack of, support (Maguire 2000). Buckman (2005) adds to this list, including fears of our own mortality and fear of being blamed, among others. Many of these fears and beliefs, when looked at superficially, are understandable and may well be shared by patients too. On deeper reflection they probably do not stand up to scrutiny. It is for each person to reflect on their own practice in order to understand why they might use avoiding and blocking behaviour. An essential part of being an effective communicator in palliative care is a reasonably well-developed sense of self, i.e. who you are and what motivates you. This will be looked at in more detail in Chapter 4. Avoiding and distancing behaviour is not, however, commensurate with a caring professional approach and leaves patients who need our emotional support isolated and more vulnerable.

The most valuable and pervasive learning takes place while we are doing what we do, when we are engaged at all levels behaviourally, cognitively and emotionally (Rogers 1967). With this in mind read the following poem:

Howard Soar 1948–1973
Died in hospital

I awoke at 3.00am
You name was in my head.
Later I learnt
that was precisely
the time
you died.

You hitch hiked from New Zealand
to London and demanded
pioneering surgery.
The surgeon's skill
could not match
your spirit.

How will I get
through nights
without you?
Tired from
the late night toil
of medicine rounds,
and careful monitoring
of critically ill patients.
Who will help me?
Who will comfort Niki,
when she wakes screaming
from the nightmare of her death,
that will happen soon?

Who will listen
to Jane's plans for her wedding
and children,
she can never have?

Who will hold David,
when he vomits blood and
cries?

Who will comfort me?

As the poem tells, Howard was a patient whom I nursed many years ago. In the time that he was an inpatient, he gave emotional support to fellow patients and to us nurses. Towards the end of his life he was too weak to get out of bed to comfort Niki, Jane or David. He taught us how to do it simply by explaining that patients understood we were not omnipotent. Niki, Jane and David just wanted us to hold their hands and comfort them in their pain as best we could. It was difficult for them to understand why professionals didn't do this.

HELPFUL STRATEGIES

Giving bad news – truth telling

Giving bad news was looked at in Chapter 2 from the patient's perspective. In particular it was emphasised that pace and depth of information should be sensitively given, aiming to maintain the patient's sense of control and thus help a healthy adjustment to changed circumstances. In this chapter research looking at truth telling and a strategy for giving bad news are outlined.

Historically, in the UK patients with a life-threatening illness may not have been told their diagnosis. It used to be common practice to speak with the relatives first and even collude not to tell the patient. This is still considered the norm in some cultural groups, as discussed in Chapter 2. This tradition is based on what is arguably a misplaced sense of kindness to protect the patient from a painful truth. So should we tell patients the truth?

A large study collected information preferences from a heterogeneous sample of patients attending outpatient clinics in the UK. Over 34 hospitals were involved in the study. Inclusion criteria comprised adults who were about to see a medical, clinical or surgical oncologist about their cancer treatment, diagnosis, prognosis, tests or routine follow-ups; 2331 patients participated in the study. The results were as follows:

• 87% (2027) wanted all possible information, both good and bad news
• 95% (2203) preferred to know whether or not their illness was cancer.

The results from this very large study provide conclusive evidence that a vast majority of patients with cancer want a great deal of specific information about their illness and treatment. The researchers note that failure to disclose such information on the grounds that a significant number of patients may not want to know their diagnosis is therefore untenable (Jenkins et al. 2001).

A meta-analysis of the literature on truth telling and psychological distress was conducted. Of 681 abstracts from around the world, 14 studies from 8 different countries represented the best available evidence. The analysis concluded the following:

• There is good evidence that open disclosure had a positive effect on outcomes
• Evidence and trends to suggest patients prefer open and full disclosure
• Non-informed patients had increased psychological distress
• Ambiguous conflicting information increased anxiety.

Wilkinson et al. (2005)

There is a consensus in the literature that honest information about diagnosis serves the patient best. However, it can be complicated by patients fluctuating between wanting to hear the truth and wanting to hide from the truth. Truth is important in building trust in a relationship (Macdonald 2004). It is synonymous with treating patients with dignity and respects their autonomy (Randall and Downie 2006). However, all these authors are also experienced clinicians in palliative care and they stress the importance of communicating in such a way that the patient is encouraged to participate and be active in directing the flow, rate and depth of the news being communicated. This is in line with maximising the potential for promoting a healthy adaptation to the truth.

It is a generally held belief that patients like to hear the diagnosis of their illness from their doctor. Certainly the person delivering bad news, if not the doctor, should be the patient's clinical nurse specialist. Where possible, the patient should know that the consultation will be about the diagnosis and be invited to bring someone with them if they want. The strategy outlined here emphasises in particular the verbal content.

Giving bad news

We tend to associate bad news with telling the patient their diagnosis; however, there are many other occasions when bad news is given, e.g. it may not be possible for a patient to die in their place of choice, hoped-for financial benefits may not be forthcoming, a respite admission may not be possible. In broad terms the steps laid out here to tell someone of their diagnosis can be applied to all occasions when giving bad news. The overall aim is to help patients remain the experts on themselves by giving the information at the rate and depth dictated by them. The model discussed is the six-step protocol proposed by Buckman (2005) (Table 3.1).

Table 3.1 Six-step protocol for giving bad news

1. Getting the physical context right

2. Finding out how much the patient knows

3. Finding out how much the patient wants to know

4. Sharing information (aligning and educating)

5. Responding to the patient's feelings

6. Planning and following through

It is important that the meeting between the patient and professional can be in a private place and that there are no interruptions by telephone or bleep. Ideally the meeting should be prearranged and the patient given an opportunity to bring someone with them. Advise them to bring a pad and pen so that, if need be, notes can be made. The patient should know that the meeting is to discuss the diagnosis and be encouraged to write down any questions that they have in advance. It is important to adhere to the principle of good non-verbal behaviour by ensuring that everyone is seated and properly introduced before starting. Having said all this, listen to this:

> My sister was told that my mother had died in the middle of a busy hospital corridor. The bleep of the doctor informing her was going off. He was shifting from foot to foot clearly needing to answer the call. He said, 'I am so sorry to have to tell you but your mother has just died. She had a cardiac arrest; we did everything we could. I so wanted her to recover because she had such spirit. And now, I'm so sorry, I must go as I am needed in theatre. Sister will look after you.' My sister remembers this as a positive experience. She felt that the surgeon cared for our mother by acknowledging her spirit and saying he wanted her to recover, and respected his need to be elsewhere.

The six step protocol for giving bad news

Find out how much the patient already knows or suspects

The following may need to paraphrased with a sentence explaining that you have all the facts and results; however, *it is useful to know exactly what you are making of things and we can build on that.*

Some phrases that can be useful in determining what the patient already knows are:

> 'What did the previous doctors tell you about your illness?'
>
> 'When you first had symptom X what did you think it might be?'
>
> 'What did Dr X tell you when he sent you here . . . ?'
>
> 'Did you think something serious was going on when . . . ?'
>
> Buckman (2005)

Find out how much the patient wants to know

This can be paraphrased with a statement such as: 'I don't want to overwhelm you with too much information and nor do I want you to feel that things are being held back that you would rather discuss now. So I need your help here and, do remember, we will be meeting again; this is not the only opportunity to discuss things.'

Some phrases that can be helpful in establishing how much information patients want are:

'Do you like to know exactly what is going on or would you prefer me to give you just the outline?'

'Are you the sort of person who would like to know exactly what's wrong or would you prefer just to hear about the treatment plan?'

Would you like me to give you the full details of your illness – or is there somebody else whom you would like me to talk to?'

Buckman (2005)

Sharing information

Here Buckman (2005) suggests that you start this part by *aligning* yourself with the patient, i.e. that you begin by reinforcing the correct parts of the information that the patient has shared with you, using their words as far as possible. You then go on to share the information that you have at a pace determined by your constant observation of the patient's response. If there is a big gap between what the patient thinks and what is, then *a warning* is considered helpful, e.g. 'I'm sorry but the situation is really quite serious . . .' and then pause before going on. Try to grade the information gradually, assessing the patient's response at each point. Useful phrase here are:

'Am I making sense?'

'Do you see what I mean?'

'This must be a bit bewildering, but do you know roughly what I'm saying?'

Clearly, throughout it is also important to invite questions as information is shared. The key ingredients are steady observation and continued gentle guidance on the direction of the interview rather than sudden lurches (Buckman 2005, p 161).

Responding to the patient's feelings

This is crucial in the process. The meeting is paced to give the patient time to express shock, anxiety, fear and indeed their unique response to the news. A useful way of doing this might be:

'I can see what I have told you has made you very distressed?'

And, after a pause:

'Can you bear to tell me exactly what is making you distressed?'

Here the patient is being told that there is no assumption about why this news should upset them; the patient's own fears are important here. Also the question is presented so that the patient can choose not to talk about their feelings at this point (Maguire 2000). If the patient is able to express fears and anxieties they should be summarised and checked out with the patient. It is also important to add here that, if the patient responds by denying, this should be respected.

Planning and following through

At the end of the meeting the main points including the anxieties raised should be summarised clearly and mutually agreed between the patient and professional. After the summary, check if there are any questions that the patient still wants to ask. If there are any positive supportive suggestions that can be made for the immediate future, this should also be done. However, the health-care professional should avoid the 'We can fix it all mode'. There should be a clear understanding between the patient and professional about what the next step will be, when another meeting will take place, and who can be contacted in the interim if the patient wants more information or to talk things through.

This is a very brief overview of a crucial stage of a person's illness experience. Students are advised to read the two texts referred to in this section for a more detailed account.

Tape-recording consultations

In recent years some centres have introduced the practice of audio-taping patient–doctor interviews and giving the patient the audio-tape for reference. Bruera et al. (1999) audio-taped conversations for a study that included 60 palliative care patients who were also receiving written information. In this study patients were significantly more satisfied with their clinic appointment than patients not receiving a tape. The tape was also valued by relatives and friends. McHugh et al. (1995), in a similar study, highlighted that, although recording aided retention of information, it could be unhelpful in terms of psychological distress, particularly when the patient had a poor prognosis. The implications here are that more research is needed and also consideration given to recording information about discussion of prognosis.

Denial

The concept of denial has been discussed in Chapter 2. As a reader, ensure that you have read this before going on. People use denial as a coping mechanism when the truth is too difficult for them to bear. Unless denial is causing complications, e.g. emotional distress to the patient, or preventing help-seeking behaviour, there is broad agreement in the literature that health professionals should not challenge denial.

> Patients use denial as a defence when the truth is too painful to bear. So it should not be challenged unless it has created serious problems for the patient or relative.

Maguire (2000, p 299)

Denial is undoubtedly a common and effective coping strategy which enables many patients to survive emotionally by ignoring unpleasant facts or absorbing them over time at their own pace. If this approach best satisfies the patient's own need then this should be respected.

Macdonald (2004, p 68)

This view is also supported by Stedeford (1985), Vachon (2005) and Kübler-Ross (1970); the last adds that it is important that we do not encourage or embellish denial, but be gently supportive of the person in denial. Vachon (2003) adds that it is not a good enough reason to challenge denial if the professional feels that it is desirable that the patient and the family accept what is happening. This sort of responsibility is a misguided assumption of responsibility.

Randall and Downie (2006) agree that denial should be challenged only if it is causing emotional distress to the patient or causing them to refuse beneficial treatment. They disagree with challenging denial for the benefit of the family, as has been suggested by others, e.g. Maguire (2000). They state that this approach, aimed at benefiting the family, may in turn harm the patient.

It can be important, however, to establish if this is a *true denial* or whether it is a situation that has been *socially constructed* in some way and is being called denial (see Chapter 2), or indeed whether the patient has had the diagnosis explained.

Assessing for denial

Start by asking patients to tell you about their illness now and how they feel about what is happening to them. You may find from this that, in fact, they are not in denial but perhaps just avoiding talking about their illness. They may be trying to protect relatives from painful truths. However, if the patient does seem to be denying the seriousness of the illness, a useful question at this assessment may be 'Would it be helpful to have more information about your illness?' (Kaye 2003). If the patient says no to this, leave things as they are. Kaye (2003) recommends that doctors ask patients at each visit: 'How do you feel things are going for you at the moment?' Multidisciplinary teams should clearly document significant conversations to avoid repeat assessments that could be distressing for the patient.

Challenging denial

If this is to occur, it should be done by someone experienced in psychological care, either a professional in mental health or an experienced nurse or doctor, who has preferably been trained to advanced communication skills level. Maguire (2000, pp 299–300) gives useful suggestions on how to approach this, e.g.

Ask the patient to give an account of their illness exploring how they felt at each key point, e.g. when the first symptoms appeared, when they had results of tests.

Gently explore what they think is wrong. There may be glimpses of doubt here, e.g. 'I am certain it's nothing serious; at least I am pretty sure'. Reflect back the glimpses of doubt, e.g. *pretty sure*. This could prompt the patient to say 'Well, maybe I have cancer' or indeed to say the opposite, e.g. 'Yes I am sure it's not serious'.

In this instance it is best to leave it for now. Sometimes, instead of a clear-cut answer to the *pretty sure* reflection, patients may show some ambivalence about whether they want to face reality, e.g. they may just shrug their shoulders and say 'I don't really know . . .'.

> It might be useful here to gently confront, e.g. it sounds as if part of you believes it's not serious and another part might be willing to consider it is. Which part of you should I relate to?

In this instance be guided by the patient's response. Another strategy is to look for a window in the denial, e.g.

> Is there ever a moment when you think things may be more serious?

Maguire (2000, p 300)

Respect the patient's answer.

Patients in denial may apparently not be open to new treatments. Inclusion in a drugs trial, for example, may require the patient to sign a consent form that indicates that the treatment has been discussed. One solution in the circumstance is to present the patient with a hypothesis:

> Supposing you were in a very difficult situation and there really was no alternative, are you the sort of person who would like to consider some very new experimental treatment? The patient may say, 'Well yes I suppose I would if I had to' and then discussion about the treatment could be gently led by the health professional. They may however say 'No I am not going to be a guinea pig'. It would probably be best to leave it there.

Macdonald (2004, p 68)

Interpersonal and intrapsychic denial

Connor (1992) puts forward the notion of *intrapsychic deniers*. He describes this as a denial that helps to preserve a weak ego and occurs when people feel, consciously or subconsciously, overwhelmed by a serious threat. He describes *interpersonal* deniers as people who use denial to preserve interpersonal relationships. It is used to protect others from the emotional distress that they might feel as a result of open disclosure. He believes that *intrapsychic* deniers constitute a small percentage of terminally ill individuals. His beliefs are based on his clinical experience with hundreds of hospice patients.

Connor conducted a study on 24 patients who he considered to be *interpersonal* deniers. The experimental group (13) were interviewed, with the aim of creating an opportunity for exploring and gaining insight into their own coping processes. Questions were direct but sufficiently open-ended for patients to be able to choose their own level of self-disclosure. Both the experimental group and the control group (11) filled in psychological assessment tools designed to measure denial in terminally ill patients, e.g. the Defence Mechanism Inventory Reversal Scale (Ihilevich and Gleser 1986). Both groups were tested twice, the experimental group before and after the interview. The data indicated that 'in the absence of psychological dysfunction, patients using interpersonal denial may respond favourably to sensitive psychological intervention' (Connor 1992, p 9). Connor found that denial increased in the control group.

Connor notes in his discussion that it was difficult to recruit to the study. Direct contact by him, the researcher, was the most effective approach. He states that his extensive experience in working with terminally ill people may have been a variable in conducting the research and may have influenced results. He stresses that any efforts to replicate this study should consider the abilities of the investigator. Connor's motivation for challenging denial is that he believes this leads to a more open communication between patient and family members. In his write-up he does not include any qualitative data of subsequent communications or details of follow-up interviews with patients or their families.

Holmberg (2006) is a professor in education from Sweden. She presents a case history of the communication between her and her dying 36-year-old son. She writes:

> When my son, through gentle guidance from the palliative care team, finally realised that he was dying, he stopped denying and took control over his last days. The communication between us was again open, honest and warm and we could share the grief.

> Holmberg (2006, p 15)

It is always difficult to make blanket policies, which is a shame, because, as a rule, they feel very safe. Challenging denial is a huge responsibility and needs great sensitivity and expertise. There is a serious risk that the patient's condition may deteriorate while issues from the challenge to denial go unresolved. This outcome is clearly a significant harm (Randall and Downie 2006).

Dealing with difficult questions

Here, in line with a health-promoting approach, the aim is to help the patient to reflect on what is already known, recognise gaps in knowledge, fill them where possible and share uncertainties (Wilkinson and Mula 2004). In this patients remain, as far as possible, the experts on themselves, congruent with a holistic approach. The value of the verbal facilitating skills described earlier cannot be overestimated. Listening for and picking up on verbal cues are crucial. It is the skilful use of these strategies that will achieve the aim outlined.

The patient may ask 'Am I dying?'. It is impossible for the professional to know if the patient wants reassurance that death is not imminent or the truth. You can check this out by asking for an honest response, e.g.

> Can you tell me why you are asking that question now?

The answer may clarify whether the patient really wants confirmation. It is important not to give false reassurance, but if the patient gives a clear signal that the question was asked without really wanting an honest answer the professional can check this out by saying:

> You were asking about your illness. Do you want to talk more about that?

If the answer is *no* gently withdraw and leave it there (Cancer Action Team NHS 2007). However, do make a note of the conversation and be mindful in your next meetings with the patient that this may be on the agenda.

If the answer is *yes* then sensitively confirm that it is so:

> What you are saying is right . . . your illness has progressed and you are dying . . .

Expect and allow silence. It is so important here to follow the *patient's agenda*. It is tempting to rush in with an articulate well-rehearsed monologue that you feel will reassure the patient. This would take the patient, who is struggling with mortality, out of control. Added to that, in your reassurance you may raise issues that are terrifying to the patient, issues that they may not be ready to consider. Instead after a silence gently ask a question such as:

> This may feel like a strange question now, but it's important for us to try to understand what's happening from your viewpoint. Can you tell me how all this is making you feel now . . . what concerns are uppermost in your mind?

Wait for the patient's response. Use silence, acknowledgement, reflection, clarification and open focused questions to proceed at the patient's pace, providing requested information where you can, at a depth that is acceptable, avoiding the sudden lurches described by Buckman (2005) in giving bad news. Only address the issues that the patient raises; this is vital.

Before you leave the patient summarise what has been said. Invite any more questions (Wilkinson and Mula 2004). Agree any action, e.g. provision of more information, an appointment with a particular member of staff. Agree when you will see the patient again and explain who will be available in your absence to talk with him or her, and how they can be contacted. Explain also that you will share this information, unless he or she objects, with the multidisciplinary team to help with support and continuity of care.

Questions about prognosis

In practice we know that making an accurate prognosis is tricky. Glare and Christakis (2005) review the literature on predicting survival in patients with advanced disease. In their conclusion they highlight that the SUPPORT study (Knaus et al. 1995) shows that patients will change their behaviour once they understand that the chance of surviving 6 months is small. Their last sentence states:

> What ultimately may be needed is not so much an accurate prediction of time but acknowledgment of the possibility of dying, communicated carefully by the compassionate and skilled physician.
>
> Glare and Christakis (2005, p 40)

Putting a prognosis into figures, e.g. 3 maybe 4 months, is generally considered unwise in palliative care. These prognostications are usually inaccurate and can lead to considerable distress. Patients who do not reach the time stated may feel cheated.

Equally, if they do, and exceed it, they may have put everything that they have into the time they were given and, when death does not happen, it can feel very difficult. If people are bargaining for more time (see Chapter 2), it is possible that they are asking more than one person questions about their prognosis. If different people give different responses it will cause distress to the patient and may cause friction in the team. It is usually a sensible precaution that just one or two key workers discuss prognosis. For an inpatient, this is usually the doctor in charge of the case and for an outpatient the clinical nurse specialist or GP. However, this does not mean that you pass the buck immediately. You might say:

> That's a difficult question. Can you tell me why you are asking it now?

There may be a seemingly very practical reason, e.g. a family wedding coming up. Listen carefully to what the patient says using verbal facilitating skills. You might then say:

> It can be distressing if people say different things. Experience tells us that it is better if you talk with the doctor in charge of your case about this. Shall I arrange for you to see her or him?

If the patient agrees you could offer to be there as well if it is practicable. Or perhaps they would like a relative or friend to be included. If none of this is possible then suggest:

> We could meet again after that and discuss what was said if you would like.

Maguire (2000) offers a framework for talking with patients and/or relatives about a prognosis. You might say:

> You have asked how long you have. Everyone is so different and the problem is that we really cannot make accurate predictions. And we know that it is distressing when people are given timescales that can't be accurate.

Acknowledge the uncertainty:

> This uncertainty must be awful for you. I wish I could be more helpful.

The patient or relative should be given time to express anxiety. Maguire (2000, p 298) then suggests that you check whether the patient or relative wants any more information about signs that may indicate that the illness is progressing. Seek the advice of the person to whom you are talking. Let them remain the expert on themselves. You could say:

> What I could do, only if you want me to, is suggest some changes that might indicate that the illness is active and you are getting worse.

If there is a clear signal to go on, then depending on the individual's illness you may say something like:

It is likely that there would be some obvious weight loss; you may lose interest in food and some activities. You may feel very tired a lot of the time.

You can explain that as long as there are no obvious signs such as this, it usually indicates that the disease is not active and it may be wise to make the best of that time. It is important to offer continuity of care and ideally patients have a number to ring if they want to talk between appointments. Some people will not want to have these changes suggested to them. They will cope better without. Seeking permission to explain these is vital (Maguire 2000).

Patients remain in charge of themselves and you simply need to confirm the truth and seek permission to tell relatives that they are aware, and negotiate with them that they talk to each other about the illness and its ramifications (Maguire 2000). It is important, as always, to ensure continuity of care. If the patient shows no awareness you may be dealing with denial. If this is so it is useful to talk with the relatives about this phenomenon.

COMMUNICATING WITH PEOPLE WITH DEMENTIA

Kay de Vries

As global life expectancy is rising, so the prevalence of people with dementia increases, and it is important to develop confidence and expertise in communicating with such people. In the early stages of dementia, communication issues are less problematic. Early stage communication issues manifest as a result of subtle memory problems, decreased spontaneity and disorientation to time, and there may be anxiety, reflecting some insight. This is a time when it is important to develop innovative ways of managing the surroundings of people with dementia to enhance all communication processes (Allan and Killick 2001).

During the stage of moderate dementia these symptoms increase. The person has increasingly impaired judgement, language problems and abstract thinking, and at this stage will no longer be able to manage finances or medication, and will have difficulties with activities of daily living. At the severe stage, these symptoms are even more pronounced: the person may be reduced to single word communication and use stereotypical language, e.g. singing. At the end-stage there is increasing disorientation, speech may be difficult to understand but with occasional words or phrases, or they may become mute and there is increasing reliance on non-verbal communication (Bryan 2007).

Everyone can communicate no matter how severe the dementia and staff/family who say 'he can't communicate' need support (Frank 1995; Bryan 2007). Communication does not need to be just verbal, and the use of touch/human contact to communicate with people with dementia is essential. This should be based on considerations of what the person responds to as the disease progresses and can take the form of hand stroking, gentle hair brushing, taking an arm when walking. It may be necessary to get closer to the person to communicate and this can feel as if one is invading the personal space of the person with dementia, so it is important that approaches are unrushed and carried out in a relaxed manner.

Facial expression of the carer is also important. Smiling and trying to reflect any emotions that are conveyed are important when communicating, e.g. if the person with dementia looks worried, you might say that must be worrying and look worried. Making eye contact and trying to keep it is also useful and important, particularly where it is possible to understand any expression conveyed through the eyes of the person with dementia. It is useful for a carer to use his or her own voice quality to reflect any tones that are picked up from the person. Active and reflective listening is important when communicating with the person with dementia, as is the ability just to sit and be silent, and in late stage dementia just sitting and being comfortable in a 'joined silence' may be all that is possible. Overall, it is important to establish closeness through touch and to listen for tones and noises that may convey emotional information, and recognise that the person with dementia has a need to communicate with the key message being: communication is always possible (Bryan 2007).

CONCLUSION

You can work with dying people as both a generalist and a specialist in palliative care. You can be expert in your delivery of care in assisting patients with activities of daily living and helping with pain and symptom control. However, you can still fail to give gold standard palliative care. The essential for excellence in palliative care is good communication. The reasons for this have been clearly outlined in this chapter. Recently, after 36 years of nursing practice I did the 3-day Wilkinson Model Communication Skills Course as part of the national roll out. It has enhanced my practice considerably and I wish that I had done it years ago. Many of the verbal and non-verbal behaviours that are at the heart of this approach were well known to me, but practising skills with actors simulating patients was a steep and most productive learning curve. The videos used for the course vividly demonstrate the value of verbal facilitating skills. It is advisable for all professionals to take such opportunities to refresh and re-learn the essence of good communication skills. Communicating with patients with dementia presents a challenge and it is addressed in this text by Kay de Vries. Understanding blocking behaviour is also an essential element of being a good communicator, as is self-awareness and the practice of self-care. These two valuable perspectives for palliative care professionals are discussed in Chapter 4.

MAIN IMPLICATIONS FOR PRACTICE

- There is evidence that communication skills can be taught and maintained over time (Wilkinson et al. 1999b).
- Aberrant communication skills can be socially learnt and used unconsciously to protect heath-care professionals from perceived stressful conversations. As the sections on questions demonstrate, they can be very sophisticated.
- Communication skills will not improve over time unless we are self-aware and conscious of the approach that we use.

- At each new event in the patient's disease trajectory, the following steps are useful in reaching a mutual understanding of what is happening for the patient:
  Know the facts
  Ask what the patient understands about what is happening
  Ask how this is making him or her feel
  Discuss how he or she is coping in terms of internal and external resources
  How has he or she coped with similar crises in the past? What or who has helped? (Wilkinson and Mula 2004)
- Without mutual understanding between patient and professional of the illness and events surrounding it, we stand little chance of connecting with and being helpful to our patients.
- Many patients simply want us to be there for them and listen to their expressions of pain. They do not necessarily expect us to answer their existential questions and they will appreciate our attempts to listen and encourage free expression, even if they seem clumsy.
- Communicating with people with dementia is an important part of care.

SUGGESTED FURTHER READING

Heaven C, Maguire P (2003) Communication issues. In: Lloyd Williams M (ed.), *Psychosocial Issues in Palliative Care*. Oxford: Oxford University Press, 13–34.

Maguire P (2000) Communication with terminally ill patients and their relatives. In: Chochinov HM, Breitbart W (eds), *Handbook of Psychiatry in Palliative Medicine*. Oxford: Oxford University Press, 291–301.

Vachon M (2005) The emotional problems of the patient in palliative medicine. In: Doyle D, Hanks G, Cherny N, Calman K (eds), *Oxford Textbook of Palliative Medicine*, 3rd edn. Oxford: Oxford University Press, 961–84.

Wilkinson S, Mula C (2003) Communication in care of the dying. In: Ellershaw J, Wilkinson S (eds), *Care of the Dying: A pathway to excellence*. Oxford: Oxford University Press, 74–90.

Chapter 4
Self-awareness and self-care

KEY POINTS

- **Saving a life versus stealing a death**: the true story of Eva Marie illustrates the impact of an unplanned approach to end-of-life care. Sometimes in trying to save a life we steal a death.
- **Facing death**: death anxiety: health professionals will invariably have a level of anxiety about death, their death, the death of someone close to them. Failure to be proactive in recognising these fears can lead to a breakdown in communication with the dying person and their family and friends.
- **Making space for decision-making**: decisions regarding resuscitation active treatments and/or introducing a palliative approach should be made in a robust systematic way. These decisions need protected time. Where possible the junctures to discuss critical issues should be built into hospital policies and treatment protocols.
- **Self-awareness**: death anxiety should be addressed in the curricula of health-care professionals. Increasing self-awareness through a process of guided reflection allows individuals to *find their own pace* in exploring death anxiety.
- **How much did Nicky impact on my life?**: 30 years on Nicky is still a vivid memory. How far is our decision-making about our own lives influenced by the experiences at work?
- **Self-care**: reflective practice can be a big part of this: health-care professionals can marginalise compassion fatigue by making the choice to care for themselves.

SAVING A LIFE VERSUS STEALING A DEATH

**Eva Marie dies in the intensive care unit
and leaves her daughter Sarah alone in the world**

Rhythmic hiss of a ventilator
breathes life into
Eva Marie.
Her swollen eyes
need tape to keep
them closed.
A life monitor squeaks
like a terrified mouse.
A green light flashes
erratically,
and warns of
her failing heart.
A sour fermenting smell of decay.
'Mummy, why are you so cold?'
'Sarah, she will never feel warm again.
She is dying'
'Who will I live with then?'

This is the story of Sarah's mother, Eva Marie, whose death was defined by the death anxiety of the health-care professionals responsible for the management of her care. Sarah was ten when her mother was dying. Sarah was caring for her alone at home in between going to school. It was their secret.

My daughter announced at the dinner table one evening that Sarah's mother was dying. From the look in her eyes I knew my daughter believed this to be true. When I couldn't raise Eva on the phone the next day I decided to visit. I wanted to reassure Kate that all was well.

Sarah answered the door when I knocked and at first refused to let me in. The smell from the house alerted me that all was not well and I insisted on entering. Just one look at Eva confirmed to me that she was dying. She was deeply jaundiced, and had gross ascites and very oedematous ankles. She was too weak to move. She had had a large haematemesis at one point and a melaena stool. The floor was littered with over-the-counter analgesics. She had, she said, excruciating back pain and had been trying to ease it. She also said that she thought she had cancer of the bones. This was never confirmed. She said that she was dying and asked that I look after her daughter. Sarah nodded, confirming her mother's statement about her death. Sarah, Eva said, knew what to do about the funeral. Sarah nodded again.

A GP was called, symptoms listed and a brief history given. On arrival, he spoke briefly to Eva and then turned to Sarah and said, 'We will send your Mummy to hospital to make her better'. There was pain in his face. That is what he genuinely wanted to happen. I found it impossible to be assertive at that point, although I had affirmed with Eva that I too thought she was dying. Eva said, 'I would rather go to a hospice'. No one listened.

Eva was admitted to hospital where a diagnosis of liver failure was made. She was also in heart failure. The plan was to transfer Eva to a leading liver unit for a transplantation. The referral was refused. The glimmer of hope that I may have had when the GP talked of making her better had long since evaporated. The reality of the situation was that a young single mother who was estranged from her parents and any other family members was dying. There was no one to look after her daughter. No father available.

In spite of the refused referral for treatment at the liver unit the medical team continued to treat Eva actively. This included drugs and blood transfusions for her bleeding oesophageal varices. As well as a central line, she also had a peripheral line, cardiac monitor and continuous oxygen via a facemask. The presence of this technology made physical contact with her daughter almost impossible. Sarah visited three times a day. Often she had to stand aside while nurses recorded vital signs and doctors visited. There was no privacy. When Eva spoke she simply said 'I wish I could have gone to the hospice'.

Each time that we visited the concern and pain in the eyes of the health-care professionals when they looked at Sarah were almost palpable. They seldom addressed her or spoke to her. This happened only in the last 2 days of Eva's life. By now two guardians (old friends of Eva's) had been appointed in the event of her death. They assumed the role of next of kin, although neither could visit the hospital because of work pressures and location.

I did gently challenge the senior registrar on the second day after Eva had been refused for a liver transplantation. I expressed concern that Eva was dying while receiving acute care. I politely questioned the wisdom of futile care. I expressed concern that it was making it impossible to share quality time with her daughter. The doctor was very kind and listened; however, she seemed to be saying that they should not give up trying. As she spoke her eyes wandered and fixed on Sarah who was visiting and was visible through the window into her ward; she was visibly very upset for Sarah.

On the fourth night Eva had a respiratory arrest. I was telephoned in the morning as Sarah was staying with us. The night sister (someone whom I knew professionally) said, 'The doctors were there when she arrested so they thought they should go ahead and intubate'. Was she trying to say that it was fear of litigation that underpinned the decision to intubate? Had this replaced the overwhelming emotional pain felt for her daughter as the driving force in decision-making in the care of Eva?

Eva spent the last 6 days of her life on a ventilator in the intensive care unit with the usual accompaniments of dopamine infusions, muscle-paralysing drugs and monitoring machines that whirred and buzzed erratically. I wonder if she could hear them. She showed no signs of life; however, we will never know if she could think or feel during that period. She was cold to touch. She developed gross exophthalmos and oedematous eyelids. Eventually her eyelids were taped down to keep them closed.

Resuscitation and intensive care serve a valuable function for those with acute reversible illness and for people needing specialist care after major trauma and surgery. However, it was clear to me, an experienced nurse that Eva belonged to a group of patients for whom resuscitation and intensive care acted only to prolong suffering and deny personal space to have last conversations, precious moments with relatives and friends. It is a striking paradox that doctors who are so immersed in a scientific approach will continue with treatment in the face of futility. Is this their defence against the anxiety of helping people to face their death? Is it still somewhere deep-rooted in medical psyche that death is a failure? There is no deeply held ethical base in medical practice about giving care when cure is no longer possible (Higginson 2002; Kafetz 2002).

And why wasn't I more assertive? Why didn't I insist that the doctors listened to Eva's requests for a hospice admission? I will never know what conversations she had with the doctors or who led them. Menzies-Lyth (1988) states that, when protecting ourselves against anxiety, as nurses, we will cling to the familiar even when it ceases to be appropriate or relevant. Perhaps this is what I did, and here the familiar was the medical hierarchy.

This chapter now looks at death anxiety among professionals and returns to the narrative of Eva in the discourse.

FACING DEATH

Death anxiety among health-care professionals

There is an abundance of literature on communication skills but less on the subject of death anxiety among health-care professionals. The potent fear of death among young health-care providers, many of whom may not have seen anyone die before entering health care, coupled with the lack of education about attitudes to death, is a recipe for disaster (Neuberger 2003). In a death-denying society much of the interaction of health professionals with dying people will be reactive and unlearnt – as in the case of Eva.

Anxiety can manifest itself in different ways. It is generally agreed that this may include behavioural signs as well as distorting thought patterns and interference with a person's ability to function effectively. Tomer and Eliason (1996) describe the concept of death anxiety as being about fears of the process itself – ceasing to be – and concerns about what comes after death. If we have not examined our own thoughts and fears about dying it does not mean that we do not have them. Our failure to face the fear of our own death is an important reason why we find it so difficult to help dying and bereaved people. This view, expressed by Richard Chartre, the Bishop of London, in his president's lecture to the King's Fund in June 2003, is one that is shared by palliative care experts (Parkes 1985; Buckman 1993b; Kübler-Ross 1993; Faulkner and Maguire 1994).

The higher the level of death anxiety experienced by health professionals, the more likely is the professional to exhibit negative behaviour towards dying patients. These behaviours include evasive treatment, withholding information, and avoiding and distancing themselves from the patient (Eakes 1985; Farrell 1992). By the use of reflective practice health professionals can gain insight into the layers of their emotional reactions and interactions with dying patients. If there is no education about death anxiety in the curriculum, and in the absence of reflective practice, it follows that death anxiety occurs as a reactive emotion when we are caring for the dying person, or someone whom we know dies, or when we are dying. The inevitability of our own death is of course inescapable. Death anxiety and the barriers that it creates between patients and professionals remind me of a beautiful poem called 'The Elephant in the Room'. In it the author, Terry Kettering, compares the inability of people to talk about painful things to being in a room with an elephant. The elephant takes up all the space and leaves no room for a meaningful relationship, and the result is trivial chatter. In the last lines of the poem the person with existential pain pleads not to be left alone with the elephant (Grollman 1993).

However, while we wrestle with death anxiety and the accompanying emotions and behaviours, conscious and subconscious, people die. In many instances, as in the case of Eva, we rob them of their dying, *of a good death*. At least of their last chance to say 'I love you . . . In the future I hope that you . . .'. We must ask ourselves, 'Whose agenda is being followed? Ours or the patient's?'

The wounded healer

This chapter may seem unsympathetic towards the health professionals involved. It is not meant to. However, being a fly on the wall in the unfolding story of Eva Marie and Sarah has been a haunting one. In this instance the professional carers cared enormously. The look of sorrow and despair in their eyes when Sarah visited is part of the haunting. On leaving the hospital after Eva Marie's death I saw one of the staff nurses who had been looking after her that day walking down the corridor. Although I could see only his back I recognised his posture of abject despair – a familiar posture of despair that had often been mine when I worked in critical care. I am not sure if this is what Kearney means when he talks of the *wounded healer* but those were the words that sprang to mind.

Kearney (2000) draws upon Greek mythology and practice. He highlights that Hippocratic medicine is evident in its ability to diagnose and treat illness and physical pain. He talks about the potential for healing if modern medicine could combine the Hippocratic approach with Asklepian medicine. Asklepian medicine is concerned with the healing of suffering from within and depends upon both the patient and the carer using inner senses of emotion, instinct and intuition. Historical evidence suggests that the twin systems of Hippocratic and Asklepian medicine worked together for the well-being of the sick and disabled in the ancient world (Kearney 2000).

As modern medicine has evolved the Asklepian approach has diminished. The result is often a failure to use the inner senses of instinct, emotion and intuition in spite of modern health-care professionals often being bestowed with the emotional integrity, maturity and desire to do this. Losing the Asklepian way results in existential pain for both the patient and the carer.

If the health-care professionals caring for Eva Marie and Sarah had invited their stories they would have realised that the dying emotions had started a good while before they met this pair. They could have helped and supported Eva Marie and Sarah through this. They could have cried and laughed with both of them. Although they may have been sad when Eva Marie died, the absolute despair that is so wounding may have been avoided. It is hoped that they could also have felt a sense of privilege and professional pride in sharing this experience with Eva Marie and Sarah.

MAKING SPACE FOR DECISION-MAKING

- In the case of Eva there was a sense of vital decisions being made in a reactive way. In some situations, this has to be – patients' conditions change unexpectedly and health-care professionals have to make huge ethical decisions, usually about resuscitation, in a split second. It is not surprising that professionals will err on the side of wanting to give the patient the best possible chance of survival and so instigate an active approach. A hospital policy that stated that, in the event of an unexpected change or of refused referral, a meeting to discuss the implications of continuing active treatment or considering a palliative approach instead would provide a space for busy professionals to stop and think. Such a meeting could include senior professionals from acute and palliative care, as well as the patient or patient's advocate. There would need to be a willingness of staff to be flexible and attend these meetings at short notice. In Eva's scenario, it would have been time well spent. She may have been transferred to the hospice. She might at least have been given a side room with a TV and open visiting hours.
- Such meetings could also be useful for the management of patients with a diagnosis of a chronic illness for which a cure is not possible, e.g. heart failure or liver cirrhosis. It could be written into treatment protocols that, after a first life-threatening episode, patients should be seen, their understanding of their situation assessed and options for care looked at. This does not preclude further active treatment but rather introduces the idea of palliative options that could run alongside acute care. Introducing the palliative team to patients receiving chemotherapy and radiotherapy has long been a tradition in good oncology care. There is a planned approach to comfort and well-being as well as cure. Patients for whom cure is no longer possible thus already know the palliative team.
- Just as patients can benefit from well-constructed decision aids (see Chapter 5), so can professionals. The Resuscitation Council (2001) provides a framework for making decisions about 'do not attempt to resuscitate' orders. A 'do not attempt resuscitation' order should be made only after appropriate consultation and consideration of all relevant aspects of the patient's condition. These include:
  – the likely clinical outcome, including the likelihood of successfully restarting the patient's heart and breathing, and the overall benefit achieved from a successful resuscitation
  – the patient's known and ascertainable wishes
  – the patient's human rights, including the right to life and the right to be free from degrading treatment.
- The Resuscitation Council (2001) also states that views should be sought from all members of the medical and nursing teams in primary and secondary care and from people close to the patient. A useful addition to this would be a palliative physician or clinical nurse specialist (CNS). In this way a viable palliative approach and plan could be outlined. However, in the absence of a palliative representative the options that could be built into the meeting outcomes would be to place the patient on the Gold Standards Framework or the Liverpool Care Pathway. This should be within the scope of generalists in palliative care.
- Prognostic scoring systems are available for use in critical care and provide a further decision aid for physicians. The APACHE III score (Knaus et al. 1991),

for example, was developed from a database of over 17 000 patients (Ridley 1994). They give health-care providers important information to help inform decisions on treatment and prognosis (Ohno-Machado et al. 2006). No one seems to be suggesting that decisions should be made by using just the scoring system. According to Ridley (1994), prognostic scoring systems are not widely used in the UK. It is also important to remember that stopping active treatment does not preclude the medical team correcting what is correctable, e.g. electrolyte imbalance. Use of an objective scoring system in the case of Eva may have helped the doctors to focus on, and face up to, her survival chances, and thus could have been helpful in making a decision to provide a palliative approach.

- In discussion with colleagues from critical care, they expressed the opinion that, by use of prognostic indicators to aid a decision to stop active treatment, they may blight the chances of the patient who survives despite all the odds being stacked against them. For anyone who has had the experience of caring for someone in critical care who suddenly wakes up, it is indeed a truly powerful experience. In practice, we must ask is it really tenable to continue active resuscitative treatment, for someone whose survival chances are not considered viable, on a *just in case* basis? Could this be regarded as an unwanted infringement of patient autonomy (Dunphy 2000) as well as an infringement of human rights (Resuscitation Council 2001)?

Making critical decisions in a quagmire of conscious and subconscious emotions is not conducive to making decisions that are in the patient's best interest. Use of decision-making tools as aids, e.g. prognostic indicators, will help objectivity. Being flexible and attending ad hoc meetings to discuss the viability and ethics of treatment will share the responsibility, and help to ensure that all the appropriate people are consulted. Finally, the presence of a palliative representative at such meetings gives support to the acute professionals and can offer a support and planned palliative approach to care for the patient, where in the past it may have been felt that we had nothing more to offer.

Death anxiety and education

There is no doubt that all universities providing education for health professionals should be addressing subject areas of death in society including the many cultural and spiritual influences. In particular the issue of death anxiety and its impact on patient–professional relationships and effective communication should be addressed. Empirical evidence supports that this is not a simple process (Boyle and Carter 1998). It is imperative that education around death anxiety is conducted within an atmosphere of support and acceptance. An understanding of the concept and an examination of the evidence base for death anxiety is a good starting point. It is important for students to examine their attitudes to death and give some thought to their own death, although how this is achieved is debatable. Overt experiential exercises that invite people to plan their own funerals, for example, may produce unwarranted distress for those who have suffered bereavement. In a multicultural society where increasingly people seek asylum and new starts against a backdrop of violence, *death exercises* may evoke vivid and horrifying memories. Studies that have investigated the effects of death education on participant stress and anxiety levels do indicate a reduction in death anxiety where respondents have to some extent given consideration to their own death (Hutchinson and Scherman 1992).

SELF-AWARENESS

The emergence and popularity of reflective practice may hold the key to health professionals exploring death anxiety to reduce the incidence of the avoiding and distancing behaviour that occurs in clinical practice. Boud et al. (1985) cite motivation and open-mindedness as prerequisites for reflective practice.

Self-awareness is both the starting point and the journey in reflective practice. Self-awareness is about knowing and understanding oneself, about examining personal beliefs, values, attitudes and motivations, and understanding how these impact on our personal and professional relationships. It can be a surprising process as we learn new things about ourselves. It can be uncomfortable as we face aspects of our personality of which we are not proud. By analysing feelings, knowledge and experiences in practice, a new concept of self and how you impact on patients, relatives, friends and colleagues will emerge and more questions will be posed.

In palliative care health-care professionals aim to sit beside the patient as they live their final chapter. Wherever the setting – intensive care unit, acute wards, hospice, care home or home – knowing and managing oneself within the relationship is a vital component to being able to support the dying patient (Johns 2006a).

> To be available to the other I must windscreen wipe my own concerns in order to see the person in terms of their experience and manage any resistance I may have towards the other person, for whatever reason, in order to flow with them. Naturally I need to be mindful of these concerns in order to manage them skilfully. Only then can I truly listen to the other person's story and connect with the other person in terms of their experience. If I am driven by my own concerns, these concerns will distort my viewing lens and consequently jeopardise my ability to wholly connect with the person.
>
> Johns (2006a, p 257)

Reflective practice

Practising reflection regularly requires commitment and self-discipline. More enlightened health studies curricula build reflection as a continuing thread throughout the course, often also forming part of a continuous assessment theme. The mentorship model of teaching now used in nurse education provides an opportunity for reflective practice to occur between mentor and mentee. Sound education in use of a reflective approach for mentors and students is clearly fundamental. Health-care organisations would do well to give protected time for reflective practice to occur.

Guided reflection is a process of self-enquiry to enable the practitioner to realise desirable and effective practice within a reflexive spiral of being and becoming (Johns 2006a). Reflection can be seen as almost an abstract concept, and probably as a response to this a number of models have been devised to aid the reflective process, e.g. Gibbs (1988) and Boud et al. (1985). Without a model the reflective process is in danger of becoming an introspective one with all the subconscious and conscious prejudices that we have and behaviours that allow us to avoid analysing uncomfortable emotions.

Johns' model for reflection has been developed over some years and has been changed and refined as a result of continually using it in dialogue with practitioners. It is as follows:

- To what issues does it seem significant to pay attention?
- How was I feeling and what made me feel that way?
- What was I trying to achieve?
- Did I respond effectively and in tune with my values?
- What were the consequences of my actions on the patient, others and myself?
- How were others feeling?
- What made them feel that way?
- What factors influenced the way that I was feeling, thinking, feeling or responding?
- What knowledge did inform me or might have informed me?
- To what extent did I act for the best?
- How does this situation connect with previous experiences?
- How might I respond more effectively given this situation again?
- What would be the consequences of alternative actions for the patient, others and myself?
- How do I *now* feel about this experience?
- Am I now more able to support myself and others better as a consequence?
- What have I learnt?

These cues form the model for structured reflection (Johns 2002).

These cues are not a prescription for reflection; rather they provide a guide to help access the mystery of experience (Johns 2006a). In the light of previous discussion of the impact of death anxiety on our relationships with dying people, the words 'the mystery of experience' are very apt here. Johns (2002) recommends that, for deep learning to occur, guidance for another person is required. Reflective practice can evoke internal conflict. A second person as guide, challenge and support will aid the process of exploring anxiety rather than rationalising and protecting against it. Johns (2002) also highlights, simply because we see things differently, that it does not necessarily follow that we can act differently and that, on occasions, we may feel relatively powerless to change aspects of self. Perhaps on these occasions we can value the insights that we have as increasing our level of self-awareness.

The frequency of reflection will vary with individual motivation. Johns reflects after each shift. It is important to keep a balance with reflection. There is a temptation to reflect only when we feel some disquiet about an occurrence. However, it can be surprising what we learn from reflecting on the ordinary day and the things that go well. The process of guided reflection (with another) is something that Johns seems to practise once or twice a month.

HOW MUCH DID NICKY IMPACT ON MY LIFE?

Can I ever know myself?

I joined a writing course recently and was challenged to write a poem, which is something I have not done for 40 years. I was amazed that, on sitting down to write a poem, Nicky Wilde filled my head. I wrote the following poem about him in 10 minutes. I have often thought of him in the past 30 years but will probably never understand what impact he may have had on my life.

Nicky Wilde (1956–1972)
Died One Night in Hospital
Bleached hair once spiked
now flaccid
frames a motionless mask
called face.
Laughing eyes,
now express fear, sorrow
and shame.
Sixteen, on the brink of an adventure,
called life.
Eager to captain his own ship.
Bloated belly,
dark yellow skin and
monotone voice,
end his dreams.
Long sleepless nights,
his music and Maggie May
his solace.
I was his nurse
and his Maggie.
Rod sings
'When I fall in love this time, it's gonna last forever'.
Nicky's forever is almost
over.
Friday night.
Party time.
Sticky crimson blood, lots of it
splatter the banana white walls in a side room.
Nicky dies
while Maggie parties.

Nicky had been on an adult medical ward for some weeks. He had a rare liver disorder called Wilson's disease. As a result he had cirrhosis of the liver and also parkinsonian symptoms. He had just started an active social life when the symptoms began. He loved music and girls.

I was asked to step in and do a block of eight night duties when a colleague went off sick. I agreed but explained that I could not do the seventh night as I was hosting a party with my house mates. I got to know Nicky well during those nights. It was clear that he was very frightened. We brought his bed to the nurses' station each night so that we were with him between tasks. He played his music and we held his hand when we could. He loved Rod Stewart.

I had the seventh night off for the party. When I came back on night eight he was gone. He had died while I was partying. He had asked for me as he vomited blood and died.

The questions I ask myself now are:

- Why did I within a year of his death go to work in an acute liver unit where, of course, I met lots of other Nickys?
- Why have I been drawn to palliative care?
- Is it possible that that brief experience with Nicky helped to shape my professional life?
- How much can our subconscious motivate our decision-making?

SELF-CARE

A vital part of caring for ill and dying people is also caring for yourself. It is only in recent years that this concept has been on the agenda in health care. Wright (2004) replaces the term 'burnout' with 'compassion fatigue'. Burnout suggests irreparable damage. Compassion fatigue, he feels, more accurately portrays what happens to health professionals. He equates the following sayings, often used in his stress workshops, with compassion fatigue:

'No energy for it anymore.'

'Emptied, nothing left to give.'

'Too many questions, not enough answers.'

All health-care professionals can make a choice whether or not to care for themselves. Individuals can marginalise compassion fatigue by being proactive about self-care. Many organisations offer staff support programmes ranging from a paid series of counselling sessions, opportunities for complementary therapies to protected time for clinical supervision. Some organisations offer very little or nothing. If you work in an area where support is available, it is wise to take advantage of it. If you work in an area where nothing exists, it is probably best to move on, as the message of undervaluing staff is clear. However, whether or not there is support, it is still important to take responsibility for your own self-care. What follows are some pointers to self-care but it is by no means a comprehensive guide.

Value yourself

It is important that you value yourself and what you do. Do not always rely on others to boost your morale. Sometimes, in health care our work seems so mundane that we forget the value of it. However, for example, I am proud that I can help someone to the toilet, wipe their bottom and know that, as far as it is possible, I have left them feeling dignified and cared for.

If you have been involved in a difficult scenario at work and you find it difficult to stop thinking about it, be proactive in reflecting on it in a structured way or, better still, reflect with a guide or mentor. You can make a choice to stop thinking about the issue until you have space to reflect on it. You may sometimes find that, on reflection, the part that you played was fine – it was the situation that was difficult. If that is so, value your contribution. If you could have done things differently to have achieved a better outcome then learn from it. When things go wrong train yourself to think of the things that went well.

Self-talk

Social psychologists will tell us that we talk to ourselves a lot of the time. Some of the talk is very obvious – we may have conversations in our head. However, we also talk to ourselves in attitudes and feelings. Here are some examples:

- You may go into work and your manager walks past you without acknowledging you. You may think, 'now what have I done?' or 'she really doesn't like me'. Actually she may have been deep in thought and not seen you.
- You may say that you cannot do something when in fact what you really mean is that you have never tried to perform a particular task. For example, you may say that you are hopeless at embroidery. A more accurate description might be: 'I have never tried my hand at embroidery. I expect I could be quite good at it.'
- It is easy to get things out of perspective. Your train may be cancelled. It is easy to think 'Just my luck – it always happens to me.' On analysis that theory may not stand up and it could be that it has been late just once out of many times catching a train.
- Learn how to take compliments. Accept a compliment with a thank you rather than saying 'it was nothing'. This will have a negative impact on the person paying the compliment as well as you.

This kind of negative self-talk can lead to poor self-esteem. When self-esteem is low it is difficult to find the confidence to deal with stressful situations. This can lead to a lack of confidence in our abilities. We need confidence in ourselves to support dying people.

Making choices

It is important to know that we can make choices about how we react to situations. For example, people will often talk about the 'emotional labour' of caring for dying people in terms that indicate that they are exhausted by it. If we choose to work in health care, particularly palliative care, then clearly being close to sadness and strong emotions is inevitable. Emotional labour does not have to be exhausting. Knowing that I have given good nursing care alongside a kind and caring supportive approach to patients, relatives and friends in a dying scenario gives me a professional satisfaction that is nurturing and not at all exhausting.

Being assertive

It can be difficult when we do not have the skills to say when we are unhappy about something. This may lead to a spiral of grumbling or complaining about something or someone, which is damaging to self-esteem. It is kinder to colleagues and will contribute to a healthier working environment if you develop the skill of being assertive so that, when you are unhappy with someone, you can raise and discuss it in a non-threatening professional way. It is important to distinguish between being assertive and being aggressive. Here are some simple steps to guide you in being assertive:

- First look very carefully at what the issue is and decide what you hope to achieve by discussing it.
- Prearrange a time with the person with whom you want to raise the issue. Explain briefly what you want to discuss.
- You may be nervous, so before the meeting check out your non-verbal communication which should be neither too aggressive nor too passive.
- State the issue objectively and clearly. You may need to repeat yourself.
- Do not be side tracked into talking about anything else; stay with the original concern.
- Listen to what the other person has to say. He or she has a valid point of view and just because you are being assertive it does not necessarily mean that you are right.
- Aim for a win–win outcome. You are discussing an issue cooperatively and resolving it with compromise, where possible, helps each person to feel that something has been achieved.

Self-nurture

It is important that you have protected time to nurture yourself. Be proactive in this. Make a list of all the things that you enjoy doing, people with whom you enjoy being, places you like to be and activities that you do that help you to chill out. It might also be useful to think of a time when life was not good and remember what it was that helped you to get through this difficult period. Finally, you should end up with a personal profile of what nurtures you or, another way of saying it, what helps you to avoid compassion fatigue. Now make a care plan for yourself. Do not wait until you are tired or feeling exhausted from the emotional labour of life and work. Build nurture into your daily/weekly routine. You may find when you reflect on your usual routine that you look after yourself well already. However, if you find that you are not looking after yourself, then it is time to make a care plan for yourself. If you have not done this before, avoid being over-ambitious and planning a timetable of nurture that would be impossible to achieve.

Guided reflective practice

Finally, please do take time to indulge in reflective practice. Not only can you improve your practice, but you grow; although growing can sometimes mean facing anxieties and examining them, the net result is one of feeling more confident and thinking more highly of yourself. Guided reflection with a trusted colleague and friend can also feel like a special social occasion. This section is by no means a complete guide to self-care. You would do well to attend a course on handling stress.

Finally, dying is not a dress rehearsal. It is only ever going to happen once in a lifetime. As such, it deserves a process of scrupulous decision-making and attention to detail. Futile treatment at the end of life is more about the professional's anxieties than the patient's best interest and is unacceptable. Self-awareness and self-care are fundamental ingredients for professionals to sit beside patients as they navigate their death. With this formula, caring for the dying person and family and friends can be a rewarding and enriching experience.

MAIN IMPLICATIONS FOR PRACTICE

- It is important to make protected time for decision-making in health care.
- It is important to use objective data and also decision aids, where they exist, to help professionals make a decision about treatment plans.
- The patient's input must be sought when possible. Advance directives should be part of the process if available.
- Health-care organisations should draw up policies that include guidelines in making crucial decisions.
- Policies should also indicate when a crucial decision should be considered.
- Specialist palliative care services should support crucial decision-making in acute care.
- With no proactive approach to decision-making, often crucial decisions are made emotionally by health professionals. This can have dire consequences for the quality of death of some patients.
- A good degree of self-awareness and understanding of one's own attitude to death is a prerequisite for objective decision-making about discontinuation of treatment.
- Self-awareness is a dynamic beast and can be promoted by reflective practice, preferably with a guide, i.e. a structure and another person. Ideally it should be done regularly, e.g. twice monthly.
- It is important to take responsibility for caring for your own psychological well-being. Be proactive in self-care.

SUGGESTED FURTHER READING

Benner P, Wrubel J (1989) *The Primacy of Caring, Stress and Coping in Health and Illness.* Reading: Addison-Wesley Publishing Co.

Bond M (1986) *Stress and Self Awareness: A guide for nurses.* London: Heinemann Nursing.

Capacchione L (2001) *Living with Feeling: The art of emotional expression.* London: Rider Books.

Johns C (2006) *Being Mindful, Easing Suffering. Reflections on palliative care.* London: Jessica Kingsley Publishers.

Johns C (2006) *Engaging Reflection in Practice: A narrative approach.* Oxford: Blackwell Publishing.

Kearney M (2000) *A Place of Healing: Working with suffering in living and dying.* Oxford: Oxford University Press.

Chapter 5
The sick role and partnership working

KEY POINTS

- **Introduction**: there is a tension between the traditional culture of the health service and policy and expectations of contemporary society. Health-care managers need to be proactive in supporting a cultural change.
- **Partnership care**: partnership working is non-hierarchical. The health-care professionals are experts in diseases and their management, patients the experts on themselves. Continuing negotiation between the patient and health-care professionals is needed to maintain partnership.
- **The sick role**: historical and contemporary research and experience highlight that patients feel vulnerable. This hampers patients feeling equal in the partnership.
- **Face-to-face partnership**: good face-to-face partnership needs professionals to start every significant conversation by checking the ground rules.
- **Information giving**: the key to partnership working is effective information giving. Professionals cannot consider information to have been successfully imparted until they have evaluated what the patient has understood. Thinking that is out of the box is needed so that information giving has the time and priority that it needs.
- **Written information**: this complements verbal explanations. It should be of good quality and cater for all ages and special needs. There are organisations that will help to ensure that good quality information is delivered in a variety of ways. Professionals should use these.
- **Decision aids**: a variety of decision aids is currently available. Many are not evaluated. Research on a few suggests they are helpful to patients and increase patient participation. Quality control is important and professionals should recommend only reputable aids.

INTRODUCTION

The NHS Cancer Plan (Department of Health or DH 2000b) and the *Manual of Cancer Services Standards* (DH 2000a) both direct that patient involvement and consultation be integrated into the provision and evaluation of cancer services at all levels, thus building on directives from the Calman–Hine report (Calman and Hine 1995), which emphasised that NHS services should be patient centred and that at all levels decisions made should take account of patients' views and preferences. Other political directives over the past 20 years have encouraged the public to take charge of maintaining their own health, e.g. *Promoting Better Health* (DH 1987) and *The Health of the Nation* (DH 1991a). *The Patients' Charter* (DH 1991b) encourages people to complain if standards and targets are not met. The foundations for working in partnership with patients are in place. This theme remains high on the government's agenda and is elaborated on in *Building on the Best: Choice, responsiveness and equity in the NHS* (DH 2003a) and *Our Health, Our Care, Our Say* (DH 2006).

As a student nurse in 1969 I cared for someone called Peter Smith, who had had a myocardial infarction. He was in his late 50s. I had initiated a successful resuscitation attempt on him. Some days later he tried to give me £2 (a lot of money in those days). When I refused the gift he shook his head saying, 'You can't know what being in hospital means to me'. He then went on to tell me the story of his sister, Emma, who died at the age of 13. He was 11. She had pneumonia. His family could not afford a doctor although, as her condition worsened, his parents asked him to run to the doctor's house. Despite running faster than ever before and the doctor responding immediately, Emma died within minutes of the doctor's arrival. He did not charge on this occasion.

Peter Smith's experience would have taken place in the 1920s. In 1946 the National Insurance and National Health Service Acts were passed and health care was set to become a right and not a privilege. Peter Smith, a grateful recipient of health care, personified the public attitude towards the NHS in the mid- to late twentieth century. Undoubtedly the culture within health care has come a long way since the days when many families kept money in a jar on the mantelpiece to pay for seeing a doctor (Tony Blair, in the foreword to *The NHS Cancer Plan* – DH 2000b). However, achieving partnership working, both in face-to-face communication with patients and at an organisational level, will not happen simply because the legislation says that it should. For these legislative initiatives to become a reality they require, in the main, a cultural shift on the part of both the general public and health-care professionals.

The traditions of health care in this country, as in many, are rooted in a religious culture. As the health service culture in the UK evolved, the relationships that developed mirrored those of a religious Victorian household: the doctor, the father figure in control and somewhat formidable; the matron, the household manager who commanded respect; the patient, the passive child (Bowman and Thompson 1995). This has translated in practice to a paternalistic approach on the part of health-care professionals to patients.

Morgan (1990) explains that culture refers to a group's system of knowledge, ideology, values, laws and day-to-day rituals. He comments that culture at work may well be more influential on a person's behaviour than culture at home and in their community. Organisationally, and now in the health service, we have a change in ideology and values. However, the ideology, laws and values embedded in the day-to-day rituals of health caring and the systems of knowledge, custom and practice that exist are deep-rooted and complex. The cultural change required by all parties to achieve successful face-to-face partnership working, as opposed to a paternalistic approach, will not occur just because we want it to; rather it will evolve.

For this evolution to progress successfully, it may require educators, managers and leaders at grass roots to be proactive in adopting a process for achieving a cultural change. Dyer (1984) provides a seven-point plan for this:

1. Conduct a cultural audit by ascertaining what beliefs and values are considered dominant in an area. Monitor any differences between what is done and what has been said to have been done.
2. Assess the culture in the light of this and the need for change.
3. Assess the risk to the existing cultural values.
4. Ensure support from senior management.
5. Unfreeze the cultural pattern if there is serious resistance. This may need a leadership change.
6. Decide how to introduce the change, e.g. methods of education, social learning.
7. Monitor and evaluate.

Even with this proactive approach it may take years before partnership working will become the predominant culture. It will also require an understanding from professionals that different models of care will need to be employed for different individuals. Some patients will still want to take a passive role (Sheldon 2003).

In Chapter 3 communications between patients and professionals were looked at in some detail. This good face-to-face communication between professionals and patients is highly valued by patients (National Institute for Health and Clinical Excellence or NICE 2004a) and will form the basis for partnership working at an individualised patient care level. These individual relationships are particularly important when a potentially fatal diagnosis is made and choices about treatment options have to be made in a limited space of time. Patients are shocked and may also feel in awe of professionals who have access to detailed information about them and, at this early stage anyhow, most probably more knowledge of this illness that is suddenly theirs!

In Chapter 4 it was identified that health-care professionals may well have insecurities too. The articulate, assertive, well-educated patient or the angry, defensive patient may provoke a feeling of awe in the professional. We all have experiences of fears and insecurities that are part of our daily working life. To add to the conundrum, we will almost certainly regularly get a skewed idea of what patients feel about the care that we give. In their efforts to please us, patients will say thank you with cards and chocolates when they really mean 'Could do better'. I know, I was one of those patients. It is a mistake to underestimate the hostage effect of being a patient. *It is important to have read Chapters 3 and 4 before continuing any further.*

PARTNERSHIP CARE – WHAT DOES IT MEAN?

Successful partnerships are non-hierarchical and the partners share decision-making responsibilities. Within the doctor–patient relationship, the doctor is the expert on diagnosis, treatments and options. Only patients know about their personal experience of illness, habits, beliefs, attitudes and preferences, i.e. are experts on themselves. Both types of knowledge are needed to manage illness successfully (Coulter 1999). Patients may need support from friends, relatives and professionals to use their personal experience in this partnership, because of feelings of shock at the situation, communication difficulties or special needs, e.g. learning disability. People who need this help may not be immediately obvious. My friend was head of English at a local university when she was diagnosed with cancer. She says that, for the first 3 months of her illness, she was unable to take on board fully any information given. Although she read good-quality information, she simply could not comprehend it. She relied on her partner and a close friend to help her maintain a partnership with health-care professionals.

The emphasis on sharing responsibility for decisions needs to be in skilled hands and tempered with common sense. Speck (1998) highlights that the pendulum can swing too far, too soon. Patients who are presented with choices of treatment or non-treatment and provided with statistical odds for outcomes and side effects can feel isolated and disempowered if the professional withholds the benefits of their own experience.

Partnership requires attention to, and explicit discussions about, the relationship. In other words, ground rules for the partnership should be made and reviewed. An example of this happening has been highlighted in the strategy for giving bad news, i.e. enquiring about the level, depth and involvement that the patient wants at that point. It is advisable to use this strategy at any key conversation with the patient, and this will provide the explicit discussion needed to maintain a partnership relationship. When patients are admitted to hospital it is important to discuss with them ground rules for communicating, e.g. they will receive most attention when requiring physical care. This also provides an opportunity to ask questions and request interviews with named people. It is important that it is emphasised that staff are available to talk on request, and patients are also told times of ward rounds. A relationship is dynamic and will need partners to adapt to changing circumstances. Health professionals may take a less active role in the partnership when a shocked patient *collects him- or herself* and takes the reins in the illness. Sometimes, later in palliative care, patients become more passive as their illness fatigues them. It is within a sound partnership relationship that emotive issues, e.g. around resuscitation, artificial feeding and hydration towards the end of life, can be discussed in advance, and advance directives can be made so that the patient's opinions are clear when they are no longer able to communicate them.

THE SICK ROLE

It is important to have insight into the culture of being a patient to be able to understand the shift that may be needed by health professionals and patients to achieve partnership care. Some health-care professionals will have been patients and some honest reflection on this may be helpful to their practice.

The sick role was first described by the sociologist Talcott Parsons (1951). A central part of being sick is to seek medical advice, cooperate with medical experts and want to get well as soon as possible. In return for fulfilling these obligations, the patient is exempt from social responsibilities and, to an extent, self-care that can be delegated to a relative or friend. However, until the doctor diagnoses you as sick, *you are not sick* in the eyes of society. Therefore, if feeling sick and not fulfilling your usual obligations, you may be met by a lack of sympathy from relatives and employers. So at the start of an illness the person's autonomy is threatened. Furthermore, when certified sick, sympathy of others is threatened if the patient fails to demonstrate that they want to get well as soon as possible.

Charmaz (1983) gives valuable insights into the experience of illness from her qualitative research involving 57 patients with varied diagnoses. She describes patients as scrutinising encounters with others for hints of negative reflection on them, of being painfully aware of changes in close relationships as a result of physical dependency. Patients also reported feelings that, if they openly displayed their suffering, or showed self-pity, anger or guilt, they may estrange the people who still take an interest in them. In a society that emphasises doing rather than being, they felt that their life seemed less meaningful.

Morrison (1994) took an existential phenomenological approach to facilitate interviews with 10 hospitalised patients. Nine of the patients were anxious that any comments made were not to be interpreted as criticism of the staff. One of the major themes was that patients experienced feelings of crushing vulnerability. These manifested in feelings that nursing staff were not interested or supposed to get close to patients and reports of feeling like an object and being forgotten. Lack of privacy and being talked about as if they were not there increased feelings of vulnerability. Patients coped by presenting themselves in a particular way:

- Becoming obedient and compliant
- Conforming to ward rituals and routines
- Putting on a brave face and being outwardly cheerful
- Being honest and open with personal information
- Not asking questions although they wanted to.

Perhaps one of the most significant findings was an overriding reluctance of the patients to criticise the staff.

Warren et al. (2000) were participant observers in a ward where they also interviewed 11 patients. Two rules taken for granted among the patients were that they must *put on a brave face* and *not be a bother*. Being grateful and not complaining were also important *feeling rules* that emanated from the hidden curriculum of the ward culture. Some patients, so as *not to be a bother*, restricted their fluid intake, ignoring medical advice, to reduce the need to be taken to the toilet. Patients often displayed a light-hearted approach, joking with staff and other patients. Thus, they were praised for their courage by staff, i.e. for putting on a *brave face*. This particular phenomenon is an echo of earlier work done by Coser (1965). Again, through participant observation in a ward setting, Coser observed that a subculture developed to which the patient was admitted only if his or her misfortune became the subject of a joke. Medical and nursing staff joined in with this.

In Stockwell's (1972) observational study carried out in different ward settings, she identified some patients as being deemed unpopular by the nurses. This report made the national press. It was published at a time when nurses were considered by the public to be almost angelic. The thought that they might regard some patients as unpopular was unfathomable. In this report, similar behaviours to those described by Morrison (1994), Warren et al. (2000) and Coser (1965) were observed. Furthermore, patients who cried or complained were punished by being ignored by nursing staff. Other studies show similar findings to the ones cited here. The theme of patients feeling vulnerable is one that has endured for several decades. In my contemporary work with patient education groups I regularly hear stories that echo these findings.

These feelings of anxiety and vulnerability can clearly negate the patient being able to enter into a partnership role concerning their own care. In Chapters 3 and 4 the feelings of inadequacy and anxiety of professionals were discussed, and the subconscious use of the resultant distancing and blocking behaviours highlighted. Thus the potential for partnership working is in danger of being stifled by a cradle of anxiety. The professionals are the experts in the health-care arena. We want patients to have the opportunity, if they choose, to become experts on themselves. The aim of these three chapters has a very practical application. By having more understanding of the insecurities of patients, and by reflecting on our own feelings about relating to seriously ill people, we may feel better equipped to take the lead in promoting a more honest, open and helpful relationship with patients. The alternative can amount to play-acting, and is time wasting and destructive to partnership care.

FACE-TO-FACE PARTNERSHIP: ATTENTION TO INFORMATION GIVING

For the patient, particularly when newly diagnosed, the vulnerability in partnership is generally about a knowledge deficit, about something that is a central part of their life. Experiences of treatments and relationships with health professionals along the way can shape styles of coping with their vulnerability.

Giving bad news was discussed in detail in Chapter 3. *It is essential to have read this to maximise the learning potential from the rest of this chapter.* The emphasis is put on giving information at the rate and depth indicated by the patient, thus laying the foundations for partnership care.

A review of the literature by Mills and Sullivan (1999) concluded that the six functions of information for patients are: to gain control, to reduce anxiety, to improve compliance, to create realistic expectations, to promote self-care and participation, and to generate feelings of safety and security. Looking at the six functions of information giving against the sick role research, emphasising vulnerability, it clearly demonstrates the role of good information giving as being a key to partnership care. This approach complements the belief that good communication is the cornerstone to good palliative care.

Understanding the information that is being imparted is clearly fundamental, particularly if the patient is in a position where choices need to be made. Recent focus groups with cancer patients suggest that people experience a dearth of information, although theoretically much is available (Smith 2000). A quote from a female cancer patient sums this up:

They were all very wonderful but I realised afterwards that nobody told me anything.

National Cancer Alliance (1996)

Health-care professionals need to be aware that patients are often unable to recall a great deal of information that is given to them. It is well documented that people often emerge from consultations with incomplete understanding of what is happening (Muss et al. 1979). Very early studies indicate that outpatients often could recall only about 30% of what had been said to them immediately after an appointment (Ley and Spelman 1967). Over the years things have not changed dramatically. Recall among hospital patients for medical information was rated as poor, with a mean of 54% of information being retained (Ley 1988). Recall for patients receiving a cancer diagnosis falls to approximately 25% (Dunn et al. 1993). In cases when life-changing news is unexpected, patients are often unable to absorb any further information (Maguire and Faulkner 1988).

A review of the literature was inconclusive in being able to predict which patient characteristics may hamper or aid recall of information. No consistent relationships were found among age, intelligence, social class and mood states (Fallowfield and Jenkins 1999). However, the literature reveals that the interview structure can aid recall in a number of ways. Patients remember facts given at the start of the interview more readily. Topics that they regard as more relevant are more easily recalled (these may not coincide with what the health professional deems most relevant). More statements made by the doctor equate with the patient remembering less. Items that patients do recall do not get forgotten over time. Sometimes they have verbatim recall of what they think the doctor has told them (Fallowfield and Jenkins 1999).

Time needs to be given to information giving, just as time has to be given to physical examinations and investigations to aid diagnosis and assess fitness for anaesthetic, for example. We know that inadequate communication is distressing for patients and professionals and personally unrewarding for health professionals (Fallowfield 1993), so it needs attention. It would be good advice to all readers to take an advanced communication skills course if you have not already done so and keep a reflective diary concentrating on communication skills.

Information giving cannot be regarded as a one-off event. It is a process, and health-care professionals need to think creatively about how to achieve this. This is particularly challenging when time constraints are in place, e.g. as with a diagnosis of cancer where surgery is needed. The process of giving information is not complete until the health professional has some evidence that the patient has understood the information. The process followed by Hayward (1975) has been demonstrated to be successful. Hayward's process took three meetings with the patient. All meetings were prearranged and the objectives of the meetings made clear:

1. **The first meeting** established what the patient already knew and what the patient wanted to know at this point. The health professional will fill in gaps as appropriate. Even if patients have indicated that they want a more passive role, e.g. 'just get on with the treatment and I will ask questions as I go along', there will still be information that will be necessary to give, e.g. about organisational and experiential details of treatment plan. *Here please refer to the section in Chapter 3 on giving bad news.* At the end of this session main points are summarised and the patient is given an opportunity to ask questions. Hayward left patients with written information highlighting the main points of the interview. Jones et al. (1999) found that patients preferred to have written information based on their own medical records rather than general information. So a quick handwritten

summary at the end of the interview or a pre-prepared computer written summary highlighting the main points for individual patients could be very helpful. The practice of audio-taping consultations was discussed in Chapter 3 and, although some research indicates that it is very helpful in aiding information retention (Bruera et al. 1999), some demonstrated that it caused distress when discussion of prognosis was recorded (McHugh et al. 1995). More research is needed here. At the end of the first meeting, a second meeting should be arranged and patients and the relatives/friends also invited to bring a prompt sheet with any questions that they want to ask on it.

2. **The second meeting** is to assess what patients have understood and what they feel about what is happening to them. Ideally the interview should start with patients being invited to summarise what they understand and having an opportunity to put questions to the doctor or clinical nurse specialist (CNS) in terms of information. Again, the professional fills in any gaps in knowledge and clarifies any issues that may be confusing. If decisions have to be made about treatment this would be the time to discuss choices.

3. **The third meeting**, in Hayward's study, was an evaluation of what the patient had understood. Ideally, at this stage the patient is clear about the diagnosis and treatment plan and is able to explain this to the health professional with reference to relevant details regarding, for example, pre- and postoperative procedures, pain relief plans and individual treatment plans. Depth of knowledge about diagnosis and whether prognosis has been discussed in detail will be individual to each patient.

Perhaps health professionals need to think out of the box to come up with ways of incorporating this process into a constrained time frame. Claiming that there is just no time and that the outpatient appointment system does not allow sufficient time identifies a problem that needs to be addressed. I often hear people on the advanced communication skills course saying that they cannot give the time to information giving that they would want because appointment slots are short. The same professional may also comment that he or she spends a lot of time dealing with anxious people on the telephone. Being more proactive about information giving may reduce the incidence of time-consuming telephone calls.

My mother visited a cardiac outpatient department. She was told that the results of her angiogram suggested that she needed an urgent triple coronary artery bypass operation. She was shocked and anxious. She had no idea that she was so ill. The surgeon told her that it would be performed within 2 weeks and in that time she had two opportunities to find out more about the operation and events surrounding it. Each Tuesday, the cardiac unit held a study day for pre-surgery patients and their relatives and friends. My mother not only met other people who were going to have the operation but also members of the multidisciplinary team. Each member of the team explained what his or her role, in relation to a coronary artery bypass, was and what was expected of the patient. So, for example, the ward nurse explained about the admission procedures and the reasons for fasting, as well as the monitoring that would occur after surgery, and how pain relief was managed. The physiotherapists taught leg and breathing exercises and explained their importance. This procedural and experiential information is precisely the information that Hayward

(1975) found, in his study, helped to reduce experiences of anxiety and pain and promote recovery after surgery. The surgeon did a slot on the anatomy and physiology of the operation, which was optional. This, too, is in line with Hayward's research. Not everyone is reassured by being told precise details of the anatomy of the surgery. Some may find this terrifying. On this occasion, two patients who had previously had the operation talked about their experiences and there was an opportunity to ask them questions. Preoperative assessment investigations were also built into the day for those whose surgery was imminent. The last session of the day was led by a ward nurse and the physiotherapist and it was an MCQ (multi-choice question) test on what had been taught. This was accompanied by lots of laughter. Each patient was given a small booklet produced by the team condensing the main points included in the day. The day was invaluable for my mother and an example of excellent practice.

As a result of earlier directives, cancer networks are probably ahead in forming partnership groups with patients. A survey in 2005 demonstrated that 30 of the 34 cancer networks had formed partnership groups with patients. Three of the five core elements that commonly underpin the aims of the groups are influencing policy and service, providing a voice for service users and improving patient care (Richardson et al. 2005). Organising and administering a day such as the one experienced by my mother could well be within the remit of such a group; input from professionals could be minimal, e.g. a 40-minute slot. This sounds like good use of time if it reduces phone calls from anxious patients. A partnership group with which I was involved was keen to provide a buddy system for newly diagnosed patients. The professionals in the group, taking a paternalistic stance, vetoed this opportunity. We must question if professionals should 'game keep' in this way. Effectively they robbed future patients of an important choice and undermined the concept of partnership working by not exploring this offer more seriously. Although it would be important to ensure good quality buddying decisions, organisation of such a service should surely be a shared responsibility.

As well as the individual health-care professional's challenge to meet individual information needs there are also organisational challenges. These encompass: treating information needs as a core activity; ensuring adequate funding, space and time devoted to patient information; implementing and reviewing guidelines on patient information; and auditing methods of working (Jones et al. 2000).

WRITTEN INFORMATION

Written information is clearly not a substitute for verbal information; it complements it. As previously stated, patients have a preference for written information that is tailored to them. A personal information file is currently undergoing trials in cancer networks. The file is in two parts: one contains general information about cancer, e.g. making a diagnosis, tests and treatments, and this can be added to; the second part is a personal diary where a record is kept of personal health care, including test results and transcription of consultations.

Good-quality written information is vital. A study looking at 50 different information leaflets used the SMOG (simple measure of gobbledegook) and Flesch tests to assess readability of each booklet. The SMOG test selects 10 sentences from the start, middle and end of the text and counts the number of words with three syllables. The Flesch test works on a similar method. The reading age of material can be pinpointed when the number of words per sentence and per 100 words is known. All but 2 of the 50 booklets in the study were written at a reading age of 15–16 years. Only one breast care booklet was written at a reading age of 14. It cannot be assumed that written information will be understood. In a study of written information, it was concluded that material written at a reading age of 15 is likely to be understood by 54% of the population (Ley and Florino 1996). They highlight that tabloid newspapers, which account for 70% of newspapers sold in the UK, are written at a reading age of 12.

The Plain English Campaign is an international organisation that aims to ensure that any documents, leaflets, booklets and websites are easily understood by the public. It provides writing guidelines and will also test material for clarity. Documents that reach the required standard are able to display the Crystal Mark logo on their material. This is a service that is now being widely used (Plain English Campaign 2006). The King's Fund in London also provides a guide for writing information for patients – *Practicalities of Producing Patients Information* (Dunman and Farell 2000). DISCERN is a validated system for judging the quality of written information on treatment. A study looking at 57 participants attending online DISCERN workshops found that at follow-up most (89.6%) reported that their attitude to consumer health information of all types had changed, mostly becoming more systematic and critical. It was concluded that it is possible that DISCERN can provide users with simple flexible skills for dealing with a wide range of treatment information available (Charnock and Shepherd 2004).

DECISION AIDS

Helping patients to make informed decisions is key to partnership working. The sorts of decisions to be made, for example, include initial and later treatment options, continuing treatments when disease is progressing and advance planning as disease progresses. The availability of decision aids is expanding, with some now available on the internet. Decision aids such as video and audio-tapes, interactive computer programs and leaflets using a question-and-answer format, are designed to help patients understand their options, consider the benefits and harm to their personal circumstances, and then participate in decision-making. The use of decision aids in this way is economical in terms of professional time and allows patients, relatives and friends to consider options without the pressures of immediate time constraints, and with the people with whom they feel easy. However, few decision aids have been evaluated. O'Connor et al. (2003), in a systematic review, identified 200 decision aids; 30 of the aids were evaluated in 34 randomised controlled trials and another trial evaluated a suite of 8 decision aids. The review of the trials found that decision aids improved people's knowledge of options, created realistic expectations of the benefits and harm, reduced difficulty in decision-making and increased participation in the process. They did not seem to have an effect on satisfaction with decision-making or anxiety. More research is needed (O'Connor et al. 2003).

There is a problem with selecting good sources of information. Professionals need to be able to direct the patient to high-quality information. This involves carefully monitoring leaflets and booklets and ensuring that they have been written to meet Plain English Standards and/or appraised using some of the published guidelines and checklists currently available. Using a patient group to evaluate the finished product is routine for some organisations, e.g. Macmillan Cancer Relief. The internet is a growing source of information to which many patients now have easy access. Gateway services are now being offered by several providers. This is a selective process that includes only information that meets certain criteria.

SPECIAL NEEDS

As already mentioned, there is a variety of information sources available: audio-tape and video-tape cassettes for those with reading and sight problems. Many of the big charities have telephone information lines managed by well-trained people to give information and listen to problems. The associated major websites have chat rooms for patients and relatives as well as giving information. The charity Cancer-BACUP publishes information and provides audio-tape cassettes in 13 different languages, although this does seem to be exceptional and hopefully a template for other organisations. There are organisations that make information more accessible for people with learning disabilities. Interactive computer programs are often attractive to younger patients, e.g. teenagers. A list of different sources of information can be found at the end of the chapter.

CONCLUSION

Partnership care will not *just happen* in most circumstances. It requires a good level of self-awareness and high-quality communication skills from health professionals to be proactive in achieving what is still a huge cultural shift in health care. Partnership care is largely about shared decision-making, with the professional being, at least initially, the expert on their illness and patients the experts on themselves. However, the partnership is dynamic and all concerned may need to adjust to shifts in the nuances of the balance of responsibilities in making decisions. In their sincere efforts to create partnership, working professionals should not overlook their responsibility to provide the patient with the benefit of their experience and knowledge. Professionals should also take responsibility for initiating conversations that are about advance care planning. Ensuring that patients have access to high-quality information to aid decision-making is also an important organisational responsibility.

MAIN IMPLICATIONS FOR PRACTICE

- Patients are the experts on their own individual beliefs, habits, attitudes and preferences. The doctor is the expert on the diagnosis and treatment options. Both types of knowledge are needed to manage illness effectively.

- Research looking at the sick role demonstrates that people often feel very vulnerable as patients. A relationship needs to be built with the patient towards offering choices and sharing decision-making.
- Patients being asked to make decisions about their care with insufficient experience or knowledge to do so may feel disempowered.
- Ground rules for sharing information with patients should be made with them.
- Information giving is a process. The professional should never feel that information has been given until they assess what the patient has understood.
- Information giving needs protected time, just as aspects of physical care do.
- Written information needs to be accurate and clear. It is wise to follow recommended approaches, e.g. Plain English Campaign guidelines.
- Use approved decision aids to help patients make choices.
- Health-care professionals should think out of the box with regard to giving information study days for patients.

SUGGESTED FURTHER READING

Johns C (2006) *Being Mindful and Easing Suffering.* London: Jessica Kingsley Publishers.
Monroe B, Oliviere D (2003) *Patient Participation in Palliative Care: A voice for the voiceless.* Oxford: Oxford University Press.
Royal College of Nursing (2004) *Caring in Partnership: Older people and nursing staff working towards the future.* London: RCN.

Websites

www.plainenglish.co.uk
www.discern.org.uk
www.literacytrust.org.uk/campaign/smog

Chapter 6
Hope and spirituality

KEY POINTS

- **Introduction**: a feeling of hopefulness is a unique state named by the individual feeling it. The feeling of hopefulness can be nurturing even if the hoped-for state is unattainable.
- **Hope research**: research studies looking at the hope of a patient receiving palliative care have identified similar themes. Hope-fostering characteristics are concerned with affirming relationships, setting goals and maintaining independence, finding meaning, using inner resources and feeling valued. Hope-hindering conditions include feelings of abandonment, devaluation of personhood and having uncontrolled physical symptoms.
- **Intuitive practice**: aspects of care that we know to be good practice nurture hope. Sustaining hope is an intuitive part of human nature and caring practices.
- **Spirituality**: this has been described as giving us a sense of personhood and uniqueness. It acts as an inner source of power and energy.
- **Personhood**: using Cassell's parts of personhood, it is possible, on reflection of my practice and that of some of my students, to identify spiritual aspects of care that occur as a natural part of practice.
- **Expertise**: there are times when the expertise of people with more advanced skills is necessary to help with spiritual pain, e.g. mental health practitioners, chaplains and those with advanced communication skills training.
- **Religion**: spirituality is broader than religion. However, for many people their religion is a central part of their spirituality. A brief look at what is important as death nears is included for Buddhism, Christianity, Hinduism, Islam, Judaism and Sikhism.
- **Competencies for spiritual care**: the Marie Curie spiritual and religious care competencies for specialist and palliative care are outlined in line with the NICE guidelines.

INTRODUCTION

The word 'hope' has commonly been associated with cure, so patients receiving palliative care have no hope because there is no cure. In parallel with this, treatments aimed at helping patients to feel better or slow down progression of an illness, e.g. palliative radiotherapy and chemotherapy, have been equated with giving patients false hope. This is a very superficial and inaccurate view of the multidimensional concept of hope. A working definition of hope put forward by Farran et al. (1995, p 6) captures its contradictions and its durability:

> Hope constitutes an essential experience of the human condition. It functions as a way of feeling, a way of thinking, a way of behaving and a way of relating oneself to the world. Hope has a way of being fluid in its expectations, and in the event that the desired object or outcome does not occur, hope can still be present.

Another definition of realistic hope that complements this working definition is: 'Realistic hope is thought to have the potential to change human existence for the better without reaching for the unattainable' (Jones 2005, p 28). A feeling of hopefulness is a unique state that is felt and named by the individual feeling it. In the main it is not accurate or helpful for others to make assumptions about the quality and dimensions of that hope.

HOPE RESEARCH

Written with Professor Kaye Herth, based on her original Hope Study

Until recently there has been limited research on the concept of hope in those with advanced terminal illness (Herth and Cutcliffe 2002). Early articles focus on hope as being energising in situations of adversity and are almost synonymous with finding meaning, e.g. Korner (1970) and McGee (1984) document strong relationships between hope and survival in Nazi concentration camps. Frankl (1946), a psychiatrist, writes about his experiences as a prisoner in such a camp and the significant impact of maintaining hope even in such dire conditions. These early accounts have been interpreted as demonstrating that having hope endows people with psychological and physical energy in adverse conditions.

Over the past decade studies on hope have been primarily concerned with individuals in the advanced stages of cancer or human immunodeficiency virus (HIV) infection (acquired immune deficiency syndrome or AIDS). Quantitative studies have concentrated on the relationship between hope and psychosocial variables such as age, activity and fatigue levels across the dying trajectory. Qualitative studies have sought to elucidate the meaning of hope for terminally ill people and how hope is maintained and engendered.

Cutcliffe (1995), Flemming (1997) and Urquhart (1999) focused on the meaning of hope for palliative care patients. Hope was described as being an inner power or strength that can enrich lives and enable individuals to look beyond their pain, suffering and turmoil. Herth (1990a) was the first person to conduct research that aimed to define hope in patients receiving palliative care and to identify strategies that foster and hinder hope. These strategies are important to nurses who often assume a primary role in the care of terminally ill people and are in a strategic position to foster or hinder hope (Herth 1990a).

Buckley and Herth (2004) replicated Herth's (1990a) study, which was then the only published study to use a longitudinal design combined with method triangulation to research the terminally ill patient population. Herth's (1990a) study explored hope in a convenient sample of 30 patients receiving hospice care. It identified seven hope-fostering categories and three hope-hindering categories. The replication study, carried out in the UK as opposed to the USA, involved 16 palliative patients (Buckley and Herth 2004). It demonstrated almost identical results. Several qualitative studies have appeared in the literature since the study by Herth (1990a). Post-White et al. (1996) conducted a qualitatively descriptive study exploring meanings of hope and strategies used to sustain hope in 32 patients with cancer. Five themes were identified. These themes are similar to those described by Herth, with the exception of light-heartedness, affirmation of worth and uplifting memories, all of which were not specifically identified (Table 6.1).

Flemming (1997) conducted a qualitative study and interviewed four dying patients. She focused on meaning and identified three specific areas that influenced hope:

1. The maintenance of the disease as it existed at the time of the interview, underpinned by hope of a cure
2. The existence and presence of significant family members and an anticipated future with them
3. The maintenance of positive interest in the individual by health-care professionals.

Bezein et al. (2001) conducted narrative interviews with 11 patients with cancer receiving palliative care. They concluded that a tension exists between hoping for a cure and living in hope that encompasses 'reconciliation and comfort with life and death'. Living as normally as possible and experiencing relationships in which a patient's terminally ill status was acknowledged were important to a patient's hope. However, the person is valued for whom they are and not categorised by the disease.

In a study of 10 elderly palliative care patients, Duggleby and Wright (2005) add the dimensions of positive reappraisal and leaving a legacy. Positive reappraisal refers to people's ability to find meaning in their life as progressive illness changes their situations, expectations and goals. Their participants also explored the importance of leaving a legacy. Life review is focused on the individual whereas leaving a legacy is focused on others. This is a very similar concept to mature hope. Hinds and Martin (1988), in a study involving 58 adolescent oncology patients, found that they had the ability to hope for others, e.g. their family and friends after their death – thus termed 'mature hope'. This feeling of hopefulness was sustained and nurturing to the participants in their study.

There is a consensus between the earlier anecdotal accounts and the later qualitative research that hope is associated with finding meaning and using one's inner resources, as well as being a source of psychological energy. In all six studies in palliative care settings, affirming personal relationships and relationships with caring staff emerged as central to maintaining hope.

Table 6.1   Categories that foster and hinder hope

Buckley and Herth (2004)	Herth (1990a)	Post-White et al. (1996)
Hope-fostering categories and subcategories		
Love of family and friends Meaningful relationships and being loved and giving love	**Interpersonal connectedness**	**Affirming relationships**
Spirituality/having faith Strong Christian faith, faith in God and family, and the spiritual world – life after death	**Spiritual base**	**Anticipating survival**
Setting goals and maintaining independence Attainable; unattainable	**Attainable aims**	**Finding meaning**
Positive relationships with professional carers Helping relationships with regard to illness and being treated with courtesy and respect	**Affirmation of worth**	**Living in the present**
Humour Camaraderie with other patients Laughing with professional carers and laughing as an inner resource	**Light-heartedness**	**Using inner resources**
Personal characteristics Determination and being a fighter	**Personal attributes**	
Uplifting memories	**Uplifting memories**	
Hope-hindering categories and subcategories		
Abandonment and isolation Spouses that will not or cannot support patients psychologically Poor communication with professional carers	**Abandonment**	
Uncontrollable pain and discomfort Loss of independence and control	**Uncontrollable pain and discomfort**	
Devaluation of personhood Offhand, flippant remarks Apparent lack of interest from professionals	**Devaluation of personhood**	

Setting goals and working to reach these goals are components of hope. These concepts might be transferable to other settings, which could include long-term care residences for older people, some of whom will have experienced 'social death' associated with breaking ties with the past and giving up their home, and also younger people facing progressive chronic illness.

The tension between mortality and immortality is a recurring theme. There is a cognitive acknowledgement of the prognosis but not always an emotional recognition that hope and dreams for a future may be curtailed. This phenomenon was noted by Kübler-Ross (1969) and more recently highlighted by Copp and Field (2002).

The remainder of this section details the results of the replication study on hope, looking at hope-fostering and hope-hindering categories identified by 16 dying people (Buckley and Herth 2004).

Categories that foster hope

The participants identified categories that foster hope as helping them to remain hopeful in the event of facing their mortality. As in Herth (1990a), seven hope-fostering categories were identified and three hope-hindering ones.

Love of family and friends

All 16 participants acknowledged family and friends as being important to fostering hope. Five talked of meaningful relationships being directly helpful. One said: 'I couldn't cope with dying without R [husband], he keeps me hopeful.' Being loved and giving love were cited as important to 13 participants. Just being with family and close friends was important to the hoping process. Participants particularly mentioned children and grandchildren as fostering hope. One said: 'Seeing my granddaughter in the Brownie uniform – that's hope to me.'

Some people enlarged on this and expressed hopes for the future of their children and grandchildren. This has been described as mature hoping by Hinds and Martin (1988) and seems to be as psychologically nurturing as hoping for a personal future. One participant said: 'I really hope my grandson will become a professional foot-baller, he has set his heart on this.' It might be, as Herth (1990a) suggests, that the human presence of family and friends restores human-centred dignity and affirmation of being, which are necessary for the emergence of hope.

Spirituality/having faith

Of the 16 participants, 15 felt that having faith in a spiritual world encouraged hope. Five identified a strong Christian faith as being extremely important to them. Seven talked of their faith in God, linking it with their families. One said: 'In this crisis, basic Christianity is coming back and the love of my family is a big part of that.'

Three people did not have a religious faith; however, they believed in a spiritual world incorporating life after death. They also emphasised the importance of having faith in others. One said: 'You have got to be able to have faith in people who are treating and helping you.'

One person claimed to have no spiritual beliefs and felt that death was 'the end'; the researcher visited him a second time when he was in the hospice days before his death. He was restless and appeared frightened. His family did not visit him and he turned his friends away. He said hope was still important to him but it was becoming 'less and less accessible'. For most of the participants, faith was important: faith in God, faith in an afterlife, faith in family and friends, as well as faith in professionals. The concept of faith was central to their hoping and the expression of their faith was unique for each person.

Setting goals and maintaining independence

For 11 of the 16 participants, hope was linked with working towards self-set goals and achieving these was a source of pleasure. For some patients the goals were clearly not attainable. A 58-year-old patient, who was bedridden, said in July: 'My next trip will be at the end of October to Fiji and then, if I can get rid of these swollen legs, I'll spend Christmas in Sydney, Australia, with my son.' He was still alluding to a future of some months hence, although his prognosis was expressed in terms of days. For others, as their condition deteriorated, their goals were refocused and became less ambitious. One said: 'You always have to have goals. These days I do small things. Now I'm determined to keep on dressing myself each day.'

Positive relationships with professional carers

A positive relationship with professional carers was mentioned by 13 of the 16 participants. Some mentioned specific people with whom they had an ongoing relationship. One said: 'If I'm low, I tell her [clinical nurse specialist or CNS] and we talk. It helps.' Some mentioned specific incidences, e.g. when bad news was broken. Other participants highlighted particular wards where they felt that the overall attitude of the staff helped them to remain hopeful. Some cited both. The striking aspect of this category was how much the 'little things' matter, e.g. patients cited the importance of carers 'bothering' to find out what name they preferred to be called by, being courteous and willing to answer questions.

Humour

Six participants mentioned humour when talking about maintaining hope. Two people had received radiotherapy on a daily basis. Both valued the camaraderie that developed between them and other patients receiving similar treatments. The other participants were part of support groups and described the ability to laugh together about shared misfortune as being very important to maintaining hope. Four of the participants referred to humour as being an important inner resource. One said: 'Mixing in the right company, which makes you cheerful, that helps. Their cheerfulness keeps you going.'

Personal characteristics

Personal characteristics were mentioned by 12 of the participants. Being positive and determined to maintain optimism in the face of deterioration was the theme of these comments. One said: 'I'm the sort of person who always keeps going no matter what.'

Uplifting memories

Although patients did not directly identify uplifting memories as an element that fosters hope, some lapsed into recalling good memories as they spoke. In several instances the memories recalled concerned their children when they were young, e.g. happy memories of family holidays. Remembering 'youth' seems to be important to hope.

Hope-hindering categories

Patients had little trouble identifying times when they had felt hopeless. Herth (1990a) found the same phenomenon and suggests that one reason why periods of feeling hopeless come to mind so quickly may be because they are times when patients feel frightened and out of control. Analysis of categories that hinder hope in this research matches Herth's (1990a) supposition. As in Herth's (1990a) study, the hope-hindering categories were uncontrollable symptoms, e.g. abandonment and isolation, pain and discomfort, and devaluation of personhood.

Abandonment and isolation

This related to instances when patients felt unable to share their fears and anxieties with relatives, friends or health-care professionals. One woman said that her husband was good and loving but he had never allowed her to talk about her illness. She intimated that she would rather he was absent on occasions when she wanted to talk. Similar comments were made by participants in Herth's (1990a) study. Herth comments on this stating that emotional withdrawal while remaining physically present was worse than physical withdrawal. However, there were also examples of married couples who had not talked together about dying and that was acceptable for them. They intimated that words were not really necessary; they both knew and understood that death was going to part them physically.

Uncontrollable pain and discomfort

Losing independence was an important issue for most participants. One woman lost hope dramatically as she lost the use of her legs. She said: 'I envy anyone who can walk six steps.' In situations where symptoms could be controlled, the loss of hope was transient and relatively easy to put to one side. Ten participants could remember days when pain or nausea was so bad that they 'wanted to die'. One man said: 'I was in so much pain at the time that it really would have been a relief to slip away, then the next day you feel better and wonder "why on earth did I feel like that?".'

Devaluation of personhood

Just as small gestures, such as being courteous and ready to engage in conversation, could provide hope, offhand and non-caring remarks could hinder it. In eight examples, the news of a cancer diagnosis being delivered in a perceived non-caring, offhand manner caused feelings of hopelessness. The patients were made to feel like a 'non-person' (Herth 1990a) at one of the most significant events in their life.

Discussion

The implications of this study are extremely important for health-care professionals in all care settings. Traditionally, 'caring' is seen as the nurse's role, and nurses have sustained contact with patients. Herth (1990a, p 1258) highlights 'nurses can serve as catalysts to create internal and external conditions that foster caring relationships between terminally ill people and their families and friends and professional caregivers'.

This research highlights important areas for all members of the multidisciplinary team involved in caring for dying patients. The important and positive aspect of this work is that the implications for practice are not new. Aspects of care that we know intuitively to be good practice nurture hope. Sustaining hope is an intuitive part of human nature and nursing practice. Caring practices are the essence of good care.

Love of family and friends emphasises the importance of extending care to family and friends. Particular emphasis on the importance of children and grandchildren was evident. Seeing children and grandchildren inspired hope in patients. In the past it has not been uncommon for parents and professionals to try to protect children from the death of family members by not including them in discussions and not telling them the truth. Exclusion leads to isolation, leaving children unsupported in their feelings and unprotected from their fantasies (Munroe 2003). Dyregov (1991) concurs with Munroe that children have the same needs as adults in wanting to know what is happening and should be given the opportunity to express their feelings and ask questions.

The task for the multidisciplinary team is not only to welcome children as visitors but also to give help and direction to parents in supporting children to cope with grief. This first step is to reassure them that children should be included in the family scenario when someone is dying. They should be supported in visiting dying relatives and be given honest information about what is happening. Children should not necessarily be excluded from family discussion and meetings with members of the multidisciplinary team. Creating child-friendly areas in wards is a good starting point. Welcoming and supporting children associated with the dying person not only helps patients to feel more hopeful but also encourages a more positive experience for children.

Considering spirituality in its widest sense and supporting the individual's faith are vital. The National Institute for Health and Clinical Excellence (NICE) guidance on cancer services (NICE 2004b) stresses the importance of all those involved in assessing patients' needs to be highly tuned to the spiritual dimension of care, particularly as some patients might express their needs only once.

Patients identified that it was important to have faith in those caring for them. Inadequate and thoughtless communication was reported to hinder hope. It is imperative for all members of the interdisciplinary team to have good communication skills to maintain a hopeful state. The NICE (2004b) guidance stresses that patients and carers frequently comment that the communication skills of health-care and social-care professionals are poor. The guidance recommends intensive training in communication skills for health-care professionals as in courses developed by Fallowfield et al. (2002). Their research, involving 160 oncologists, demonstrated that such courses could significantly improve key communication skills.

Maintaining independence for as long as possible is important for the hoping process, e.g. using models of nursing that encourage a partnership approach, which gives control to patients. Helping patients to use their inner resources to optimise their quality of life and make a healthy adaptation to facing mortality is central to the holistic approach (Buckley 2002a). When people are weakened by fatigue the challenge is to find a balance between helping and nurturing independence.

Being able to foster empathic relations with patients based on trust promotes hope, as does courtesy and respect. For patients who feel abandoned and isolated, hand or foot massage can bring psychological warmth and comfort (Buckley 2002b). Two quasi-experimental studies demonstrated the positive effect on morale of massage and aromatherapy massage in dying patients (Corner et al. 1995, Wilkinson et al. 1995). Busy ward staff could enlist the help of trained volunteer complementary therapists to provide this service in the absence of therapists being available as part of the multidisciplinary team. Teaching relatives and friends how to give a hand and foot massage can provide an intimacy that illness may have precluded. Parkes (1991) suggests that being able to contribute to the care of dying patients might help relatives and friends to cope with the grieving process.

Remembering precious moments in dying people's lives can also promote hope. Relatives and friends can support patients by participating in remembering the important events of their life and the good times that they shared. Reminiscence can be aided by use of photographs and looking at them together. Leaving the photographs on the patient's locker will enable staff to join in this activity. One patient whom the researcher nursed benefited from his son making an audio-tape of his favourite music. The patient would play the music when receiving nursing care and recall important aspects of his life as he listened.

Dying people maintain a sense of humour and being able to share that with them can be enriching for patients and carers. Herth's (1990b) study of 14 terminally ill patients concluded that humour is as essential during the terminal phase of an illness than at other times during illness and health. Self-help groups, formed by two participants in this study, worked well and, in particular, both talked of the importance of humour in that group. The authors believe that more exploration of the nurse's role in supporting humour within and outside of self-help groups needs to be undertaken.

Good pain and symptom management is essential to maintain a hopeful state. Health-care professionals should continue to develop skills of assessment, aiming to anticipate and minimise potential problems in these areas. Historically, a palliative approach has been pioneered in cancer care as part of the hospice movement. Professionals working in specialist palliative care now have a role in helping to ensure that the body of knowledge that guides good pain and symptom management is shared with colleagues practising as generalists in palliative care.

Sometimes listening to patients, 'being there' and demonstrating empathy can be challenging, as can facilitating caring relationships in families. Self-awareness is a valuable asset to health-care professionals. Wakefield (2000) recommends that palliative care nurses should practise relentless self-care so that they can continue to support dying patients. Dunniece and Slevin's (2002) qualitative study stresses that the experienced nurse's practice of caring, and his or her commitment to sharing a patient's journey towards his or her mortality, is vital. Therefore, looking at self-awareness and self-care should be an integral part of training in communication skills to help support staff caring for dying patients.

Conclusion to the Hope Study

The meaning of hope in these participants was equated with the love that they felt for family and friends, their own inner resources and spirituality. Central also to hope was being goal focused and maintaining independence. As disease progresses, so goals are 'scaled down'. This adaptation seemed to evolve with surprising ease in most participants. In three terminally ill patients, as activities of daily living became more limited, so 'bedside nursing' became more important. Being courteous and friendly, able to laugh with patients and maintaining good levels of 'basic' care are paramount to the ability of patients to maintain a feeling of hopefulness. For many, the hope becomes a 'mature hope' (Hinds and Martin 1988), i.e. hope for others in their family rather than a personal hope. This study also concurs with Bezein et al. (2001) in that hope for a cure seems to be inexhaustible in terminal illness.

This study, similar to Herth's (1990a), has confirmed that hope is important to the terminally ill population in both America and England, and losing it increases psychological pain and distress. In all instances in this study the loss of hope was transient. Sustaining hope is closely associated with sustaining a caring relationship with dying patients and facilitating relationships between the terminally ill person and their family and friends.

SPIRITUALITY

The approach to medicine in the western world has been highly successful in terms of preventing, curing and managing a whole range of diseases that, at the dawn of the twentieth century, were fatal. This has been achieved by a scientific approach that has concentrated on the disease as opposed to the person. A rapid expansion in knowledge and technology was stimulated in part by the two World Wars. Scientists and medical doctors wanted to match the war efforts of the foot soldier in terms of the treatment and rehabilitation that could be offered in the face of hideous injuries and rampant diseases. Ironically, Walter (1994) sees World War II as diminishing the role of spirituality in the dying. Spirituality, although not confined to culture or religion, has been associated historically with the presence of the clergy. In the face of countless atrocious deaths the clergy were humbled and public health workers and doctors have supplanted priests at the bedside of those who are dying (Walter 1994).

Life is full of cycles. Many patients now feel that they have become lost in the scientific approach to their disease, and find diagnosis and treatment an alienating process (Daniel 2001b). This theme echoes in part Dame Cicely Saunders' motivation for the hospice movement. She writes that as well as good symptom control there should be emphasis on family and the patients' inner life. There should be group understanding together with an ability to make sense of the inner concerns and values of a person (Saunders 2006d).

The NICE (2004b) guidelines for palliative care state that the needs of patients for spiritual support are frequently unrecognised by health-care and social-care professionals who may well feel uncomfortable broaching spiritual issues.

It may be that we feel under-confident to support patients spiritually because its many different definitions and interpretations give spirituality an almost intangible and elusive mantle. In the main the thought of supporting someone with existential pain can make us feel humble and inadequate. Helping someone with physical pain, a more concrete concept, can have exactly the opposite effect, making us feel helpful and efficient as we give the treatment and explain the purpose to our patients. It is hardly surprising then that we turn away from the spiritual. Unless we are self-aware we will always graduate to what is our comfort zone regardless of the patient's pain.

Spirituality has been described as giving us a sense of personhood and uniqueness. It acts as an inner source of power and energy, which helps us 'tick over' as the person we are. It is an intangible dimension that motivates us to be connected with others and our surroundings. It drives us to establish positive and trusting relationships with others and to strive for meaning and purpose. Our spirituality can give us peace and tranquillity through our relationship with 'something other'. It can be an important source of wisdom, inspiration and meaning. Spirituality comes into focus at critical junctures in our lives, perhaps when we feel emotional stress or physical illness or near death (Sherwood 2000; Narayanasamy 2001; Swinton 2001).

Highfield and Cason (1983) used Cassell's framework of religious existential needs on which to base their study. The four spiritual needs that they identified were:

1. The need for meaning and purpose in life
2. The need to give love
3. The need to receive love
4. The need for hope and creativity.

Religion

In our health-care system in the past spirituality has been closely associated with religion. Many of us remember an enquiry about a person's religious affiliation as being our only concrete contribution to the 'spiritual care' of our patients. For many people religion is associated with worship, places of worship and life rituals, baptisms, funerals and weddings. Religions in literature are described as being about a supernatural or divine force and about a system of beliefs, ethical codes and philosophy, which provide a framework for living (Narayanasamy 2006).

It is generally agreed that spirituality is much broader than religion. However, for some people their religion is a central part of their spirituality. Religion, like spirituality, will often come into sharp focus for people in times of illness or crisis. Spirituality is more of a journey, and religion may become the transport to help us on that journey. Some people may be highly spiritual in nature but not necessarily religious, whereas others may be religious without being spiritual (Narayanasamy 2006). In a multicultural society it is very important that health professionals are mindful to support and help facilitate the many diverse religious practices that may form a vital part of end-of-life care. An important part of an initial assessment of new patients is to enquire about their religious practices and, if appropriate, discuss how worship for them can best be facilitated. It would be both respectful and reassuring if the professional demonstrated some insight into the person's religion. However, people are often very patient with professionals and provided that we take steps to inform ourselves more fully, as well as contacting relevant religious leaders and arranging the physical environment for worship, if appropriate, ignorance need not damage a relationship. Later in this chapter some different religious approaches to death are highlighted.

Spirituality: a practical approach

In spite of many years' experience as a nurse and a good deal of reading about spirituality, I was still left wondering if, apart from obvious occasions, I had addressed patients' spirituality in practice. Then one day a colleague/student handed in her assignment looking at suffering and spirituality using Cassell's (1991) framework of personhood as a foundation. After reading the assignment, I reflected on my own experiences using Cassell's (1991) framework and identified occasions in practice that I believe were addressing spiritual care. Cobb (2001) also links personhood to spirituality and he adds that spirituality, similar to health, is enigmatic and its familiar presence seldom registered unless it is challenged or dislocated.

The parts of personhood (Cassell 1991)
A person has a past
A person has a family
A person has a cultural background
A person has roles
A person has relationships
A person is a political being
A person does things
A person has a body
A person has a secret life
A person has a perceived future
A person has a transcendent dimension

Here follow memories of care giving in relationship to personhood. On reflection much of this is spiritual care given unconsciously, naturally, as part of the 'usual' routine approach. I draw on my own experience and that of my students.

A person has a past

As I was assisting an elderly married woman with her hygiene needs she asked if she could talk about her first husband. Her first husband had been killed in action in World War II. She and her second husband were married shortly after the war. Her second husband's first wife had also been killed in the war. When they married they had made a pact not to talk about their first marriages at all.

Thereafter, whenever I was with her she talked about her first husband. She described his physical looks and personal characteristics. She told me about how they first met, when he proposed, and shared some precious memories of their short time together. All this as we went about the business of helping her to get up and ready for the day. Each time I left the room she smiled and put her finger to her lips indicating 'don't tell' – I would mirror the same back to her. It felt easy and special to listen to her memories. She said that she had never been able to talk about her first husband in that way since he died.

A person has a family

John was in his 60s and dying. His long history of alcohol abuse had put an enormous strain on his family relationships. Although he had been estranged from his family for some time, when they heard that he was dying they visited him regularly on the ward. John had been restless and irritable when arriving on our ward. An enthusiastic staff nurse had noticed that he enjoyed music and, after acquiring a list of his all-time favourites, had asked her 'DJ' husband to compile a tape-recording of his favourite songs.

The tape served as a medium to find some peace and relive happier memories with his family. I was in the room one day when his daughter, who had been particularly cold and distant with him, laughed and hugged him when hearing the Hollies sing 'When you walk in the room'. Apparently he used to sing that to her.

A person has a cultural background

An elderly man was dying at home. As he came close to the end of his life, a Marie Curie nurse was brought in for night duties. She was alarmed at the amount of pain that he was in. He was not on opioids and her experienced background was such that she felt sure that she could advise the GP appropriately to control the pain. The man refused her suggestion. He went on to explain that, as a Buddhist, he wanted to be conscious when he died. He also explained that he felt it important to feel the pain. His daughter had died 30 years previously of cancer and died in 'agony'. As her father he felt that he too should feel pain like her. The Marie Curie nurse respected his wishes and he accepted her offer of a hand to hold until morning.

A person has relationships

An elderly man was dying at home. He was confined to bed, not eating or drinking, and had a syringe driver administering diamorphine. He was slipping in and out of sleep, sometimes aware, sometimes not. The community nurse was just finishing his care when she heard children arrive. Almost immediately they were told to be quiet because of granddad. She went downstairs and asked what was happening. The sick man's wife said 'they were whistling – I didn't want them to disturb their granddad'. The community nurse explained that he would probably enjoy their voices. The children said, 'we were whistling – granddad taught us to whistle'. With the permission of their grandmother the nurse took the children to their granddad's room and asked them to whistle as loud as they could. They did and granddad smiled.

I think they reminded this dying man, who had necessarily relinquished almost all his roles in life, that he had had and still had a very special relationship with his grandchildren.

A person has roles

I was visiting a woman in her 40s at home. She was dying, now confined to bed with a syringe driver. She had young children of 6 and 9 – the same age as my own children. We had talked about them together in the past. She and her husband had planned how he would manage the future for the children without her.

As I was changing her syringe driver she asked if I could give her extra drugs so that she could die that day. I asked why she was saying that now. She explained that her children no longer asked for her, they called for their father. She said it would be better for them when she died so that they could get on with living without her. A long silence followed. She broke the silence by saying that, no, we could not do that, as how could her husband face the children knowing that she had deliberately ended her life. We sat in silence then for a while and she quietly slept. I massaged her feet before I left. She died a few days later.

A person is a political being

Patrick was a young man of 35 who was dying. He had been a very successful businessman in London, used to managing people, and seeing his plans for business come to fruition. He was a bachelor and lived alone. As his condition weakened he sold his flat in London and moved in with his mother on the south coast. Accepting help was difficult for him and we all worked to help him stay as much in control of his own days as possible. He had been an avid rugby player and his rugby club in London was having a special celebratory weekend. Patrick was determined to go. A friend was to pick him up. His blood count was low. He said that if he could have a blood transfusion he felt that he could manage the weekend. He had a blood transfusion and had a good time with his friends at the rugby club. He arrived back home on Sunday evening and died later that same week.

A person does things

Jill was a woman who liked to be busy. She had always worked full time as a catering manager while bringing up her young family. Her motor neurone disease fairly rapidly and severely limited her mobility. In the hospice day centre she started to paint. In spite of her new disability she discovered a creative talent that she did not know she had. She said to me one day 'I wonder what would have happened if I had started sooner'. Her paintings were displayed. Later when her hands were weak, she created computer graphic images. She was delighted that she could leave this unexpected legacy to her family.

A person has a body

Niki was 18 and she was dying of cancer of the colon. As a child she had been overweight. The weight loss resulting from her cancer, she felt, suited her and indeed she did look good. Her parents helped her to buy new clothes, which she greatly enjoyed wearing. She talked about her illness and impending death in an easy way. Towards the end of her life her legs became very swollen and she was jaundiced. This upset her greatly. I visited daily and massaged her legs, which she felt helped. She would be sleepy after the session. I taught her mother to do this and, after my morning session, she would repeat the massage three or four times a day. She said that, as she massaged Niki, they talked about things that they never thought they would and this was very special. Niki died 2 weeks after the onset of jaundice and oedema.

A person has a secret life

An elderly woman with a large family was within days of dying. While helping with her hygiene needs, she talked to me about her illegitimate son whom she had had some 70 years before. He had been taken away for adoption and she had no idea where or with whom he had lived. No one now alive in her family knew. She talked of the pain of losing him and of how, when she had been busy with the four children whom she had subsequently had in wedlock, sometimes months went by and she thought little about him. Now she was dying, she thought of him every day and longed to know what had become of him, but knew it was impossible. I sat with her for a while. I massaged her hands. She thanked me for listening to her secret.

A person has a perceived future

Mr Jones was 58 and dying of cancer. Earlier in his illness he had talked of his great disappointment at not having a period of retirement. He and his wife had worked hard to save for their retirement and they had made many plans. He talked sadly and sometimes bitterly about his loss. Within weeks of his dying he began to make plans again for the future that he had once acknowledged he would never have. He would spend happy hours with his wife planning elaborate holidays. This fluctuation between denial and acceptance was first noted by Kübler-Ross (1969) and has been more recently highlighted again by Copp and Field (2002). In this case, making plans for a future, which at some time in the same day or week he would acknowledge that he had not got, served to nurture and help him cope at a very difficult time. We were able to explain this to his wife, who once she understood made a choice to enjoy his hopes and dreams with him.

A person has a transcendent dimension

Cassell (1991) says that everyone has a transcendent dimension – a life of the spirit, however expressed or known. Perhaps to the dying person this is about leaving a legacy, a legacy of spirit in terms of what they have meant to people.

Niki, the 18-year-old young woman dying of colon cancer mentioned earlier, wanted to feel that her death could help her family. She had a large extended family. Colon cancer is unusual in a person so young. As a result of her talking with her GP and gastroenterologist, Niki died knowing that her whole family would have regular screening for colon cancer. A short article about her case was written for a medical journal and she knew that this was in progress when she died.

Personhood is not about reductionism

Cassell (1991) is very keen to highlight that people cannot be reduced to their parts so that they can be better understood. However, the nature of spiritual pain in its widest sense may be better understood by this theoretical approach to personhood. From the examples of spiritual care highlighted here it will be seen that often the care is about 'being with' the person and listening to their expressions of spiritual pain; providing a presence that is enabling in terms of empowering and enabling others to change, grow, accept and die peacefully is what health-care professionals, particularly nurses, do every day (Goldberg 1998).

In their study Dunniece and Slevin (2000) suggest that 'being there' for patients is about listening, explaining, giving information, answering questions and being present without speaking. Added to that, being present and giving a gentle soothing massage can do much to ease the suffering of spiritual pain.

In a study looking at 20 patients with end-stage heart failure and 20 patients with inoperable lung cancer (patients were interviewed in-depth every 3 months for a year), Murray et al. (2004) found that spiritual issues were significant for many of the patients. They noted that health professionals may lack the skills to uncover and address these issues. Creating the opportunity to listen to patients' spiritual distress requires highly developed communication skills. Indeed, although I have high-lighted how we can provide spiritual support as part of our daily work, there will be times when more expertise is needed. This is recognised in the spiritual and religious competencies of specialist palliative care (Box 6.1). Access to professionals with a mental health qualification and ministers of religion may be necessary to provide more complex spiritual care. Dealing with difficult existential questions is addressed to some extent in Chapter 3 and should also be within the remit of someone who has attended the national advanced communication skills course.

RELIGIOUS PRACTICES CONCERNED WITH DEATH

As previously stated, for many people their religion can be an important part of their spirituality. Enquiries should always be made of patients to see if this is so. Reference material in the ward library outlining different customs and practice is a good resource. Knowledge of how to contact ministers from all different religious organisations should also be available. It is vital that health professionals never assume that they know what is the best way to help meet a person's religious spiritual needs, but that they always assess with the patients what is required.

Buddhism

Buddhism is rapidly growing in the west and there are many different schools of Buddhism. The Buddhist does not have a god. A Buddhist is expected to make his or her own way to a form of nirvana, which is perfection, perfect peace and freedom from suffering. There is a belief in rebirth in Buddhism, but not necessarily in human form. The body is seen as a temporary vessel.

Traditionally, a dying Buddhist needs space, peace and quiet for meditation. A dying Buddhist may want a monk or teacher to talk and chant scriptures with. Traditionally and ideally dying fully conscious and in a calm state is important. A fellow Buddhist may chant with the patient in the absence of a monk or teacher. Different schools of Buddhism may have different traditions regarding the care of the body after death. It is useful to contact a monk or teacher from an appropriate school for advice. Buddhists are cremated or buried according to local tradition.

Christianity

The Christian religion is based on the belief that Jesus was born 2000 years ago in Bethlehem. Jesus is the human embodiment of a loving, just and personal

Box 6.1   Spiritual and religious care competencies for specialist palliative care

Level 1
All staff and volunteers who have casual contact with patients and their families/carers
This level seeks to ensure that staff and volunteers understand that all people have spiritual needs and distinguishes between spiritual and religious needs. It seeks to encourage basic skills of awareness, relationships and communication, and an ability to refer concerns to members of the multidisciplinary team.

Level 2
All staff and volunteers whose duties require contact with patients and their families/carers
This level seeks to enhance the competencies developed at level 1 with an increased awareness of spiritual and religious needs, and how they may be identified and responded to. In addition to increased communication skills, identification and referral of difficult needs should be achievable, along with an ability to identify personal training needs.

Level 3
Staff and volunteers who are members of the multidisciplinary team
This level seeks to further enhance the skills of levels 1 and 2. It moves into the area of assessment of spiritual and religious need, developing a plan for care and recognising complex spiritual, religious and ethical issues. This level also introduces confidentiality and the recording of sensitive and personal patient information.

Level 4
Staff or volunteers whose primary responsibility is for the spiritual and religious care of patients, visitors and staff
Staff working at level 4 are expected to be able to manage and facilitate complex spiritual and religious needs in patients, families/carers, staff and volunteers. In particular, they will deal with the existential and practical needs arising from the impact on individuals and families of illness, life, dying and death. In addition, they should have a clear understanding of their own personal beliefs and be able to journey with others, focused on people's needs and agendas. They should liaise with external resources as required. They should also act as a resource for the support, training and education of health-care professionals and volunteers and seek to be involved in professional and national initiatives.

Reproduced with the permission of Marie Curie Cancer Care (2003).

god. There are different denominations of Christianity and they all believe in an afterlife.

Some Christians will want Holy Communion while they are in care institutions. The taking of bread and wine is associated with the body and blood of Jesus and accompanied by prayers for the forgiveness of sins. As death becomes imminent some Christians will want to be anointed with oil. This is traditionally called the last rites. The anointing is associated with repentance and forgiveness of sins in preparation for the afterlife, usually referred to as heaven. There are no special requirements in terms of handling the dead body. Either burial or cremation is acceptable.

Hinduism

Hindus have different schools and their beliefs and customs can be very different. Hinduism is an ancient religion and there are three supreme gods: Brahma the creator, Vishnu the preserver, and Shiva the destroyer and regenerator of life. As such they are in a sense all one and the same (Neuberger 1999). Hindus believe in reincarnation, which is a return to earth in a better or worse form. Traditionally death itself is not feared but the process of dying may be.

Hymns and readings from the Hindu holy books may be a source of comfort while dying. A Hindu priest may be called to perform holy rites. Traditionally a dying Hindu will want to be given Ganges water and the sacred Tulsi leaf by mouth from a relative. Ideally a Hindu should die with the name of god being recited.

Usually the family will want to attend to the body themselves. If this is not possible health professionals should wear gloves and not remove any jewellery or religious objects. Traditionally, Hindus are cremated with the exception of children under 3 who are buried.

Islam

Followers of the Islamic religion are called Muslims. Islam was revealed by god (Allah) to the prophet Muhammad in Mecca (now in Saudi Arabia). Muhammad was born in AD 570. Muhammad was an ordinary man. His teaching was that all men and women were called to Allah's service and they should try to live a perfect life following the Quran (Neuberger 1999).

Devout Muslims believe that death is part of Allah's plan and to struggle against it is wrong. The acceptance of terminal illness as Allah's will mean that Muslim patients will often want less in the way of pain relief and more in the way of opportunity for prayer (Neuberger 1999).

A dying Muslim may want to face south-east – towards Mecca. Other Muslim friends and family may want to join the dying person and recite verses from the Quran. A declaration of faith is said when death is imminent and the dying person responds by affirming that there is no 'God but God' and Muhammad is his messenger.

After death the body must be kept covered. Traditionally same-sex Muslims will perform a ritual washing of the body. For non-Muslim health professionals they must obtain permission to touch the body and, if granted permission, wear disposable gloves. Postmortem examinations are not accepted easily. Muslims are buried, not cremated, and this is carried out as soon as possible.

Judaism

Judaism developed from the religion of the ancient Israelites as recorded in the Tanach or Five Books of Moses (Old Testament). Orthodox Jews believe that the whole of the law was given as a single entity by God to Moses on Mount Sinai, involving also the legal codes of the Mishnah and Talmud as 'oral law' (Neuberger 1999). Judaism is practised in different ways by different groups and in different areas of the world. Traditionally orthodox Jews believe in an afterlife, a world to come. The life-affirming strand in Judaism is strong. Life is a gift to be valued and preserved for as long as possible.

As death nears, traditionally a Jewish person should not be left alone. A rabbi may be called to pray and recite psalms with the dying person. The dying person should recite the Shema (the Declaration of Faith) as they are dying or before death. After death occurs it is customary to stay by the body for 8 minutes while a feather is left over the mouth and nose to ascertain that breathing has stopped. Traditionally, the body is then placed on the floor covered in a sheet, with the feet facing the door, and a candle beside it. Washing and preparing the body for the funeral are considered to be a great honour and often carried out by men or women from the Jewish congregation. The body is not left alone until burial.

Non-Jewish health workers should seek permission to handle the body and do so as little as possible, just covering with a white sheet. Traditionally, the Jewish Burial Society may collect the body and perform a ritual wash before burial. Post-mortem examinations are disliked, and burial is within 24–48 hours if possible.

Sikhism

The Sikh religion was founded in the sixteenth century by Guru Nanak. Its male adherents are recognised by wearing a turban and also the four other signs of Sikhism:

1. The *Kesh*, uncut hair, usually worn in a bun by both men and women. The bun is covered by the turban in men and also in a few elderly pious Sikh women.
2. The *Kangha* is a comb worn in the hair and should always stay with the person even if they cannot wear it in their hair.
3. The *Kara* is a steel bangle that a Sikh wears on a wrist.
4. The *Kirpan* is a symbolic dagger.

The Sikhs were warrior people and so a *Kirpan* was, traditionally, the sword that a Sikh had ready for military action. Now either it is worn as a symbolic brooch or it is a blunt instrument a few inches long. Also there is the *Kacha*, which are special under-garments. Sikhs never completely remove their *Kacha*. They will shower or bath with one leg in the old pair before putting on the new pair. It is imperative, when caring for Sikhs, to show respect for their religious symbols (the *Kesh*, *Kangha*, *Kara*, *Kirpan* and *Kacha*). Traditionally, they will want to keep the symbols on their person at all times and it is important that health professionals are creative in helping this to happen.

It is possible that many members of the Sikh community will want to be together at the bedside of the dying person and read the *Gurugranth Sahib* with them.

Some Sikhs may want *Amrit*, holy water, in their mouth as death nears. A Sikh person traditionally should die with the name of God, *Waheguru* (wonderful Lord), being recited.

After death health professionals should not trim hair or beard. The 5Ks (*Kesh, Kangha, Kara, Kirpan* and *Kacha*) must be left on the body. The body should be covered with a plain white cloth. The family may wish to bathe the body themselves. Sikhs are traditionally cremated as soon as possible.

Spiritual support services

Spiritual care has in the main been poorly understood and as a result perhaps underdeveloped. However, we do more in our everyday caring approach of importance to an individual's spirituality than we realise. This mirrors the research on hope (Herth 1990a; Buckley and Herth 2004). Intuitive caring practices can nurture both the hope and the spirituality for the dying person.

The NICE supportive and palliative care guidelines state, in key recommendation 11, that patients and carers should have access to staff who are sensitive to their spiritual needs. Multidisciplinary teams should have access to suitably qualified authorised and appointed spiritual caregivers who can act as a resource for patients and carers and staff. Staff should also be aware of local community resources for spiritual care. Finally, the NICE (2004b) guidelines suggest that Commissioners and workforce development confederations should be mindful of the spiritual and religious care competences for specialist palliative care developed by Marie Curie Cancer Care.

CONCLUSION

On the face of it, hope and spirituality can appear as complex existential concepts. Certainly the psychological impact of hopelessness and spiritual troubles can be hugely painful. However, an intuitive, caring and honest approach and an ability to listen actively can in fact be very helpful in restoring some hope to those living with spiritual pain. We often cannot do anything but listen and be kind; it does not fix the existential pain but it is important not to minimise the nurture of this supportive approach. It is important to remain aware of the value of the positive impact that attention to seemingly small details and a few kind words can have.

MAIN IMPLICATIONS FOR PRACTICE

- Feelings of hopefulness are nurturing. People may hope for the unattainable. Although health-care professionals should not encourage this, it is perhaps unwise to address this as false hope.
- Patients can feel hopeful in the face of no cure. They feel hopeful while maintaining independence and sharing good times with family and friends.
- Research demonstrates that individuals find hope in everyday events. It is attention to detail concerning all aspects of care, be they physical or psychological, that can help people feel hopeful. It is the small things that really count.
- By helping with pain and symptom control, communicating effectively and kindly, and helping patients and friends and relatives in their communication, you will help to promote a feeling of hopefulness.

- Spirituality is hard to define; however, a person's spirituality and/or religious beliefs come into sharp focus when someone is dying.
- Intuitive caring practices can help people in spiritual pain. See the text for examples of this using Cassell's concept of personhood.
- Different religious practices can be important to people as they die. It is important that health professionals are mindful of this and respect the wishes and practices of the patient and family.
- People suffering overwhelming spiritual pain will need referral for more help from mental health services and/or ministers of religion.

SUGGESTED FURTHER READING

Frankl V (1946) *Man's Search for Meaning*. London: Hodder & Stoughton.
Farran CJ, Herth KA, Popovich JM (1995) *Hope and Hopelessness: Critical clinical constructs*. London: Sage Publications.
Narayanasamy A (2006) *Spiritual Care and Transcultural Research*. London: Quay Books.
Neuberger J (1999) *Dying Well*. Hale, Cheshire: Hochland & Hochland Ltd.

Websites

www.actualizations.com/quotes/hope
www.alberta.ca/hope
www.flyingcolors.org
www.passthison.co
www.rainbowconnextion.com

Chapter 7
Finding resilience together

KEY POINTS

- **Resilience in health care**: the concept of resilience has attracted increasing interest over the past few decades. Health researchers are now turning their attention to what a resilient approach can offer health policy and research.
- **Helping patients to find their inner resources**: the challenge for health professionals is to learn from, and support, individuals as they use their inner resources to develop strategies for coping – in other words, nurturing resilience.
- **Patient groups**: in groups patients share coping experiences as well as anxiety; group work is enjoying a revival. Since the late 1970s the benefits of improving coping skills and quality of life and more in patient groups have been demonstrated in research.
- **Psychoneuroimmunology**: the mind can influence physiological response. The study of psychoneuroimmunology (PNI) demonstrates that, when people are supported in mobilising their own coping strategies, it has a positive effect on the body's physiology and psychology. Research studies demonstrating this are reviewed.
- **The elements of successful groups**: these are highlighted from a meta-analysis by Calde et al. (2002). They are: education, homogeneity, clearly defined interventions, supportive environment and those that teach coping skills and stress management.
- **The expert patient – tapping a valuable source of experience**: this is derived from the chronic disease self-management programme and builds on the concept that knowledge and experience held by patients have for too long been an untapped source.

  Not everyone wants to belong to a group; however, given the research reviewed in this chapter, both generalists and specialists in palliative care should look to developing patient groups as a choice for dying people.
- **Patient groups need clear objectives and facilitators need expertise and access to supervision**: support groups that emphasise a positive approach need to be cautious. Optimism, with no structure, reality or depth, can be counterproductive and result in terminally ill individuals feeling guilty and blaming themselves for disease progression.
- **Patients in well-run groups can resolutely face their death and die with dignity**. Witnessing the death of others in the group may bring them closer to the people who care for them as they gain new insights into the experience of grief (Spiegel et al. 2000).

RESILIENCE IN HEALTH CARE

Resilience is defined in the *Chambers Twentieth Century Dictionary* (Kirkpatrick 1983) in the following way: recoil: elasticity, physical or mental. And being resilient as: elastic physically or mentally. The concept of resilience has attracted increasing interest in the past few decades. Early work has focused on the resilience of children and their abilities to withstand extremely adverse, social deprivation and family disadvantage and avoid delinquency. Later work was concerned with avoidance of depression and anxiety after war and natural and manmade disasters (Bluglass 2003). Health researchers are now turning their attention to what a resilience approach can offer to health policy and research. In health care the term 'resilience' is applied to both the status of adapting or reacting positively to adversity, and the social processes and practices that seem to foster these positive reactions (Research Unit in Health and Behaviour Change or RUHBC 2006a).

Traditional approaches to illness have been to focus on the disease process rather than the individual's ability to adapt, or perhaps even to thrive, in the face of adversity. Health-care professionals have traditionally been seen as the experts in disease and disease management. Historically the patient has assumed the role of a passive receiver of care.

Illich (1975) defines health as a process of adaptation and raises the concept of a 'healthy death'. He states that health:

> ... designates the ability to adapt to changing environments, to growing up and ageing, to healing when damaged, to suffering and to the peaceful expectation of death. It also embraces the future and therefore includes anguish and the inner resources to live with **it**.
>
> Illich (1975, p 167.1)

Inherent in this definition is empowerment of individuals to control their own destiny. This idea is indeed echoed in current health promotion strategies in the UK. Viewing health as a process of adaptation rather than simply an absence of disease, or a reaction to a disease, creates a positive, active approach for the delivery of palliative care. The challenge for health professionals is to learn from, and support, individuals as they use their inner resources to develop strategies for coping and adapting – in other words nurturing their resilience.

Using inner resources is something that is at the heart of holistic care. We often use the word 'holistic' to denote that we are thinking not only of the physical but also of the social, psychological and spiritual. A definition of holism that fails to address the concept of inner resources can sound disabling. It is imperative that the health professional's approach is an enabling one. In this way reactive sources of resilience (something that someone does as a direct response to a difficult circumstance) will be encouraged and may flourish.

The second half of the twentieth century has been a period in which more people have lived into their 70s, 80s and 90s. This greater longevity has brought with it an increase in terms of managing long-term illness, e.g. cancer, strokes, arthritis, mental illness and other conditions. The predominant pattern in most developed countries now is managing long-term illness in an ageing population (Department of Health or DH 2001). The demographics also highlight that there will be a dwindling pool of young people going into the health professions, so we are going to need to look at new ways of working. Home visiting by clinical nurse specialists, for example, is both time and financially uneconomic compared with nurse-led clinics and working with patients in groups.

PATIENT GROUPS

Group work is enjoying a revival in contemporary society. This is in part because the public have organised groups for themselves, in the form of a wide variety of help and support groups, e.g. the Self Management Training for Manic Depression (SMIP) is user developed and user led. The programme design encourages confidence in individuals' abilities to take control of their own lives. It was developed from a course that originated in Ohio, and early research suggests good outcomes, including improvements in mood sustained 3–6 months after completion of the course.

Professionally organised groups now also seem to be flourishing and this may be as a result of public demand or conscious/unconscious reactions to time and money constraints. Since the late 1970s, research has consistently shown the benefits of groups in improving cancer patients' quality of life, e.g. improving mood, coping skills, relieving psychophysical distress and improving physical function (Chochinov and Breitbart 2000). A group situation multiplies the potential opportunities for learning new ways of coping by the number that is in the group. Thus, together patients nurture resilience in each other in a most natural way. Importantly, health professionals involved in running such groups are exposed to rich learning experiences that they can take to new patient relationships.

PSYCHONEUROIMMUNOLOGY

In the 1970s, Dr Candace Pert isolated endorphin, an opiate naturally occurring in the brain. Since the discovery of this neuropeptide, over 200 other similar chemicals have been recognised. These substances are secreted not only in the nervous system but also in all other parts of the body (Daniel 2001a). The effects of stress on the body are well recognised and accepted, e.g. raised pulse and blood pressure, excessive cortisol. There is a growing body of research that demonstrates the opposite. When people are supported in mobilising their own coping mechanism it has a positive effect on the body's physiology and psychology (Spiegel et al. 1989; Walker et al. 1997).

Research studies in PNI

Fawzy and Fawzy (1994)

Fawzy and Fawzy (1994) looked at the effect of a structured group intervention over 6 weeks for 38 patients with newly diagnosed melanoma. The group work focused on health education, coping skills and managing stress. The group had six weekly sessions of 1.5 hours. When compared with a control group of 28 individuals, the experimental participants had significantly lower levels of depression, fatigue, mood disturbances and confusion. They also had higher levels of vigour, as measured by the profile of mood states. This group was also described as being more likely to use active behavioural coping techniques. On immunological testing, the experimental group had an increase in the percentage of large granular lymphocytes. This trend persisted for 6 months after the intervention. At 6 years the death rate was significantly greater in the control group than in the experimental group. The hypothesis of the study was that those who received the health-promoting intervention would cope better than those who did not. The increased survival time was a surprise result.

Spiegel et al. (1989)

Spiegel et al. (1989) completed a prospective randomised study with 86 women with metastatic breast cancer. Women were randomly assigned to an experimental or a control group. The experimental group took part in weekly support sessions for a year. In the group fears of dying were discussed and also ways of living the remainder of their lives as richly as possible. Discussions of family relationships and improving doctor–patient communication also featured. The group was taught hypnosis to control pain and other distressing symptoms. At the end of the year it was found that the 'treatment' group had significantly less mood disturbance, fewer phobic responses and half the pain of the control group. A follow-up study revealed that the survival time of the psychosocial treatment group was 36.6 months and that of the control group 18.9 months. This has been described by Spiegel's team as being clinically and statistically significant and, as in Fawzy and Fawzy's (1994) study, was an unexpected result.

Walker et al. (1997)

Walker et al. (1997) studied 80 women with locally advanced breast cancer. The study assigned women randomly to parallel groups. The aim was to evaluate the psychoimmunological effects of relaxation therapy and guided imagery. Women in the experimental group were asked to practise relaxation and visualisation at least daily during chemotherapy and to keep detailed records of practice. The control group had a similar amount of staff contact in the unit and received a high level of support. Blood was taken from all women at trial entry and before the first, second, fourth and sixth cycles of chemotherapy, after surgery (lumpectomy or mastectomy) and 4 and 12 weeks after radiotherapy. Psychometric tests demonstrated that patients in the experimental group were significantly more relaxed and easy going, less emotionally suppressed and reported a better quality of life than those in the control group. The authors concluded that, even in patients who were receiving immunosuppressive treatments, such as chemotherapy, surgery and radiotherapy, it was found that relaxation and imagery produced immunological changes that might have clinical relevance.

Berglund et al. (1994)

Berglund et al. (1994) carried out a randomised controlled study involving 199 patients with cancer. The intervention group of 98 took part in a programme called 'Starting Again'. The programme consisted of 11 structured 2-hour sessions run for a period of 7 weeks by an oncology nurse specialist, assisted by experts in various fields. The contents focused on physical training and information and coping skills training. Outcome measures included a modified HAD (Hospital Anxiety and Depression) scale (Zigmond and Snaith 1983), a physical strength and activity scale of 21 items, and the Mental Adjustment to Cancer scale (Watson et al. 1988). Patients in the 'Starting Again' programme improved significantly over controls in respect of physical training, physical strength and appraisal after having received sufficient information and coping skills training.

McCain et al. (1996)

McCain et al. (1996) compared the effectiveness of a 6-week stress management training programme with standard outpatient care for 45 HIV-positive men. Outcome measures included measuring stress levels, quality of life, psychological distress and CD4 and T-lymphocyte levels. After 6 months participants in the intervention group had an increased well-being dimension in quality of life. After 6 months the intervention group had a relative decline in HIV-related intrusive thinking. The implications are that stress management may have buffered illness-related distress over time.

Cruess et al. (2000)

Cruess et al. (2000) ran a 10-week course of group cognitive–behavioural therapy for 30 HIV-symptomatic gay men. Salivary cortisol measurements were taken and mood assessment was carried out, just before and 45 minutes after each session. Participants also recorded their stress levels and compliance with daily relaxation practice. Pre-session cortisol levels decreased across the 10-week period and were related to decreases in global measures of total mood disturbance and anxious mood.

Meta-analysis of cancer support groups

Zabalegui et al. (2005)

Zabalegui et al. (2005) did a meta-analysis of randomised controlled studies evaluating support groups for cancer patients. Original studies from 14 databases published over the last 20 years from peer-reviewed journals were selected. Twenty studies with a randomised clinical trial design were included in the final analysis. Methodological quality of studies was checked using the Jadad Scale and the Checklist of Consort Statement Demographic Data was analysed using the SPSS program. The heterogeneity calculation and effect size were analysed using the Rev-Man 4-1 Metaview Program.

The findings demonstrated clearly that participation in a support group is indeed associated with significant improvement in a patient's emotional state (depression and anxiety), illness adaptation, quality of life and marital relations. Zabalegui et al. (2005) concluded that nurses should promote participation in support groups as a crucial part of patient care.

A critical evaluation of successful groups in clinical trials

Calde et al. (2002)

Calde et al. (2002) looked at 11 studies that either have found incidentally that psychosocial interventions could prolong life or had set out to investigate that question. They concluded that although the studies, one of them Spiegel's own, that demonstrated increased survival were compelling, the literature is divided; they concluded that it would not be definitively concluded that survival can be prolonged by psychosocial interventions. However, they also state that the studies have made examination of the relationships between quality and quantity of life in relationship to psychosocial intervention a respectable scientific question.

In their analysis Calde et al. (2002) identified the elements shared by groups in studies with the most positive outcomes. This is valuable data for professionals or patients initiating a new group. The components are as shown in Box 7.1.

Groups other than cancer and HIV

There is far less literature looking at the efficacy of group interventions in patients other than those with cancer and HIV infection, although it is starting to emerge.

Coronary heart disease support group

A large study was conducted looking at coronary heart disease support groups in Scotland (RUHBC 2006b). In the main members spoke positively of the groups and would strongly recommend others to join. Health benefits included the promotion of confidence to move on and live a full life. Facilitated exercise also provided confidence and there was a camaraderie that facilitated the monitoring of the health of other members. Members were particularly positive about meeting others with heart disease and this reduced their feelings of isolation. Attendance at meetings was associated with fun and had a mood-boosting effect. Members valued health practitioner involvement as a source of medical reassurance, monitoring of health studies or fast tracking into the formal health-care system. However, dwindling membership was a considerable dilemma for some groups.

THE EXPERT PATIENT

A commitment to the Expert Patient Programme was first proposed in the government's White Paper *Saving Lives: Our healthier nation* in 1999 (DH 1999a). A further commitment was made in *The NHS Cancer Plan* (DH 2000b).

Box 7.1   Elements shared by groups in studies with the most positive outcomes. Calde et al. (2002)

1. Education
Education was often very structured and included information about cancer and behaviours thought to improve compliance. Also information about hospital, diagnostic procedures and treatment issues was included, as well as aspects of nutrition, exercise, risk factors and warning signs. Some studies gave leaflets to back the written word.

2. Homogeneity
Some groups were homogeneous for disease types and some for disease stage. In disease-staged homogeneous groups, members talked about the family withdrawing from them, and so building relationships with someone in similar circumstances was viewed as highly beneficial and, ultimately, beneficial for family and friends. Not only did the homogeneity of groups alleviate feelings of being the only one, it also maximised the potential for participants to problem solve with each other, pass on coping skills and provide empathic support.

3. Clearly defined interventions
All studies that were successful had very clearly defined goals and structured content. Some used a highly structured cognitive–behavioural model. A well-defined agenda about information and support is crucial. Both Fawzy and Fawzy (1994) and Spiegel et al. (1981) have created manuals that can be used to replicate their studies.

4. Supportive environment
In successful studies participants received support from group members, their leaders or both. There is an explicit component in the model (Spiegel 1991) used where patients give support to each other and the leader is an additional source of support.

5. Coping skills and stress management
Coping skills have been defined as reducing harmful environmental conditions, enhancing prospects of recovery, helping patients tolerate and adjust to negative events and realities, and helping them maintain satisfying relationships with others (Leszcz and Goodwin 1998). Learning about their disease and how it was treated helped patients to cope with their fears and anxieties and increased feelings of control. Patients learnt coping skills from each other. Stress management input and self-hypnosis for pain and other symptoms were deemed helpful.

The Expert Patient Programme is built on the concept that the knowledge and experience held by patients has for too long been an untapped source. Health professionals have long observed that many patients with long-term disease understood their disease better than them. Not only can they teach the professional about their disease as part of a patient group, they can also teach each other, thus increasing individual resilience. Research in North America and the UK shows that today's patients with long-term disease need not merely be recipients of care; they can be actively involved in decision-making and have greater control of their lives (DH 2001).

The Expert Patient Programme is derived from the Chronic Disease Self Management Programme (CDSMP), which was developed at Stanford University after some 20 years of work with people with arthritis. People with 'chronic' illness became professionally trained instructors and led highly structured courses over six consecutive weeks of 2.5-hour sessions (DH 2001). The aim of the programme is to enable patients to develop their communication skills, manage their emotions, manage daily activities, interact with health-care systems, find health resources, plan for the future, understand exercising, healthy eating, and managing fatigue, sleep, pain, anger and depression.

Expert patient programmes in the UK are available in eight different languages, including Greek, Bengali, Hindi, Punjabi and Turkish. Work has gone into engaging with minority ethnic groups in deprived areas and bilingual trainers have been recruited and trained to deliver the course.

Children also suffer chronic illness, e.g. cerebral palsy, cystic fibrosis, ME (myalgic encephalopathy) or chronic fatigue syndrome, congenital heart disease, sickle cell anaemia. After an approach by the Children's National Standards Framework a programme has been piloted comprising three 1-day workshops targeting young people who will be making the transition from being looked after by their families to a very independent life. This course is run by teenagers. A programme for the parents of these children has also been developed.

A programme for carers, called 'Looking after me', is also running. In Bristol a course for people with learning disabilities has been piloted. For people who cannot attend a course a 6-week online programme requiring only minimum computer skills is in preparation (www.dh.gov.uk 2007/TheExpertPatientProgramme).

The important thing about the Expert Patient Programme is that it, like the End-of-Life Programme, is being nationally coordinated and evaluated. Early evaluations are encouraging. Self-reported data from 1000 participants in the Expert Patient Programme are as follows:

- 45% felt more confident that they would not let common symptoms, e.g. pain, tiredness, depression and breathlessness, interfere with their lives
- 38% felt that such symptoms were less severe 4–6 months after finishing the course
- 33% felt better prepared for consultations with health professionals.

Course graduates also reported a reduction in use of services. These are:

- 7% reduction in GP consultation
- 10% reduction in outpatient visits
- 16% reduction in accident and emergency attendance
- 9% reduction in physiotherapy use.

Added to this, 94% of those who took part in the evaluation felt supported and satisfied with the course. The results are consistent with other bodies of evidence on self-management programmes.

The impact of the internet on patient education: support increasing resilience

Many of the large charities provide excellent information for patients explaining their illness and suggesting ways of coping. Often the advice is based on experiences of patients living with the same illness. Some also have provision on the internet for patients to chat to each other online – an opportunity to share experiences of coping with each other. For many and particularly housebound patients, this camaraderie can be very important to morale as well as informative. Often patients will say that they can cope with a chronic illness most of the time; however, when they go to bed and the lights go out they become alert and often frightened of their thoughts. I remember one patient, Sally, telling me how cathartic it was in these instances to visit her chat room and write her thoughts down. She also found some solace in the fact that others online understood and, indeed, had very similar fears to her own.

CONCLUSION

Not everyone wants to belong to a group. However, the research and experiences reported here suggest that belonging to a group is something that, in an ideal world and given the potential value, should be offered to all people with life-limiting disease. To ignore or dismiss the work described here could be argued as being a breach of the ethic of beneficence, i.e. acting for the greater good of the person. We can be held accountable for our omissions as well as our actions (National Council for Hospice and Specialist Palliative Care Services or NCHSPCS 1993).

Much of the research evidence quoted comes from groups where leaders have had a mental health qualification, e.g. psychiatrists, psychotherapists and counsellors. Given the lack of easily accessible mental health professionals in the current specialist palliative care arena (Lloyd-Williams et al. 1999a), this may pose a problem.

Ironically within generalist palliative care, access to the NHS system may be easier. Alas, care home residents may find this access problematic. It is important that groups are well run and clearly defined as previously stated. Groups that cannot be led by mental health professionals should consider seeking supervision from one.

A limitation of some support groups can be their efforts and attempts to maintain a positive atmosphere, no matter what. An insistence on maintaining optimism can manifest in treating a person who expresses distress at progression as a *bad example*. This has a doubly unfortunate message. It can make the person who is becoming more ill feel excluded, and signals to the others in the group that expressing distress is not acceptable behaviour (Spiegel et al. 2000).

Support groups that emphasise a 'positive outlook' need to be cautious. Having a positive outlook and believing in medical treatment prescribed are helpful, but not a cure. Optimism with no structure, reality or depth can be counterproductive, and can result in terminally ill individuals feeling guilty and blaming themselves for their disease progression (Spiegel et al. 2000).

The very aspect that may seem most frightening about patient groups in palliative care is witnessing members of the group die. Patients in well-run groups learn that they can resolutely face their deaths and die with dignity. This experience may bring them closer to their loved ones as they perhaps gain new insight into the experience of grief (Spiegel et al. 2000). Such groups can lead to much support at a time when our social denial of death can lead to increased isolation of patients. Patient groups can increase the quality of dying as well as of living (Spiegel et al. 2000). Supporting people to find, nurture and share their resilience should be a central part of the palliative approach.

MAIN IMPLICATIONS FOR PRACTICE

- Patients should be made aware of local groups that exist to help support or educate them about their illness. They should know how to access information about these groups.
- Health-care organisations should consider forming patient groups as an adjunct to the service that they offer.
- Patients can be made aware of reliable resources available on the internet.
- Emphasise a positive approach in a group with caution and skill to avoid marginalising patients as they become more ill.
- Groups should be run by suitably qualified people and should have very clear aims and objectives that are shared with group members.
- Group leaders should enter into supervision so that the group remains true to its aims and objectives.

SUGGESTED FURTHER READING

Lewis CE, O'Brien RMO, Barraclough J (2002) *The Psychoimmunology of Cancer*. Oxford: Oxford University Press.

Spiegel D, Classen C (2000) *Group Therapy for Cancer Patients: A research-based handbook of psychosocial care*. New York: Basic Books.

Walker L, Walker M, Sharp D (2006) Current provision of psychosocial care within palliative care. In: Lloyd-Williams M (ed.), *Psychosocial Issues in Palliative Care*. Oxford: Oxford University Press, 49–65.

Websites

www.alzheimers.org.uk
www.bhf.org.uk
www.cancerbackup.org.uk
www.copdinternational.com
www.macmillan.org.uk
www.stroke.org.uk
www.worldheart.org

Chapter 8
Living with dying

KEY POINTS

- **Introduction**: facing death can impinge on all aspects of personhood and cause potential chaos and disruption for relatives and friends.
- **Social death**: family and friends often need the help of health professionals to deal with the dying of someone for whom they care. In extreme circumstances the social death of a patient can lead to their isolation and leave painful memories for relatives and friends.
- **Vulnerable groups**: there are many vulnerable groups in our society who may, for a variety of reasons, get less support from generalist and specialist palliative teams. Health professionals should be vigilant in enlisting help from statutory and voluntary organisations to minimise the risk of marginalisation.
- **Informational needs**: these need constant attention. The information belongs to the patient and carers. Any new information should be offered to the patient and carers. They should not feel that they have to seek it out. Evaluation of the understanding of information imparted is part of the information-giving process.

  Carers should feel valued: family and friends may become carers. Carers can be ambivalent about their own needs. Health professionals should be mindful of this and ensure that they are proactive in supporting the carers, in taking care of themselves and valuing their role.
- **Being heard and feeling supported**: it is vital that carers feel that they can be heard. By being heard appropriate levels of support can be offered. Carers' statutory support: carers have a right to a carer's assessment by Social Services. Carers' groups can provide invaluable support.
- **Companionship**: health professionals should take the initiative to restore companionship if collusion has interrupted this.
- **Intimacy and caring**: not all friends and relatives have the capacity to provide care. Issues of intimacy need to be sensitively dealt with.
- **Health needs**: the general health of carers is important. Professionals should take an interest in the health of carers; helping them to organise time out is a priority. Finances should be proactively addressed by professionals.
- **Difficult thoughts and letting go**: it may be comforting and useful for friends, relatives and those who are carers to express difficult thoughts.

Sometimes the people close to those who are dying may also need direction, in *letting go* of the person for whom they care. Health professionals often work intuitively in these circumstances. They need to learn to trust their intuitions, because they will usually be right. Sometimes they may get it wrong but it should not stop professionals reaching out. We can measure our success by the fact that we tried.

INTRODUCTION

Telling someone that their illness cannot be cured and that they will now need palliative care has the capacity to impinge on all aspects of personhood. The autonomous person becomes disempowered, and no longer has total control over the near and distant future. The immediate effects can by physical, emotional, intellectual, social and spiritual.

Physical reactions can include nausea, vomiting, tachycardia, fainting, weak legs and dry mouth, to name but a few. Emotionally, there may be numbness, anger, and feelings of hopelessness and frustration. Intellectually, there may be an inability to receive or understand the message given, accompanied by an inability to recall simple and well-known facts, e.g. personal telephone number. Even when surrounded by family and friends, the person may feel isolated and alone and unable to perceive these people as a resource. Spiritually there may be a loss of faith and intense distress about that. There may be a resulting overall feeling of loss of purpose and direction (Wright 1999).

Most people are fortunate enough to have a family and/or friends and the news impacts on them as well. Although a lot has been written about caring for the dying person and bereavement support, less is written about the potential chaos and disruption that the patient's family and friends are thrown into in the interim between the realisation that an illness is progressive and incurable to the actual death. In Chapter 2, aspects of facing progressive disease and death from the perspective of the patient were discussed in some detail, drawing in particular on the excellent work of Kübler-Ross (1969), and recognition of the oscillation between denial and acceptance as a familiar coping mechanism in palliative care. Chapter 3 looked at communication skills, highlighting in particular the importance of providing information at a rate and depth decided by the patient. Chapter 5 discussed partnership care and recognised that information giving is at the heart of partnership care. Information giving should have protected time, and understanding of information imparted should be evaluated as an essential part of the giving. All these chapters are relevant as a backdrop to this one, which confines itself to the important aspects of caring for relatives and friends.

Chronically ill and dying individuals have the potential to suffer many losses. Saunders (2006b) refers to this as total pain. As illness progresses, there is the loss of employment and with this perhaps also loss of role and status. The financial loss can be a severe blow to the whole family and can have many knock-on effects, e.g. increased working hours for other members of the family and increasing debts.

Within the family the role of the sick person changes as they become weaker and others may have to take over their previous functions, e.g. cooking, cleaning, organising events, bread winning, gardening. Sexual relationships may cease and/or cause disharmony as a result of illness. Later adaptations in the home may be a great help for the ill person, but may be viewed as intrusive by others. Health-care workers' visits while necessary may seem an invasion of privacy.

Body image changes, such as gross oedema and weight loss, can further damage self-esteem. Mutilating surgery and the use of a prosthesis add to the pain. Loss of energy and increased fatigue can hamper efforts to 'take more control of life'.

All this, and the rest of the family and circle of friends go about daily life pretty much as usual. The others continue to work, go to school, play, do chores and social activities while the world of the dying person shrinks. As much as the patient may love all those people he or she may feel deeply resentful that his or her usual life is precluded. Similarly, the rest of the family and circle of friends may not feel kindly towards the dying person. It is not necessarily that they do not care for them; it is just that all the changes at all levels can be difficult to accept.

The loss of an expected future, with all its associated hopes and dreams, and the fear of dying can sometimes be so acute that it remains unspoken. By not speaking about these fears, patients, family and friends may feel that they are protecting each other. There can be a tendency in the hospice world to assume that all marriages of sick people are made in heaven and all families are happy ones. We all know that this is not true. This approach can severely limit the depth of relationships and help that can be given to the relatives and friends of dying individuals.

At all times the health professional must assess the situation anew. What individuals know, think and feel about a current situation is crucial if the health professional is to be truly supportive and helpful to the family group. The reader is referred to Chapter 3 for a review of communication skills.

Extending care to family and friends can be a challenge. Towards the end of a patient's life significant others may be performing a pivotal role as an informal caregiver. A study involving 18 caregivers demonstrated that, although they recognised their high levels of stress and anxiety, they were highly ambivalent with regard to their own needs (Harding and Higginson 2001). The researchers advise that any intervention aimed at caregivers should take account of the potential for ambivalence by addressing their lack of identification with their role, enhance their existing coping strategies and ensure that any interventions are accessible and acceptable.

SOCIAL DEATH

There is the potential for the concept and process of total pain to result in 'social death'. Where possible professionals should work with both the dying person and the people close to them, to avoid this happening. Social death has been defined as a time when a person has lost his or her connection with the living world (Johnston 2004). There is evidence to suggest that, as a chronically ill person becomes weaker physically, and necessarily withdraws socially, so he or she is gradually excluded and ignored by staff and carers, who find it difficult to relate to the person socially, personally and also physically (Hockey 1990; Mulkay 1993; Sweeting and Gilhooly 1997). According to Kastenbaum (2000) the distinction between the hail and the frail, i.e. staff attempting to segregate the dying from their own and others' consciousness, has been present in almost every medical setting that she has experienced.

Family-focused risk assessment

Kissane et al. (2003) have developed a psychological assessment strategy for screening families of terminally ill patients. They use the Family Relations Index (Moos and Moos 2002), the Family Assessment Device (Epstein et al 1983), and Social Adjustment Scale (Cooper et al 1982) to assess family functioning. For families with a high level of psychosocial morbidity there is a positive association with family dysfunction. They recommend a family-focused grief therapy intervention, which is started during palliative care for those families shown to be at high risk of poor adaptation. This care is continued into bereavement with the aim of reducing the morbid consequences of grief. This innovative approach is a relatively recent development and may prove a valuable approach in the future.

VUNERABLE GROUPS

Mental health

Some diseases that result in the end of life can be perceived as carrying a stigma. Sadly, this can be a feature of mental health problems. Health professionals have a responsibility to be sensitive to this and provide support and information about the support available. In addition to the mainstream health service support, in many areas excellent and empathic support is also available for carers of people with dementia through self-help groups run by charitable organisations, e.g. Alzheimer's Society (www.alzheimers.org.uk) and Mind (www.mind.org.uk). These organisations also provide information about statutory rights and resources as well as detailed information on all aspects of caring

Learning disabilities

Friends and relatives with learning disabilities are particularly vulnerable to being sidelined when someone whom they love is dying. Research suggests that only 54% of people with learning disabilities attend their parent's funeral (Hollins and Esterhuyzen 1997). The grief and suffering of people with learning disabilities who have been bereaved goes largely unnoticed. This may well lead to further pain and difficulties not only for the individual concerned but also for the family and wider society around them (Blackman 2003). Both generalists and specialists in palliative care should be aware of the need to include and give emotional support to people with learning disabilities. This may best be achieved by liaising with local learning disability teams to share the experience of the person and the expertise in communicating with him or her. Most community learning disability teams should be able to give support from their psychology services. A national organisation that may offer help and advice is Respond – helpline 0808 808 0700).

Care homes

With the advent of the nuclear family and an increasingly elderly population, more people will die in care homes. At the turn of this century, Katz and Pearce (2003) highlighted that real choices about end-of-life care 'are not extended to residents in care homes'. In their excellent book they examine the quality of life for residents of care homes who are disenfranchised by physical and mental deterioration, and they highlight sympathetically the challenges and plight of their carers. Carers in care homes are underpaid and undervalued. The new End-of-Life Programme (see Chapter 1) is concerned that it can reach care homes. Readers are referred to Katz and Pearce (2003) to explore this issue.

Asylum seekers and refugees

These people are particularly vulnerable. Not only are they in a different country, but also they may be surrounded by people who have little or no understanding of their culture and customs. They will have left behind family and friends. They may have experienced atrocities, torture and other distressing events. Supporting a dying person may revive terrifying memories of the past. www.nationalasylumsupporterservices.

HIV and AIDS

AIDS is a disease that can also be associated with stigma and people affected often feel that they must keep this a secret. Many of these people are children. There are over 20 000 closely affected by HIV in this country. This is the story of one of them.

Clare, aged 16

I was told I was HIV+ at the age of 13, just starting secondary school. When you're told, it's like a big ton weight on your shoulders. I thought I was alone, dirty, imprisoned: Would I be accepted by anyone? Am I the only one going through this? The answer is no, there are many of us teenagers going through this in the UK. Fortunately for me there is help; hope of a real future. There is a unique group at BODYandSOUL called Teen Spirit where we don't have to feel locked in our secrecy. It is probably the only time in the week where we can be our true selves. Being with someone who knows and feels exactly how you do takes some of the weight you feel about HIV status. Teen Spirit has also educated me about my medicine better than any doctor could: given me complementary therapies which have helped and boosted my energy. I need Teen Spirit and so do other members of the group.

BODYandSOUL is the only UK charity supporting children, teenagers and their families living with or closely affected by AIDS (www.bodyandsoulcharity.org).

Many people, children included, do not have immediate access to a charity such as BODYandSOUL and so, often alone they carry 'the big ton weight' on their shoulders and are 'locked in their secrecy'.

At the end of 2005 an estimated 63 500 adults were living with HIV in the UK. In 2004 there were 1650 children diagnosed with AIDS in the UK – 75% through their mothers. There were 813 reports on AIDS and 467 AIDS-related deaths in 2004, a remarkable decrease as a result of therapies and advances in medicine. Sadly these advances and options are not available to many people in sub-Saharan Africa where it is estimated that 13 million children under age 15 years have lost one or both parents to AIDS (Help the Hospices 2005).

There was no mention of HIV in the Department of Health White Paper *Choosing Health* (DH 2004c).

Other vulnerable groups

Sadly there are many other vulnerable groups in our society, including very poor and homeless people, and prisoners. In a society that prides itself on caring for one another we as health-care professionals should strive to ensure that our services in generalist and specialist palliative care are extended equally to all members of society. *See the end of the chapter for more help and information sources.*

INFORMATIONAL NEEDS

Repeated studies (Hardwick and Lawson 1995; Ward and Cavanagh 1997; Harris 1998) highlight the importance of informational needs for relatives and friends of those who are dying. More recent research reports that there is confusion and misunderstanding about what a referral to a palliative care service actually means (Seymour et al. 2003).

Andershed and Ternestedt (2001) developed a theoretical framework concerning involvement of relatives based on an indepth analysis of four earlier studies. They identified a phenomenon of *involvement in the light* and this was characterised by the relative being well informed and experiencing meaningful involvement based on trust and confidence between staff and relatives. In Beaver et al.'s study (1999) involving 29 carers, giving advice and explaining things were among the most frequently mentioned positive comments about district and Macmillan nurses. Mok and Chan (2002), in their study of 24 family caregivers in Hong Kong, recognised that passing on knowledge skills and information helped caring to be an empowering experience for carers. Payne et al. (1999), in a study of 39 carers, found that they liked the security of regular visits where minor but niggling worries could be discussed.

The importance of information and education for carers has been echoed in more recent research. McIlfatrick (2007), involving interviews with 24 carers and focus groups with a total of 52 carers, concluded that the main needs relate to everyday social and practical aspects of care. Ekwall et al. (2007), from a postal survey involving approximately 85 carers in Sweden aged 75 and over, found that early information about alternative coping strategies and practical information might allow caregivers better possibilities to continue caring with less negative effects on their lives.

Health-care professionals in many instances need to re-think their approach. Often lack of time is given as a reason for not being available to talk with a family. Time invested in supporting and caring for the family is time well spent. It may result in care continuing instead of breaking down and needing hospital admission. It may result in preserving the mental health of the carer and it will almost certainly result in less time dealing with complaints. In view of the ambivalence of caregivers, it is imperative that health professionals take the lead on initiating consultations with carers and identifying the important role that they play.

With the permission of the patient, and preferably with the patient present, carers need to be informed of all new events. The health professional should take the lead in this. This means that on the hospital ward staff should approach visiting carers with new news and not wait for them to seek out the professionals. When visiting the home of a patient it is imperative to allow protected time to talk with the carer. As discussed in Chapters 3 and 5, information should be tailored to the individual's need, taking account of cultural background. The golden rule is to find out what is known and build on that. Establish understanding of the information given and always check how the receiver of the news feels. Information giving will be a dynamic process throughout the course of the illness. At times it will involve teaching carers/relatives about new equipment and symptom management. Patients and relatives should not feel that the information that belongs to them and information about services available are in any way being 'gate kept'.

Contact emails and telephone numbers should be given to help ensure continuity of care. Payne et al. (1999) highlighted that carers perceived telephone contact as supportive, even if it was not used as an emergency back-up, and helped to reduce feelings of isolation.

The approach outlined here is within the scope of all heath-care professionals. It is the simple everyday courtesies, being mindful of giving information efficiently and taking an interest in the carer, that is important. It would be wise to have a separate page in the patient's record, to record conversations with carers. It is easy to underestimate what a difference such a fundamental approach can make.

BEING HEARD AND FEELING SUPPORTED

Research also demonstrates that carers cope better when they feel supported psychologically by professionals. Andershed and Ternestedt (2001) concluded that an important part of the concept of involvement was a relationship with professionals that was characterised by respect, openness, sincerity and connection. Beaver et al. (1999), in their study including 29 carers, highlighted that the most frequently mentioned positive comments about district and Macmillan nurses related to support – notably that the support was not complex to deliver. Examples of comments are: 'Knowing that the district nurse will come and see you for a chat is important. They were very supportive and there when you needed them, even if it was not their field.' And: 'They were very nice and pleasant and give great support, that's what it's all about; basically, you can sit and talk to her.'

Relatives/carers will be better able to mobilise their own coping mechanisms if they can feel that they are understood and being heard. Therefore, it is important to invite them to tell their stories of the impact of the illness on their family/relationship. It is important to acknowledge and listen empathically to accounts of distress and allow ventilation of strong emotions. Sometimes, just the telling of their story can feel therapeutic. If there is any positive action that can be taken to help reduce distress this should be done. Listening to a person's story need not be time-consuming. The onus is on the professional to open this conversation by saying something like 'this must have been hard for you – can you tell me what it has been like for you?'. The importance of listening to the individual's story and showing empathic understanding of the carers'/relatives' situation cannot be over-emphasised. Whether in a hospital ward or in the home, it should form a central part of care.

Under the Carers (Recognition and Services) Act 1995, carers have a right to an assessment of their own needs. Carers' assessments are carried out by the local Social Services. They provide an opportunity for carers to discuss what they need to carry on caring, i.e. if they want to keep caring. The assessment also looks at what the carer needs to maintain their own health, and balance caring with other life and work commitments. Since 2000 there has been a national strategy for supporting carers (Carers and Disabled Children's Act 2000). Furthermore, the Carers Equal Opportunities Act 2004 promotes cooperation between carers, and requires that carers are informed of their rights to an assessment. As a result of this carers' groups are now part of many hospital, primary care, social care and palliative care services (www.carers.gov.uk).

A carers' group is a place where carers can be heard. From personal experience of running a palliative carers group, I am amazed at how quickly carers can share their pain, e.g. the previously physically strong and able husband now needs help to get in and out of bed, feelings of anger and guilt about the emotions felt when a wife and mother can no longer cook. These groups can also provide opportunities for group teachings on using hoists, washing in bed, oral care and a host of other useful chunks of information. Health professionals should know about local carer groups and provide families with details.

Carers can also find online support. The government sponsors online chat rooms for carers, as do many of the large charities, e.g. British Heart Foundation, Cancer-BACUP, Stroke Association. The Department of Health runs or supports a wide range of telephone helplines, some on a 24-hour basis and others in office hours. This information should be given to carers.

COMPANIONSHIP

Just as the ill person can feel isolated so can the relatives/carers. For many people, sharing their anxieties can make them more bearable. In a study of 12 dying patients and their spouses, all 12 spouses said that their initial reaction to knowing the terminal diagnosis was to hide their own feelings of grief and not discuss the prognosis with the dying person (Costello 1999). Although this 'business as usual' approach may be a useful initial coping strategy, prolonged use of this may interrupt the companionship between the dying person and relatives.

A study involving 20 patients with advanced cancer and 20 with advanced non-malignant disease looked at end-of-life care. The study concluded that the participants were able to judge their own health status and did not object to questions about end-of-life care (Shah et al. 2006). The implications are that those who are dying may well want to talk about their illness and prognosis. The blocks to this may come from relatives and professionals. There is a fuller discussion of this in Chapter 3.

Collusion

Professionals can be invited to collude with relatives 'not to tell the patient'. Often this is because the relatives feel that knowing will cause anguish to their loved ones. Many years of experience have taught me that, when patients and relatives can talk with each other about curtailed futures, it can help them to mobilise coping strategies together. For some people, one conversation is enough; others will talk more. The tension of protecting each other is lost. This can seem a big responsibility for health professionals. What needs to be remembered is that, although the patient and relatives are experts on themselves, the health professional represents the experience in caring for dying people. It is the health professional who needs to initiate difficult conversations and be confident in suggesting more open communication. The patient and/or relative may say no and that should be respected.

The following is a useful approach here (Wilkinson and Mula 2004):

- To acknowledge the relative as the expert on the patient and to explore why they think the patient should not know. Acknowledge and show respect for these reasons.
- Explore how it is making them feel to withhold the truth.
- Ask them if this is putting a strain on their relationship.
- It will also be useful to ask if the patient has been asking any questions and what they think the patient is making of this.
- In other words, get them to reflect on the reasons for not talking about dying.
- Get them to reflect on how not talking about death and dying is affecting their relationship.
- As a professional offer to talk with the ill person, to see what they are making of events. Suggest that they may be protecting the relative.
- While committing to not telling the person that they are dying, leave the proviso that you will answer honestly if the patient asks.
- If, after talking with the patient, you discover that they do have a good idea of what is happening, offer to mediate a conversation between the two of them, so that they can share the pain together – as companions.

If open communication is established it is useful to talk with the relative about the oscillation that may occur between denial and acceptance (see Chapters 2 and 3) and reassure them that gently supporting dreams and hopes of a future that cannot be is fine.

Sometimes, patients may want to do things before they die that seem ambitious, frequently involving foreign travel. A useful approach here is to plan for the worst and then hope for the best. Talk through the worst-case scenario with the patient and carer, and make plans for that worst scenario, e.g. check holiday insurance. If everything is feasible, go ahead with planning a good time and hope for the best.

INTIMACY AND CARING

Somewhere in a chronic disease trajectory, a relative/friend in contemporary society is called a carer. For some people this works fine. Others find being a carer more of a challenge. Whatever the situation health-care professionals need to assess carers' capabilities carefully as new aspects of care become necessary. In particular, as intimate care becomes necessary, sensitivity is needed to check out if this is possible. Gilley (1988) highlights this, drawing on her experiences as a GP. She writes of one case study when she was called out in the middle of the night. Among other issues a very weak and dying wife had been incontinent in the shared marital bed. After attending to his wife, Gilley offered to help her husband make up the spare bed. Her husband responded by saying, 'We've slept together for 50 years, I want one last night with her'. In another case history she describes a couple for whom physical intimacy was absent. The wife was distressed that her husband wanted her to comb his hair. As he became more dependent his wife – who would now be termed his carer – could not care for her husband's physical needs. He received care from the community nurses and died in a hospice.

I visited an elderly dying woman at home. She needed help with all activities of living. She had just been discharged from hospital. Her daughter Susan, a nurse, had spent a lot of time in the hospital ward with her and had been proactive in directing her care. Perhaps, as a result, ward staff had assumed that she would care for her mother on return home. She was distraught when I visited. Although she could help her mother in many ways – e.g. eating and drinking, administering medication – giving intimate care and helping with toilet needs transgressed what was possible in their relationship. I was able to arrange for community nursing support for her mother's intimate needs and Susan continued to orchestrate and be involved in all other aspects of care as was her wish.

HEALTH NEEDS

Carers need to keep themselves in good physical and mental health where possible. As previously highlighted, carers can be very ambivalent about their own needs (Harding and Higginson 2001). Often carers will be elderly and not be in good health themselves. It is vital that health-care professionals take the initiative in making sure that carers keep their hospital appointments and take medication, etc. as prescribed. Being alert to signs of depression and advising appropriately are important. The reader is referred to Chapters 2 and 13.

Whether carers are in ill or robust health, it is important to keep a check on how they are looking after themselves. In particular it is important to maximise the potential of carers for sleep. If they are not sleeping because of anxiety a discussion of pre-sleep routine and natural remedies, e.g. a lavender aroma stone to aid sleep, is a starting point. Relaxation tapes may help, as may taking an interest. Clearly not all potential helpful remedies are suggested here. However, if lack of sleep is about disturbed nights because of attending to the patient's needs, then being proactive in enlisting help from other family members or friends is a starting point. Finding professional night-sitters so that some unbroken nights' sleep are possible may be necessary.

Make checks that the carer is eating sensibly and taking exercise. It is also important to encourage carers to keep up with the usual activities that they enjoy both inside and outside the home. Sometimes professionals can be directive in this, e.g. it may be that the carer would like to go to a regular meeting but feel that the patient cannot be left. Ask the carer to think of anyone who has offered to help. Often people do, but it is difficult to accept or know how they can help. If the carer comes up with a name, suggest that they ask that person to come and sit with the patient. With a bit of luck they might do the ironing while they are there.

It is well established in the research literature that time off from caring is important; carers can manage better, on the whole, if they know that at certain times in the week they are *off duty* (DH 1999b; Banks and Cheeseman 2000; Scott et al. 2001).

Day-care centres can offer a pleasant and stimulating environment for the patient while also giving respite to the carer. As previously discussed, friends and relatives can be galvanised to give regular time to the patient, thereby relieving the carer. Hospices and care homes can give longer periods of respite, allowing the carer perhaps to take a holiday. Carers should be encouraged to pamper themselves and do something that they enjoy during 'self time' and not catch up on chores. As a health-care professional encourage other relatives and friends to do the chores. It often works. People just need a little direction.

Finances

Family finances can be a very worrying problem. McIlfatrick (2007) highlighted this as potentially one of the most worrying problems when someone is ill. Ekwall et al. (2007) also identified poor economic circumstances as being associated with increased stress for carers. This, of course, can be a particularly big issue if the main wage earner is the person dying. It is vital to enquire about this and not assume that the carer will raise this if it is a problem. Many people are embarrassed at raising financial concerns. It is important to know where and to whom to refer the patient and carer for the best possible advice. There are benefits available from central government. Many of the big charities will give one-off payments for travel expenses, equipment and even holidays.

Creative activities

Taking time to do something creative can be enormously therapeutic and rewarding. Perhaps that is why so many people love gardening. Patients in day-care units are often very creative. The charity Rosetta Life (www.rosettalife.org) uses the arts to help people record their life events, and their present thoughts and feelings, and leave a legacy of memories for their family and friends. Health professionals can encourage patients and carers together to compile, for example, photograph albums, memory boxes and videos as a legacy. Such activities can bring a very special dimension to end-of-life care.

DIFFICULT THOUGHTS AND LETTING GO

Carers may have thoughts that they find difficult to vocalise. This is probably most pronounced in a long protracted illness, which alters, or seems to alter, the nature and personality of the patient. For example, in Alzheimer's disease, where it may be that a husband or wife no longer recognises the carer and the carer feels that this is not the person whom they previously loved. It can be very comforting to invite people to vocalise their difficult thoughts. Here, often the health professional is working intuitively, responding to a feeling that the carer is troubled. It can be helpful to listen to thoughts about resentment of, and anger at, the change in the ill person, and offer reassurance that it is not unusual to feel this. Putting carers in touch with appropriate support groups, e.g. Alzheimer's disease support, can be a source of comfort. Acceptance and understanding of these difficult thoughts and feelings can help ameliorate associated guilt. Excessive guilt can be a precursor to a complicated grief pattern (Parkes 1991).

When a patient has outlived their prognosis and/or when dying is protracted, relatives and friends can have very difficult thoughts, e.g. it will be a relief when this is over. It does not mean that they will not feel upset and very emotional when death occurs – just that the waiting is difficult. I used to work weekends as a staff nurse in a hospice. I nursed a dying man with a brain tumour all weekend. His wife was exhausted. I had known them for some months – there had been other times when he was expected to die, but he had not. This time seemed different. I said goodbye on Sunday evening. When I returned the following Friday, the couple were still there. He was sitting up, looking bright. When things were quiet and her husband settled, I approached Anna. We talked quietly about nothing for a while – and then I said intuitively, 'I expect you wish this was all over'. She sobbed and I comforted her. It was a relief for her to be able to express her anguish at this protracted dying.

A student told me her story of how she acted intuitively in a situation where a wife was finding it hard to let her husband die. The wife was busy trying to 'wake her husband up' and make him eat a breakfast. Marion gently said to her, 'perhaps it is time to say goodbye to your husband'. The wife was furious with Marion and retorted that she would never say goodbye. Some hours later as Marion was going home the wife intercepted her and thanked her. She said that she had said goodbye to her husband. It had felt very special and he had smiled in his 'sleepy' state and said goodbye to her.

Marion had acted intuitively; the initial reaction was confrontational and difficult. It was only by chance that she knew the resulting value of her intervention. It is important in these circumstances to trust and act on our intuitions. Sometimes we will be rebuffed. Sometimes we will get it wrong. However, often the experienced practitioner will perceive accurately and their empathic support will be very helpful.

Sometimes as health professionals we measure our success in knowing that we tried, we reached out. Reaching out in these difficult circumstances can feel scary. What if we are wrong and we make it worse? Sometimes it will not be a good intervention for that person. However, as health-care professionals we need to accept that our successes and failures have consequences for vulnerable people. We will get it right more often than wrong if our intentions are good.

CONCLUSION

Extending care to carers is a vital part of end-of-life care. Carers may not be 'naturals' and professionals must be sensitive to this and provide support accordingly. Carers are often very ambivalent about their own needs. Professionals must respond to this by taking the initiative in ensuring that carers' information, emotional and educational needs are met. The physical health of the carer is important, particularly the sleeping, eating and exercising patterns. Recreation and time out are important for them. Dealing with collusion and helping dying people and their carers to share creative experiences can be very rewarding for professionals. Unusual and difficult thoughts should be understood and supported by good use of intuition. There are many 'hidden carers' who need the support of mainstream health care.

MAIN IMPLICATIONS FOR PRACTICE

- Family and friends often need the help of professionals to help them deal with someone for whom they care who is dying.
- Although the patient, family and friends are the experts on themselves, they will view professionals as the experts on dying and look to us for help in coping in practical, psychological and existential ways.
- Friends and relatives can be ambivalent about their own needs. Health professionals should be proactive in supporting the health of carers by ensuring that they take care of themselves.
- Friends and relatives should be offered new information as things change (with the patient's permission). There should not be a feeling that information is being 'gate kept'.
- It is vital that friends and relatives can feel that they are being heard.
- Health professionals should take the initiative to try to restore companionship if collusion has interrupted this.
- As a friend or relative slips into becoming a carer, it is important that no assumptions are made about what care they can provide. They may need education and support. Issues of intimate care should be sensitively checked out and no assumptions made.
- Professionals should be proactive in encouraging the friend or relative who is caring to care also for themselves.
- Carers have a statutory right to a carer's assessment by Social Services.
- Carers' groups can provide valuable support and carers should be given contact details of such groups.

- Useful web addresses should be highlighted to carers, as well as organisations, both statutory and charitable, that can provide useful education and support.
- Professionals will encounter carers who have difficult thoughts and problems letting go of their friend or relative. Often the professional is working intuitively here. It is important for professionals to trust their intuitions.

SUGGESTED FURTHER READING

Blackman N (2003) *Loss and Learning Disability*. London: Worth Publishing Ltd.

Gilley J (1998) Intimacy and terminal care. *J R Coll GP* **38**: 121–2.

Hanson E (2004) Supporting families of terminally ill persons. In: Payne S, Seymour J, Ingleton C (eds), *Palliative Care Nursing*. Milton Keynes, Bucks: Open University Press, 329–51.

Katz JS, Pearce S (2003) *End of Life Care in Care Homes – A palliative approach*. Oxford: Oxford University Press.

Websites

www.bodyandsoulcharity.org
www.carers.gov.uk
www.mind.org.uk
www.nationalasylumsupportservices
www.respond.org.uk
www.rosettalife.org
See also websites listed at the end of Chapter 7.

Chapter 9
Bereavement

KEY POINTS

- **Definitions**: bereavement is defined as being deprived of anything valued. Grief refers to the emotions that accompany bereavement and is a unique experience for each person. Mourning is the social face of grief and can be influenced by different cultural approaches.
- **Untimely deaths**: untimely death such as the death of a child or death by violence, suicide or accident brings a particular pathos to bereavement. In these situations any targeted bereavement care is mainly the domain of charitable self-help groups.
- **Bereavement and health**: bereavement can impact on physical and mental health in some people. Well-organised bereavement support may translate to a health promotional strategy.
- **Grief theorists**: Colin Murray Parkes and William Worden write about bereavement from the perspective of their life's works and research. Their work supports the attachment theory. A key figure in the development of the attachment theory is John Bowlby.

   Tony Walter brings a sociological perspective to grief and Margaret and Wolfgang Stroebe and Henk Schut offer a dual process model of coping with loss.

   The theorists all add something to our understanding of grief and they are not in conflict with each other.
- **Mourning customs**: a very brief overview of mourning customs for Buddhism, Hinduism, Christianity, Islam, Judaism and Sikhism is included. Fuller texts are recommended at the end of the chapter.
- **Children**: they need to be included in explanations and rituals when someone is dying. Not including children leaves them vulnerable and unsupported in their grief.
- **Old age**: this is a time when there are more bereavements in life. Many elderly people now also experience the death of an adult child. Death of friends is commonplace.
- **Bereavement and dementia**: at the heart of dementia is loss. For the relatives there may be a sense that they have lost the person while the person with dementia lives on.
- **Solitary grief**: sometimes losses are trivialised by others or seen as commonplace, and sometimes the loss cannot be acknowledged, e.g. the death of a secret love. In these situations grieving is a lonely path to walk.

- The key recommendations of the National Institute for Health and Clinical Excellence's Supportive and Palliative Care Guidance (NICE 2004b) state that provider organisations should nominate a lead person to oversee bereavement support.
- Research into type and quality of bereavement support is scant. Recent papers suggest that pre-bereavement support is important and bereavement services need to have a clear rationale. Risk assessment to identify those people most likely to benefit from support should be addressed.

DEFINITIONS

Bereavement has been defined as being robbed or deprived of anything valued, to have a valued person, object or attribute snatched away. The bereavement referred to in this chapter is confined to the loss by death of a relative or friend. Grief refers to the emotional aspects that accompany bereavement and can be regarded as an adaptation to loss. Freud (1915) was one of the first people to describe the phenomenon of grief and he defines it as the process of gradual withdrawal of the energy that ties the bereaved individual to the lost object or deceased person. Mourning is the social perspective on bereavement and can be shaped by different cultural approaches.

Our experiences of death and bereavement are much less in the western world since the mid-twentieth century. However, although less familiar, bereavement will almost inevitably be experienced by those living a natural lifespan. Grief is a unique experience. There are some deaths that may cause little grief and others that are intensely painful. Siblings can experience the death of a parent very differently. The death of a spouse can be the loss of a life-long friend and lover and, at the other end of the continuum, the loss of a life-long bully.

UNTIMELY DEATHS

Death of a child

The death of a child, whether it occurs as a miscarriage, in childhood or adulthood, is always untimely if before the death of the parent. It upsets the natural order of things. For parents, for whom one of the main tasks of parenting is to protect their child from harm, the death of a child can bring feelings of intense guilt associated with extreme grief. It is important to remember that increasingly elderly people will have suffered the loss of an adult child. In a study of 18 elderly bereaved mothers, Lesher and Berger (1988) found that they had high levels of psychological distress.

Death by suicide

Death by suicide brings an added dimension to grieving. The bereaved person may have to accept that their relationship with that person was not working as well as they thought (Penson 1990). Lake (1984) suggests that by committing suicide the dead person is forcing the bereaved to miss someone whom they did not love enough. This can lead to excessive guilt and is associated with complicated grief (Parkes 1991). Families may also feel a social stigma.

Death by violence and accident

Death by violence adds another dimension to the adjustment to loss. It is always a shocking event and it transgresses a natural trust that many have in society. It can undermine the ability of the bereaved to live comfortably in a society that has so violated their trust. Death by accident can similarly shake the bereaved person's faith in a fair society. Often there will be many unanswered questions about the accident that can bring feelings of intense anger and sorrow.

Obviously, many untimely deaths are unpredicted and so the bereaved have no period of anticipatory grief, no opportunity even to prepare to say goodbye. Sometimes last memories with the dead person may not be happy, e.g. the last meeting might have been argumentative. This brings added pain to the emotions of grief. Although bereavement care should be an integral part of palliative care, outside specialist palliative care units it is largely the domain of charitable and self-help groups. The efficacy of these groups is under-researched; however, many groups thrive and anecdotal accounts of their value are plentiful. These groups can be particularly pertinent for those experiencing untimely bereavements and a list of useful national websites is included at the end of this chapter.

Grief theorists

Many people have researched the nature of grieving and it would be an impossibility to present a comprehensive account. Kübler-Ross's (1969) seminal work has been mentioned in Chapter 2 when looking at facing progressive disease and death. Her work was done with dying patients, but is also frequently used as a grief model applicable to bereaved individuals.

This chapter is confined to discussing the work of Colin Murray Parkes, William Worden, Margaret and Wolfgang Stroebe, Henk Schut and Tony Walter. In the main it discusses what each considers to be common characteristics of grief patterns. It is my impression that these theorists are the ones most commonly referred to in the palliative care literature. The important point to highlight is that they all add something to our understanding of loss and they are not in conflict with each other (Parkes 2005). This chapter will not address, in any detail, the phenomenon of complicated grief. The reader is referred to texts by mental health experts for this detail. Before a look at the theorists the potential effects of grief on the overall health of a person are considered very briefly.

BEREAVEMENT AND HEALTH

Early papers on grief, e.g. Lindemann (1944), describe not only the psychological manifestations, but also the physical feelings associated with grief. Worden (1997) lists the most commonly reported sensations experienced by people seen for grief counselling:

- Hollowness in the stomach
- Tightness in the chest
- Tightness in the throat
- Oversensitivity to noise
- A sense of unreality
- Weakness in the muscles
- Lack of energy
- Dry mouth.

Other physical symptoms include sleep and appetite disturbances (Parkes 1972; Worden 1997). Parkes describes a tendency for people to lose weight in early bereavement. He also states that one of the first appetites to come back is that for food and often, at the end of the first year of loss, too much weight may have been gained.

In their review of 16 longitudinal studies and cross-sectional studies of the bereavement–mortality relationship, Stroebe and Stroebe (1994) concluded that bereaved individuals are, indeed, at higher risk of dying than non-bereaved people. Higher risks occur in the weeks and months closest to the loss and men appear to be more vulnerable than women. In one of these first longitudinal studies, Parkes et al. (1969) found that the great increase in mortality during the first 6 months of bereavement was for widowers dying from myocardial infarctions and other atherosclerotic degenerative heart disorders. This led to reference to the *broken heart* theory. After their analysis Stroebe and Stroebe (1994) concluded that the broken heart theory alone could not explain the bereavement–mortality relationship. Secondary changes associated with loss, particularly with stress and changing roles, are also responsible, e.g. higher incidences of death from liver cirrhosis, accidents and suicides have been linked with bereavement, as has excessive mortality among widowers from infection (Helsing et al. 1982). This might indicate an impaired immune response. Accidental deaths are significantly higher among widowed males (Helsing et al. 1982). These studies report a higher risk for other bereaved family members of dying, not just spouses. It is important to highlight that bereavement research poses many methodological challenges and ethical concerns.

Psychosocial transition

Grief arises from an awareness of a discrepancy between the world that is and the world that should be (Parkes 2005). So, for example, when a mother dies a timely death, the adult child knows cognitively that this is the natural order of things. However, emotionally it may seem like an outrage, because at the emotional level the adult child may have felt that their mother would always be there for them.

Parkes (2005) draws on the work of Brown and Harris (1978), Caplan (1961) and Rahe (1979) whose studies show that the life events that commonly precede the onset of mental illness are those that:

- require people to make major revisions to their assumptions about the world
- are lasting in their implications
- take place in a relatively short space of time.

These three criteria constitute events that can be called psychosocial transitions (PSTs). In PST the internal, assumptive world is constantly under revision. The death of someone with whom one has lived for many years can impinge deeply on all aspects of life from habitual actions, e.g. setting the table for two, to emotional support, e.g. turning to that person for advice. Parkes (2005) describes PST as a job of work to be done, drawing on Freud's (1917) concept of the work of mourning. As people are reviewing their assumptive world, they feel pain as they take stock of the present world in which they live. They review their world often at a time when their mind is in turmoil and they resist the change in a variety of ways. It will be only in very general terms that we understand individual grief. However, Parkes (2005) highlights that this does not mean that we cannot help. 'By encouraging those who are in transition to help us understand, by talking about their situation, we can help them to take stock, review and relearn their assumptive world' (Parkes 2005, p 328).

On a more positive note, Dutton and Zisook (2005) highlight that, although it is very important to be aware of the emotional, social and physical problems associated with bereavement, these difficulties are not universally associated with grief. They state that accumulating evidence suggests that resilience in the face of bereavement is the norm rather than the exception.

GRIEF THEORISTS

Attachment theory

Before discussing the work of Parkes and Worden, it is appropriate briefly to highlight the attachment theory because they both base their work on this.

To understand the impact of loss fully it is important to comprehend the attachment theory. A key figure in the development of this theory is John Bowlby. In developing his theory, Bowlby included data from control theory, cognitive psychology, neurophysiology and developmental biology (Worden 1997). Bowlby contests the view that attachment bonds result purely to meet biological needs. Bowlby's thesis is that emotional attachments come from a need for security and safety. The attachment theory is usually illustrated by citing the young animal or young child who forms strong emotional bonds with the mother or a significant other. As they grow older they leave the attachment figure for increasingly longer periods of time. However, they always return to the attachment figure for support and safety; when the attachment figure disappears, or is threatened, this can evoke strong emotions and intense anxiety. The forming of attachments with significant others is considered to be normal behaviour not only for the child but also for the adult. If the goal of attachment is to maintain, then situations that threaten this attachment, e.g. death, will give rise to strong feelings (Worden 1997).

Colin Murray Parkes

Colin Murray Parkes is a psychiatrist with an interest in bereavement. As well as working at the Tavistock Institute for Human Relations in London in the past, he has for many years been an honorary consultant psychiatrist at St Christopher's Hospice. His book *Bereavement: Studies of grief in adult life* is highly regarded and has sold widely.

Parkes (1991) talks about the nature of grief and phases of grief that are shared by many bereaved people. He is very careful to note that grief is not a linear process. When talking about phases he notes that there is a great variation between people and they oscillate between the phases.

Numbness and blunting are a phase that often accompanies the immediate loss as the person struggles to come to terms with the reality. One woman whose adult son had died suddenly said: 'the day after he died, I got up and put on my make up as usual, but I felt like a cardboard cut out, it's the only way I can describe it. I felt that for a long time and some days still do.'

Parkes (1991) describes pangs of grief as pining and yearning. The pangs of grief can also manifest in anger and self-reproach. People may feel bewildered and be in turmoil. They can feel very anxious, with no clear understanding of why, which may lead them to feel that they are 'going mad'. Helping people to understand that this is a common aspect of bereavement may be helpful. One woman said that, when she felt like this, it helped to do something physical, so she would put on her coat and walk and walk until she was tired. The realisation that the death is permanent eventually leads to a loss of the old identity and may also lead to a loss of purpose.

As the initial pain of grief may diminish the periods of apathy and despair may be longer.

Although Parkes (1991) highlights that there is no endpoint to grief, he does describe a period of reorganisation and recovery. He does not put a time limit on grief, but notes that anniversaries are often a time of renewed grieving, although once they are past they may be associated with a lightening of mood and renewed energy. He suggests that holidays, or time away, may be useful in terms of escaping from constant reminders of the loss. On return the bereaved person may be motivated to clear cupboards, redecorate – in other words, engage in activities directed to the future rather than the past, thus constructing a new internal model alongside the old.

Years after bereavement an unexpected reminder of the past can trigger the pain of loss. This can be particularly so when a person is absent, e.g. the birth of a new grandchild reminds everyone that granddad has missed this special event. However, according to Parkes (1991) many people will report that the pain of yearning has diminished to a point where it is outweighed by good times that are past, so nostalgic recollection can became one of the joys of advancing years.

In describing the nature of grief, Parkes (1991) explains that human beings share with other social animals an urge to cry and search relentlessly for the lost person. This feeling tends to recur in episodes that may be triggered by reminders of the lost person. One young student nurse whom I knew was bereaved traumatically by the death of her young husband. She describes how periodically – for a long time, e.g. 2 or 3 years – she would get into her car and actually look for him. She would slow down when she saw a group of young men and sometimes she would be convinced that she had seen him. Interestingly, she never approached the young man whom she thought might be her husband. Other times she was convinced that she had seen him on the TV news. She feels that it would have helped her to know that other bereaved people experienced this also.

Our urge to avoid or repress crying and searching is a strong social pressure in western culture. Mourning customs, which may have in the past provided social sanction for the expression of grief, have changed in the western world. Often a 'stiff upper lip' has replaced this. Clinical experience and research have shown that those who express their grief most fully at the times of bereavement cope better than those who repress it (Parkes 1991).

In reviewing and revising the assumptive world, bereaved people may tend time and time again to go over the events associated with the loss, as if looking for another explanation of events. At this time, it is common for them to feel that the dead person is near at hand and may speak to them as if they are still alive. Minimal sights and sounds may be interpreted as the dead person returning. Vivid images may occur in which the dead person is viewed briefly as if present. This has been reported in up to 50% of bereaved people. Bereaved people may interpret this as a sign of mental illness. It can be important, therefore, for someone to explain that this is a usual part of grieving.

William Worden

William Worden has over thirty years clinical and research experience in life-threatening illness. His academic appointments include being professor of psychology at Harvard Medical School, USA. He proposes that mourning, i.e. adapting to loss, can be seen as involving four basic tasks. He feels that it is essential that people complete these tasks so that further growth and development can occur. He presents tasks of mourning as opposed to phases (Parkes 1991), because he feels that this implies that bereaved individuals are then active in their mourning as opposed to mourning being a passive experience. Similar to Parkes' phases of grief, Worden (1997) highlights that, although order is suggested in the definitions of the tasks, they do not necessarily follow a specific order and a mixed bag of tasks can present in any one day.

The four tasks of mourning

Task 1: To accept the reality of the loss

Accepting the reality of a bereavement is an intellectual and emotional exercise. People often oscillate between belief and disbelief. Although one understands the spoken words 'he is dead' the emotional attachment is still strong. Searching behaviour and the desire to call out for the lost person are directly related to the accomplishment of this task.

Some people may refuse to believe that the death is real and get 'stuck' here. This can manifest itself in different ways. When a child dies the parent may keep the room just as it was on the day that he or she died. Queen Victoria had Prince Albert's clothes laid out for him every day and was often heard talking to him. Worden terms this 'mummification'. This sort of behaviour is not unusual in the short term. However, if the behaviour impinges in the long term on the person's ability to 'get on with life', it may be a sign that they need help, e.g. if the dead child's bedroom were left vacant and other children in the house were sharing a room after a long period of time, this could indicate that the bereaved person is in some element of denial.

Other signs that may indicate that someone is stuck is a constant denial of the meaning of the loss: 'I won't miss him', 'we weren't close'. This may be accompanied by jettisoning all reminders of the dead person from the house. Another sign of being stuck here is to repress the memory of the dead person, to work hard at forgetting him or her. Other people may seek the aid of a spiritualist to help them to maintain contact.

Shades of all of these behaviours may be a natural part of this task and do not necessarily mean that the person is stuck. Traditional rituals, e.g. funerals, and being able to talk through events may be helpful in accepting the reality of the loss.

Task 2: To work through the pain

Worden describes the pain of grief as emotional, physical and behavioural. He considers that it is necessary for people to acknowledge and work through the pain. Anything that allows the person to suppress or avoid the pain can be expected to prolong the course of mourning. This task can be hindered by a number of things. The bereaved person may:

- stimulate only pleasant thoughts of the dead person
- idealise the dead person and avoid unpleasant thoughts
- avoid all reminders of the dead person
- seek geographical care, i.e. taking holidays and moving around, staying with friends and family
- use alcohol or drugs excessively.

Parkes (1991) states that generally these euphoric responses are fragile and short-lived. Worden (1997) concurs with Bowlby (1980) in believing that those who avoid all conscious grieving will almost certainly 'break down' with some form of depression.

Worden notes that society may be uncomfortable with a mourner's feelings, thus giving out subtle messages not to grieve. He also notes that one of the main aims of grief counselling is to help people through this difficult task, so that they do not carry the pain throughout their life. Grief support, be it from a friend or a counsellor, is valuable in providing space for the bereaved person to talk about the deceased person and what their death means to them.

Task 3: To adjust to an environment in which the deceased person is missing

In any bereavement it is seldom clear exactly what is lost. The bereaved person may not be aware of all the roles that the dead person fulfilled until some time after the loss occurs. This tasks mirrors Parkes' (2005) theory of reviewing the assumptive world. Worden states that it is usually about 3 months after the loss that realisation begins to occur. It may mean living alone, facing an empty house, bringing up children alone, managing domestic chores, getting a job, managing finances. The list could be endless. The following are some problems that may occur in this task:

- Regression: attempts to fulfil the role of the deceased person may fail and thus lower self-esteem. Success at taking on new roles may be attributed to fate rather than to their own abilities.
- Loss of the sense of world: a loss of direction is experienced as the person's view of the world is challenged.
- Promoting their own helplessness: bereaved people may work against themselves by not developing the skills that they know they need to cope.
- Withdrawing from the world: staying in and not communicating with the 'outside world'.

This is a time when personal confidence is challenged and the bereaved person may resent having to develop new skills. However, even reluctantly developed skills can bring the bereaved person a sense of satisfaction. A friend or counsellor does well to notice these accomplishments and offer praise for efforts.

Task 4: To relocate the deceased person emotionally and move on with life

When moving towards relocation, Figure 9.1 is an example of what this might involve.

This task is not about giving up a relationship with the dead person, but more about finding an appropriate place for the dead person in their emotional life – a place that will enable the bereaved person to live effectively in the world. Worden (1997) quotes a teenage daughter who wrote to her mother 2 years after her father had died: 'There are other people to be loved and it doesn't mean that I love Dad any less.' This quote, Worden feels, articulates the grappling with emotional withdrawal and reinvestment.

Worden says that it is difficult to find a phrase that would adequately define the incompletion of Task 4, except perhaps not loving. Some people find the grief so painful that they may make a pact with themselves never to love again. Worden comments that the popular song market is replete with this theme, which gives it a validity that it does not deserve.

Talking to the person as if he or she were still in the room

↓

Thinking about what the deceased person would have said and perhaps acting accordingly

↓

Considering what the deceased person's wishes would have been before acting

↓

Finally 'the wishes' become the bereaved person's own ideas and the deceased person is no longer referred to in decision-making

Figure 9.1 Moving towards relocation.

When mourning is finished

Worden highlights that there will be many different answers to the question of when mourning is finished. He emphasises that grief does not proceed in a linear fashion and it will reappear to be reworked. One benchmark may be when the person is able to think about the deceased person with no pain. A grateful acceptance of condolences is one of the most reliable signs that the bereaved person is working through mourning satisfactorily. Worden states that grief counselling should alert the person to the fact that mourning may take a long time.

Tony Walter

Tony Walter is a lecturer in sociology at the University of Bath. He challenges what he feels is the dominant model of grief in contemporary literature, i.e. grief work through emotion, with a goal being to move on to form new relationships. His original work was prompted by two most significant bereavements for him. He argues that, while using a sample of just one person and two bereavements may sound unsound, his experience did not confirm conventional wisdom and he proposes that one defiant case may tell us more than 999 conventional cases (Walter 1996).

Walter's father died when he was 90. The address at his memorial service was given by a black Zimbabwean, who drew on his Shona tradition of living in the presence of his ancestors. He suggested that the spirit of Len Walter would be kept alive and he should be acknowledged as a continuing member of the family and village. In Shona terms the dead person is lost and then found, instead of being clung on to and then ultimately relinquished (Walter 1996). When reading the work of 'dominant' theorists thoroughly, I do not think that they would argue with this.

A study by Marwitt and Klass (1995) looks at the idea of withdrawing emotional ties from the dead. They asked a sample of students between the ages of 18 and 54 to think about a person close to them who had died and to identify a role (if any) that they currently played in their life. To their surprise no participants had any problem with this and some wrote two or three pages. In this research four kinds of roles for the deceased were identified:

- As a role model
- Giving guidance in specific situations
- Clarifying values
- As a valued part of their biography.

On a personal note, my Aunt Edith died when she was 13 years old. My father was 11, so of course I never met her. However, all our family houses displayed her photograph. Aunt Edith was kind and polite. She always did what she was told and helped her mother. She did her homework and practised on the piano without having to be told to. She was indeed a role model for all the children in the family.

Walter (1996) talks about the death of a very close friend, Corina. In arranging her memorial service he spoke to many people who knew her. He knew of many of these friends but had not met them. In talking about the Corina he knew with these friends, Walter shared memories of the same 'lovably impossible person', and he also found out new things about her that helped him to understand his relationship with her more. 'I had lost my best friend, but in a way I had found her for the first time.' Grief theorists, e.g. Stroebe (1992), refer to internal dialogues with the deceased as serving a positive function. Walter (1996) feels that it was external dialogues with others who knew Corina that was helpful to him. External dialogue can be promoted by funerals, memorial services, letters of condolence, as well as informally. Sometimes, in our 'efforts not to upset the bereaved', we do not acknowledge their loss. This is almost always a mistake and serves to protect us from thinking about mortality and has nothing to do with the welfare of the bereaved person.

Walter (1999) talks about private bonds with the dead:

- A continuing sense of the presence of the dead: Rees (1971) found that about 50% of widows and widowers experience this. This is in line with Parkes' (1991) work.
- A feeling of spiritual relationship with the dead: a study by Chambers (1997) found that women who had lost children could not talk to their husbands about the death, but could and did talk to God.
- Anecdotal evidence supports many bereaved people in Britain consulting spiritual mediums.
- Talking to the dead: there is good anecdotal evidence that people talk to the dead. Often a visit to the graveside facilitates this. A BBC TV documentary featured a man whose son had died at 19, who said that he regularly popped into the cemetery 'to have a chat with the lad'. Research by Shuchter and Zisook (1993) indicated that over a third of San Diego widows and widowers regularly talked with the deceased person, with a very small decline after 13 months.

Symbolic places and things can facilitate a private bond and be part of living with the dead, e.g. shrines, photographs, memory boxes.

Walter (1999) also addresses the public bonds, i.e. how the dead live on in everyday conversation. He looks at this in relationship to contemporary society and social mores that may inhibit these public bonds. Walter gives an interesting postmodern sociological perspective on grief and mourning. In essence there is more agreement with the 'dominant models' than dissent.

Margaret Stroebe and Wolfgang Stroebe

Margaret Stroebe (1992) challenged some aspects of contemporary grief theories. She commented that undue emphasis was put on the loss of the dead person at the expense of the subsequent changes that are likely to arise after a bereavement. As a result Stroebe and Schut (1996) presented a dual process model of coping with loss. They proposed that, when responding to loss, people need to undertake both loss- and restoration-oriented coping. Thus, the bereaved person will oscillate between the two styles of coping.

Loss orientation is about confronting the issues of grief, e.g. expressing sorrow, trying to make sense of a world without the dead person. Restoration orientation is about attending to new things and dealing with everyday life. So, sometimes the bereaved person confronts issues of grief and other times may be avoiding memories and concentrating on new things. Stroebe (1998) emphasises that adaptation to loss is about achieving a balance between these orientations. One of the refreshing aspects of this model is the 'time out' element that it highlights. During restoration focus, grief may be temporarily forgotten and the bereaved can rest from the emotional labour of it.

I think that these two statements taken from an article by Stroebe and Schut (1999) graphically illustrate their model. They document reactions to the loss of loved ones after a road traffic accident:

> There was the feeling of utter devastation at the loss of everything I loved and this led to periods of deep depression, when I wondered what was the point of going on. There was compulsive need to talk to people about the accident and how it was affecting me. Tears came often in gasping, wrenching stabs.

> Almost immediately after the accident, and while still in hospital, I had this powerful and passionate determination to get married again and to have another family. The urge motivated almost every major decision I took for the next five years and drove my social life.

> Stroebe and Schut (1996, p 85)

These statements were made by the same person on the same day, documenting his reaction to the death of his wife and two children.

Stroebe and Schut's dual process model has featured in a large study looking at the changing lives of older couples (CLOC). An analysis focused on a sample of 104 widowers and 492 widows at 6 months, 18 months and 4 years later. Bradburn's Affect Balance Scale was used as the dependent variable and the independent variables were based on Stroebe and Schut's dual process model. Analysis revealed that loss and restoration activities were important throughout bereavement (Richardson 2006).

Stroebe and Schut's model emphasises oscillation. The dominant models of grief of Kübler-Ross, Parkes and Worden may, on a superficial read, purport a linear process; however, oscillations between stages, phases and tasks are well documented in all three models.

MOURNING PRACTICES IN DIFFERENT CULTURES

Buddhism

There is a great deal of variation in Buddhist mourning practices according to country of origin. Sri Lankan Buddhist mourners, for example, may return to work after 3 or 4 days. In other Buddhist schools, mourning may last 100 days and, for a husband or father, 3 years. Japanese Buddhism mourning rituals occur during a 49-day period after death. If there was anything unsettling about the death, e.g. accidental, the mourner may state that their 49 days *are not over.*

Christianity

There is no longer any official mourning dress or period of mourning. Funerals vary and are a time for everyone to get together to show support for the bereaved people and talk about the dead person. Services now often include friends and family members voicing their memories of the dead person. After the funeral there is usually tea and cake at the house of the bereaved person or a local hall. The actions of going to a funeral in Ireland and many rituals in Scotland are as much about the living as the dead. One goes to a wake to talk about the dead person. Wakes can be very lively affairs. They can bring a strong sense of bonding and community feeling. There is no regular system of callers visiting the bereaved after the funeral in Christianity.

Hinduism

Most Hindus who die in Britain will be cremated here. Their ashes may be scattered in the Ganges later. Death among Hindus is accepted without the characteristic associated anger in western families. Mourners and friends return to the deceased house. There is a ceremony for mourners called *Sreda*, where food offerings are brought to the brahmins and rituals for the dead are performed.

In India the period of mourning and austerity is 10–16 days and culminates in rituals that enable the dead person's soul to join the ancestors. In Britain these rituals occur soon after the funeral and involve gifts to priests or charity.

Islam

Muslims are cremated and this is carried out as soon as possible. Traditionally, mourning lasts about 1 month. During this time friends and relatives visit the bereaved individuals bringing gifts of food. Conversation is centred around the person who died. It is traditional to concentrate on the good things about the dead person as opposed to their faults. The grave is visited on Fridays for the first 40 days and this is associated with alms being distributed to the poor. According to Muslim law a widow should modify her behaviour for 130 days by wearing plain clothes and staying at home as much as possible.

Judaism

Jews prefer if possible to have the burial conducted within 24 hours of the death. They feel that it is impossible to grieve properly until after the funeral. After the funeral 7 days of mourning start, called the *shiva*, and includes evening prayers at home. The community may come to join in the prayers and offer respect and comfort to the mourners. After 7 nights there is a lesser mourning for 30 days called *shloshim*. This is characterised by no festivities and daily trips to the synagogue to say *kaddish*, the mourner's prayer. After this there is a period of 11 months until the headstone is consecrated and, after a year, picking up the threads of life again.

Sikhism

After death a Sikh is cremated as soon as possible. Traditionally, the ashes are scattered in the River Sutlej in Anandpur, in the Punjab, although increasingly they are being scattered in their chosen place in the United Kingdom.

After the funeral there is usually a funeral meal at the *gurdwara* (centre of learning, prayers and hospitality). After about 10 days there is a ceremony, *Bhog*, to mark the end of a first stage of mourning. At the conclusion of mourning the eldest son is given a turban as a sign that he is now head of the family.

BEREAVED CHILDREN

For many years, adults as both professionals and parents have wanted to protect children when a death occurred in the family. It is now recognised that this form of protecting children from the truth in practice leaves them confused, unprotected from their fantasies and unsupported in their feelings (Monroe 2003).

Children can quickly sense when things are not 'right' and they will also 'pretend' that all is well with them in order to protect adults in a difficult situation. They are much more sophisticated than we give them credit for.

For professionals it is important to let parents or guardians know that it is important to ask children what they understand about what is happening. However, their capacity to understand events may be much greater than their capacity to articulate their understanding (Munroe 2003). Listen to what the child says, answer questions honestly and avoid euphemisms, e.g. 'gone to sleep', 'went away'. Here the child may feel frightened to go to sleep and/or feel abandoned. Often children have 'magical thinking' and feel that they may have caused an illness/death to happen; it is important to be alert to this. Children should be given a choice about attending a funeral and any other events connected with the death. Often, interactions with children about death are short and frequent (Child Bereavement Trust 2003). There are some excellent charitable organisations that provide very useful guidelines for supporting bereaved children, notably the Child Bereavement Trust and Winston's Wish, and their website details are at the end of the chapter.

OLD AGE

Old age is a time when there are more bereavements. Ironically, for many in old age the review of the assumptive world can seem more of a challenge than ever before. Many elderly people will experience multiple bereavements and the death of adult children or grandchildren. It is important to be aware of these aspects when caring for elderly people.

BEREAVEMENT AND DEMENTIA

Kay de Vries

At the heart of dementia is loss (Cheston and Bender 1999), and clinical observations and research have shown that people with dementia of the Alzheimer type still respond to their illness, even after their 'illness insight' has disappeared (Miesen 1997). People with dementia often experience fear and anxiety when moved from a familiar environment to an unfamiliar one and surrounded by people who are strangers (Miesen 1997, 1999; Pickard and Glendinning 2001). They may also experience a chronic trauma related to separation, loss, powerlessness, displacement and homelessness (Miesen 1997).

Bereavement can be complex for significant others in the lives of the person with dementia. If a diagnosis of dementia is not made in the early stages of the disease, there is no time to say goodbye or make preparation for the end-stage and dying stage. For relatives there is a sense of having lost the person (the person whom they were before the dementia) while the person with dementia still lives. This can lead to ambivalence about the potential death of the person with dementia, and a response of relief by relatives at the death of the person with dementia may result in a conflicted grief response by the family member.

The death of the person with dementia may be viewed with relief by the relatives for a number of reasons. The family may believe that the patient has no quality of life and that their misery is prolonged as long as they stay alive (Gessert et al. 2001). Gessert et al. (2001) found that many of the participants in their study were ambivalent about the anticipated death of their relatives and, although they believed that death would be a blessing, they did not want to appear overly receptive to death or be seen to be unseemly, advocating death. The researchers identified common challenges faced by families of people with late-stage dementia. These were: guilt associated with the institutionalisation of the family member, unfamiliarity with death in general and death as a result of advancing dementia, and limited understanding of the natural cause of late-stage dementia. They also found that the family members were unfamiliar with setting goals and making decisions on behalf of another and confusion about what actions, or inactions, might 'cause' the death of their relative. Lack of contact, and communication, with health professionals, were also identified as a barrier to family members understanding the physical changes that take place, and the care needs of the person with end-stage dementia. It is recommended that advance care planning would both improve end-of-life care for dying people with dementia and improve the experience of family members involved in end-of-life decision-making and bereavement experiences (Forbes et al. 2000; Gessert et al. 2001; de Vries 2007).

SOLITARY GRIEF

Marie Price

Life is a continual process of loss and change that requires us to adjust our lives to a greater or lesser extent. This is dependent on how we experience or categorise the event or how it is viewed by those around us, or society in general: from the seemingly trivial and potentially irritating loss of keys, when we are trying to get to work on time, to the death of a significant person with whom we have a meaningful relationship. Losses and changes necessitate evaluation and understanding. Part of adjusting often requires discussion with others in order to clarify our thoughts and put our feelings in context. Sometimes this is not possible for a variety of reasons such as where losses are trivialised or seen as commonplace, or where the loss cannot be acknowledged. Sometimes others, or society, view the grief as unnecessary, or not necessary to the degree to which the individual may need to grieve, or where the grief cannot be expressed openly.

These losses can include miscarriage where, although not an unusual event, it is significant for the person involved and includes the fathers who may be overlooked or told to keep strong. Abortion is seen as a life choice but again can have far-reaching effects for all concerned. The mode of birth can also trigger a grief reaction, e.g. birth by caesarean section can shatter the longed-for natural birth and combines birth with major abdominal surgery. Divorce and separation, not rare occurrences, possibly leave people with the idea that they must get over it. We also have typical life changes such as loss of hair or looks. These and others such as deteriorating eyesight can all produce a grief reaction and how we manage it depends on how it is seen by those around us, how secure we feel in ourselves and how well adjusted and supported we allow ourselves to be.

Then there are losses that are difficult to share with others because of the nature of the loss or the perception of others about that loss. These losses can include suicide, where the stigma may make it difficult to share thoughts and feelings, the possible guilt of not having recognised that there was anything wrong beforehand. There can be a feeling of being responsible for someone's suicide and this can never be *checked out*. There are also unknown or unacknowledged losses such as a relationship where the partner is unavailable for some reason such as already being in another committed relationship, or where the relationship is same sex and family and/or friends are unaware.

There are situations where a person has died from a disease that is feared or people are disgusted by it, e.g. alcohol or illegal-drug-induced conditions. Next we can consider refugees and asylum seekers, who may have witnessed crime and brutality towards their family and friends, and may even have experienced these things themselves. They will have lost their country, their culture and their sense of community. The attitude and language barrier in the host country may make it difficult to express these losses effectively.

The more that we are able to normalise the grieving process, starting with talking to children about feelings around loss and change, and its inevitability, the better able we will be to acknowledge situations. It will not hurt less but we will understand what is happening to us.

This section can give only a snapshot of some of the hidden losses that people experience and deal with. There are as many others as those named and they can only truly be recognised when we allow ourselves and others to explore what they are.

BEREAVEMENT SERVICES

Key recommendation 18 of the Supportive and Palliative Care Guidelines of NICE states that provider organisations should nominate a lead person to oversee development and implementation of services that focus on the needs of families and carers during the patient's life and, in bereavement, these services should reflect cultural sensitivity (NICE 2004b). The guidelines recommend that a three-component model of bereavement should be developed and implemented in each cancer network and that they should take account of the standards for bereavement care developed by the National Bereavement Consortium (2001):

- **Component 1**: many people lack understanding of grief after immediate bereavement. All bereaved people should be offered information about the experience of bereavement and how to access other forms of support. Often family and friends will provide much of this support
- **Component 2**: a more formal opportunity to review and reflect on their bereavement may be needed by some; however, this does not necessarily have to involve professionals. Faith groups, community groups and volunteer bereavement support workers or befrienders can provide much of the support at this level. However, a process of assessment should be in place to identify those people who may have more complex needs.
- **Component 3**: a minority of people will require more specialist help. This help should provide access to mental health services, psychological support services or specialist counselling/psychotherapy services. There should also be provision for the specialist needs of bereaved children and young people (NICE 2004b).

Although the subject of bereavement has been extensively researched over the years, that of bereavement support, e.g. what exists and best approaches to practice, has been less extensively researched.

In the first of two papers taking an in-depth organisational look at the English hospice bereavement services, Reid et al. (2006a) gathered data from 105 bereaved people. Data were collected via focus groups, joint interviews and one-to-one interviews. In their conclusion, they highlight three important findings:

- Pre-bereavement support makes an important positive contribution to the person's experience of bereavement. There should be continuity between pre-bereavement support and bereavement support.
- Hospices need to address the issue of risk assessment to identify those people most likely to need support.
- A clear rationale is a prerequisite for a bereavement service to develop an integrated and cohesive programme of support that can be helpful in resolving difficult decisions about individual bereavement clients (Reid et al. 2006a).

A further study by Reid et al. (2006b) looked at types of support offered in the English hospices. Semi-structured interviews and focus groups were conducted with paid and voluntary hospice staff and with bereaved people at each site. Documentary evidence was also collected. All five hospices ran events where bereaved people could meet. All also offered one-to-one support. Three types of one-to-one support were identified: counselling, befriending and support from paid bereavement staff. Although the paper concluded that overall all five hospices were offering appropriate types of bereavement support to meet components 1 and 2 of the NICE (2004b) guidelines, there seemed to be difficulty in accessing suitable sources of support for people with complex bereavement problems. The team recommended that hospice bereavement services should address component 3 of the NICE guidelines (NICE 2004b).

A comprehensive account of the organisation of bereavement services is outside the scope of this chapter. Further reading on this is recommended at the end of the chapter. Parkes (1994) highlights that carefully selected and well-trained volunteers can provide valuable support. It is important, if they have been bereaved, that they have 'come through it and . . . are not trying to vicariously solve their own

Table 9.1 Clinical presentations of complicated grief

Category	Features
Inhibited or delayed grief	Avoidance, postpones expression
Chronic grief	Perpetuation of mourning long term
Traumatic grief	Unexpected and shocking form of death
Depressive disorders	Both major and minor depressions
Anxiety disorders	Insecurity and relational problems
Alcohol and substance abuse/ dependence	Excessive use of substances impairs adaptive coping
Post-traumatic stress disorder	Persistent, intrusive images with cues
Psychotic disorders	Manic, severe depressive states and schizophrenia

Reproduced from Kissane (2005, p 1141) with permission.

problems'. Volunteers working in this capacity may support components 1 and 2 of bereavement support outlined in the NICE (2004b) guidelines.

A minority of people will require specialist interventions. It is important that all teams and organisations involved in generalist and specialist palliative care have access to mental health services. This could present a problem because research shows that employment of psychologists or psychiatrists in specialist palliative care is something of a rarity (Lloyd-Williams et al. 1999a). All this said, there are some reviews of bereavement counselling that indicate that it may not be useful for people experiencing normal grief and may, perhaps, have a negative impact (Schut et al. 2004; Jordan and Neimeyer 2003). After their analysis of four qualitative and quantitative reviews, one conclusion was that interventions are more helpful for those experiencing complicated grief. It is important also that health professionals can recognise signs of complicated grief and refer on appropriately (Table 9.1).

The use of a proactive screening tool to identify those at risk of complicated grief is recommended as perhaps offering preventive health benefits (Jordan and Neimeyer 2003).

Risk assessment

None of the five hospices studied by Reid et al. (2006a) used a formal method of risk assessment for the bereaved person, although all had processes in place to identify those whom it thought would benefit most from support. In line with a hospice approach all people were offered bereavement support; however, this is not in line with the NICE guidelines (2004a), which state that family carers should be assessed to determine their need.

The identification of risk is an important step towards prevention of ill health. Studies suggest that those most vulnerable to ill health as a result of bereavement can be recognised before or at the time of bereavement and will benefit from counselling (Parkes 1994). As discussed earlier Parkes (2005) identifies bereavement as a life event requiring PST and as such can precede mental illness.

Based on research, particularly the Harvard study of 49 widows and 19 widowers (Parkes and Weiss 1983), Parkes (1991) identifies the following aspects as determinants of grief outcomes:

- Circumstances of the death, anticipated, massive or multiple changes, brutal or violent events
- The nature of the attachment to the dead person, in terms of strength and security of attachment and ambivalence, in the relationship
- The personality and previous experience of the bereaved person, e.g. self-confidence, success or failure of resolutions of earlier PSTs
- Factors impinging after the event, e.g. social support, opportunities for new role and status
- Concurrent stresses.

Parkes has produced a Bereavement Risk Index (BRI). Subsequent studies have examined the validity of this tool and found that it discriminated between bereaved spouses at high and low risk of psychological distress before and after death (Robinson et al. 1995). Kristjanson et al. (2005) used a modified version of the BRI in their study of 150 bereaved family members. They concluded that the modified BRI demonstrated acceptable reliability and validity and was brief and simple to use. Nurses were able to use it with minimal training.

Jordan et al. (2005) developed a new instrument designed to screen for the development of a complicated mourning response in adult bereavement, called the Grief Evaluation Measure (GEM). The GEM provides a quantitative and qualitative assessment of risk factors including the mourner's loss and medical history, coping resources before and after death, and circumstances surrounding the death. Initial studies ($n = 23$ and $n = 92$), from various clinical and support settings, demonstrate good concurrent validity for established measures of bereavement trauma and physical and psychiatric symptoms, and good predictive validity for mourner adjustment a year after initial assessment. The researchers would welcome others to collaborate with research into the GEM.

Parkes (1994) comments that, as doctors, priests, social workers and nurses are likely to come into contact with people facing bereavement, they should develop the knowledge base needed to organise services appropriately. He adds that whether we like it or not we are agents of change, midwives at the birth of new identities (Parkes 1994).

CONCLUSION

Although bereavement by death of someone close to us is an inevitability of life, it is an experience that we are less used to in the twenty-first century. The nature of the bereavement may affect our ability to cope. Untimely deaths, or violent or accidental deaths may impact more than anticipated, *well-supported* deaths. Many people have written about bereavement. The works of Parkes, Worden, Walter, and Margaret and Wolfgang Stroebe have been highlighted here. Each of these adds to our understanding of bereavement; they are not in conflict with each other. Mourning customs and practices of different cultural groups are briefly outlined.

Children should not be excluded from talking about their grief and elderly people need special consideration because they are often exposed to multiple bereavements, sometimes their own adult children. Bereavement can predispose to physical and mental ill health. NICE (2004b) guidelines identify three components of confidence and recommend that individual needs be addressed through a variety of services. Identification of those most at risk of ill health is needed in order that appropriate referral to mental health services can be made.

MAIN IMPLICATIONS FOR PRACTICE

- In line with the NICE (2004a) guidelines health-care professionals should nominate a lead person specifically to focus on the needs of family and carers during the patient's illness and in bereavement.
- Services for families and carers should be culturally sensitive.
- Bereavement risk assessment and provision of a corresponding level of support may reduce the incidences of mental and physical ill health ascribed to bereavement.
- The Bereavement Risk Index designed by Parkes has been evaluated as a sound approach to risk assessment.
- The three-component model of bereavement support, as outlined here from the NICE guidelines, is what health-care organisations would do well to work towards.
- Children should be involved at all stages in the illness experience of a family member. Not to involve them leaves them vulnerable.
- People with special needs, e.g. learning disabilities and mental illness, need to be included and supported during the illness of someone for whom they care and in bereavement.
- Increasingly elderly people are outliving their children. The death of a child is always premature, whatever the ages concerned.

SUGGESTED FURTHER READING

Blackman N (2003) *Loss and Learning Disability*. London: Worth.
Neuberger J (1999) *Dying Well*. Hale, Cheshire: Hochland & Hochland.
Parkes CM (2006) *Love and Loss. The roots of grief and its complications*. London: Routledge.
Parkes CM, Laungani P, Young B (1997) *Death and Bereavement Across Cultures*. London: Routledge.
Silverman PR (2000) *Never Too Young to Know*. Oxford: Oxford University Press.
Wallbank S (1998) *The Empty Bed*. London: Dartman, Longman & Todd.

Websites

www.childbereavement.org.uk
www.crusebereavementcare.org.uk
www.winstonswish.org.uk
www.samaritans.org
www.UK-SOBS.UK
SOBS National helpline 0844 5616855

Chapter 10
Pain and other major symptoms: an integrated approach

KEY POINTS

- **Pain theories**: contemporary definitions of pain and pain theories echo an approach that considers the psychospiritual aspects of pain as well as the physical aspects.

   The main body of this text addresses the concept of chronic pain.
- **Psychological approaches**: cognitive–behavioural therapy, hypnosis, relaxation and visualisation are all therapies that have a robust evidence base but are generally under-utilised.
- **Physical approaches**: many physical approaches, e.g. application of heat, cold and transelectrical nerve stimulation, are cheap and effective. There is a growing body of evidence for the efficacy of acupuncture in helping with difficult symptoms. The expertise for these therapies is often, as the name suggests, with the physiotherapist.
- **Complementary therapies**: these are gaining in popularity in the UK, particularly in palliative care. Providing robust evidence is problematic. In the pursuit of a hard science approach we risk ignoring the collective voices of patients.
- **Creative therapies**: at the end of life the benefits of creative therapies are self-evident for those who choose them. The work of the Rosetta Life charity is exciting. Being creative at the end of life can be very special.

This chapter briefly looks at pain definitions and theories. After that, it reviews the many different non-pharmacological approaches to supporting people with pain and major symptoms. It includes both orthodox approaches, which in many instances are under-utilised, and complementary approaches. There will be an attempt to evaluate the credibility of therapies using the same evidence-based rating system as used by the National Institute for Health and Clinical Excellence (NICE), which is adapted from the work of Eccles and Mason (NICE 2004c; Table 10.1). However, by applying hard science to some approaches, e.g. complementary therapies and creative therapies, I think that we are in danger of dismissing studies and audits in which the patient's supporting voice is strong.

Table 10.1 Evidence-based rating system

Hierarchy of evidence		Grading of recommendations	
Level	Type of evidence	Grade	Evidence
Ia	Evidence from systematic reviews or meta-analysis of randomised controlled trials	A	Based on hierarchy I evidence
Ib	Evidence from at least one randomised controlled trial		
IIa	Evidence from at least one controlled study without randomisation	B	Based on hierarchy II evidence or extrapolated from hierarchy I evidence
IIb	Evidence from at least one other type of quasi-experimental study		
III	Evidence from non-experimental descriptive studies, such as comparative studies, correlation studies and case–control studies	C	Based on hierarchy III evidence or extrapolated from hierarchy I or II evidence
IV	Evidence from expert committee reports or opinions and/or clinical experience of respected authorities	D	Directly based on hierarchy IV evidence or extrapolated from hierarchy I, II or III evidence
NICE	Evidence from NICE guidelines or Health Technology Appraisal programme	NICE	Evidence from NICE guidelines or Health Technology Appraisal programme
HSC	Evidence from health service circulars	HSC	Evidence from health service circulars

From the National Institute for Health and Clinical Excellence (NICE 2004c) with permission.

In many studies qualitative interviews are used as well as quality-of-life measures. The interviews provide rich data on the experience of a therapy. Frequently they are extremely positive. There are many variables that can impact on quality-of-life scores over time, including disease progression and concurrent stresses. Patients' lives do not go into neutral because they are sick. However, unless the quality-of-life measures show a statistically significant score, the research is in danger of being dismissed. This undermines the predominant health-care philosophy that is captured in the title of the Department of Health's White Paper, *Our Health, Our Care, Our Say* (DH 2006). We should be mindful of this, particularly in palliative care when, in very simple terms, often the goal is to help people feel better about what is happening to them.

Complementary approaches

Complementary therapies are included in this chapter and their valuable place in palliative care recognised. However, because of a lack of legal regulation in this country *complementary therapists* can lay claim to expertise for which they may not have received adequate training, and this of course can be problematic. The reader is referred to the NICE (2004b) guidelines on supportive and palliative care in which a very clear distinction between complementary and alternative therapies is made. Complementary therapies are used alongside orthodox treatments with the aim of providing psychological and emotional support through the relief of symptoms. Alternative therapies, which offer a distinct alternative to orthodox treatments, are in no way recognised or recommended in this text. Health-care organisations are well advised to draw up policies that clearly identify the level of expertise that a given complementary therapist should have. *The National Guidelines for the Use of Complementary Therapies in Supportive and Palliative Care*, produced by the Prince of Wales's Foundation of Integrated Health (2003), provide invaluable information to underpin such policy-making. It is normal practice to seek the consent of the doctor in charge of a patient's care to proceed with a complementary therapy.

Different strokes for different folks

Not everybody will opt for complementary therapies or, indeed, for more orthodox approaches. This is taken as read. In an ideal world, given that this chapter is about pain and symptom management, patients should be given the choice to select an approach to pain and symptom management that they think will best suit them. In reality a paucity of resources, as a result of lack of money, and sometimes a lack of professional awareness of different therapies available, is more likely to dictate choice.

PAIN THEORIES

The International Association for the Study of Pain (IASP) defines pain as 'An unpleasant sensory and emotional experience associated with actual or potential tissue damage or described in terms of such damage' (IASP 1986). The IASP is the official world body dealing with the subject and is a multidisciplinary organisation. Members receive the journal *Pain*, and a regular update of international research findings and meetings. The IASP holds its congress every 3 years (Bowsher 1995).

The traditional theory of pain is known as the 'specificity theory'. This proposes that a specific pain system carries messages from pain receptors in the skin to a pain centre in the brain. This theory, which was popular and further developed in the first half of the twentieth century, was first described by Descartes in 1664.

As a result of research, we can have a more developed understanding of the mechanisms of pain sensations. Just as we have nerve endings that are sensitive to sound and responsible for hearing, so we also have nerve endings in the skin that are sensitive to mechanical deformations in the skin, i.e. touch. So there are also specialised nerve endings throughout the body that recognise tissue damage. These are called nociceptors. Pain results from the excitation of these specialised nerve endings and not over-stimulation of others (Bowsher 1995). The stimulation of the nerve endings is the result of a chemical substance that is released, or perhaps formed, as cells in the area are disrupted. Some drugs interfere with this process,

e.g. non-steroidal anti-inflammatory drugs (NSAIDs), and they prevent the generation of pain messengers in the specialised nociceptor nerve endings (Bowsher 1995).
Peripheral nerve fibres carrying the impulse generated by the painful stimulus enter
the spinal cord through the dorsal horn; they cross the cord to ascend predominantly in the opposite spinothalamic tract in the medulla and then to the cerebral
cortex, where the pain is perceived. Understanding this nerve anatomy and physiology has led to neurosurgery where it is sometimes possible, for example, to damage
the superficial grey matter of the dorsal horn without damaging deeper parts, thus
abolishing pain and sensation, but little else (Bowsher 1995).

The gate control theory of pain

The gate control theory of pain was first put forward by Melzack and Wall in 1965
(Melzack and Wall 1996). It complements the approach to pain taken by Dame
Cicely Saunders, Robert Twycross and their international colleagues, who saw pain
and its relief as having a psychological component as well as a physiological one.

   In the gate control theory it is proposed that pain signals that reach the nervous
system excite a group of small neurons. When the total activity of this 'pool of
neurons' reaches a certain level, a theoretical gate opens and allows the pain signals
to proceed to the high brain centres (*Mosby's Medical, Nursing and Allied Health Dictionary* – Anderson 2002). The gate can be closed, so relieving pain in two ways. It
can be pulled to from the outside by, for example, stimulation of larger peripheral
nerves, which are sensitive to touch, e.g. 'rubbing it better' or massage. It can be
pushed to from inside. This is achieved by messages descending from higher centres
in the brain. Therefore, pain may be helped by reducing patients' anxieties and/or
introducing diversional therapies, e.g. music therapy. Relaxation and guided
imagery work in this way.

Definitions of pain

The definition of pain attributed to the IASP quoted in the start of the chapter is
succinct and accurate. In the palliative care setting, the concept of total pain as outlined by Dame Cicely Saunders is one that endures and brings into focus the meaning
of a palliative approach. Dame Cicely writes that the concept of total pain was spelt
out to her in an answer given by one patient in 1963. When Dame Cicely asked her
to describe her pain, she said with no prompting: 'Well doctor, it began in my back,
but now it seems that all of me is wrong. I could have cried for injections and pills,
but I knew I mustn't. Nobody seemed to understand how I felt, and it was as if the
world was against me. My husband and son were marvellous, but they were having
to stay off work and lose their money. But it's wonderful to feel safe again' (Saunders
2000, in Clarke 2006, p 253). Dame Cicely comments on this reply in the following
way: 'Physical, emotional and social pain and the spiritual need for security, meaning
and self worth, all in one answer.' Another enduring definition that is often attributed to Beebe and McCaffery (1994) is: 'Pain is what the patient says it is and exists
when the patient says it does.' This definition, similar to the concept of total pain,
affirms that pain is much more than a physiological experience.

Pain, of course, is a symptom that something is wrong. A new pain needs investigating to decide what the problem is before it can be relieved. The pain may be caused by a septic focus and antibiotic treatment may be needed to control it. For the rest of this chapter the pain that is considered in physiological terms is chronic pain. However, before proceeding, it is important to differentiate between acute and chronic pain.

Acute pain

Acute pain is often of sudden onset. It serves the purpose of alerting the person to the presence of harmful stimuli. Its onset can be frightening and so associated with feelings of anxiety and fear. Gould and Thomas (1997) pinpoint two major manifestations of acute pain:

1. Superficial pain: superficial in that the sufferer may locate it on the surface of the body. Often it is described as sharp or pricking.
2. Deeper acute pain: usually presents as a burning or aching sensation. It originates in the deeper layers of the skin, muscles, joints, etc.

Chronic pain

This term is used in the context when patients report pain on a long-term basis. The IASP puts a figure of more than 3 months on this. The pain does not signal any new tissue injury component and so serves no known useful biological purpose. Psychological factors accompanying chronic plain can include depression (Payne and Gonzales 1996).

PSYCHOLOGICAL APPROACHES

Cognitive–behavioural therapy (evidence level A)

Cognitive–behavioural therapy offers a brief and convincing approach to people with emotional problems and there is considerable evidence for its effectiveness (Moorey and Greer 2006). The reader is referred to Chapter 7 where evidence for the use of psychological therapies in patient groups is reviewed.

The gate control model of pain highlights the importance of affective, cognitive and motivational perception of pain as well as sensory perception. In spite of this, the literature in palliative care about pain control has concentrated on direct links to tissue pathology and has been less concerned with the psychological variables (McGuire 1989). It has been demonstrated that psychological factors, including anxiety, self-efficacy and perceived control, can influence the experience of physiological symptoms such as pain, nausea, fatigue and sleep disturbances associated with advanced disease (Melzack and Wall 1996).

People will have a diverse response to threatening events and different sensations. The appraisal of the event (e.g. difficult symptom) will be influenced by the person's emotional arousal, and the behavioural response will likewise be influenced. The role of cognitive–behavioural therapy is to raise the awareness of patients that they have choices in the way that they appraise and respond to difficult sensations and situations. So the cognitive–behavioural perspective works on two assumptions: that people are active processors of information rather than passive recipients and that cognition, emotions and behaviours are to some extent causally related and people can modify the way that they view a situation affecting them (Turk and Feldman 2000). A period of assessment is necessary before reconceptualisation of a symptom can be attempted. It is important for the practitioner to establish a good relationship with the person before reconceptualisation can occur.

An example of reconceptualisation is, in the following case study, shared on a recent study day by a clinical nurse specialist working in palliative care using cognitive–behavioural therapy. The patient, Mrs A, had lung cancer. She felt overwhelming guilt as a result of her heavy smoking. Drawing a pie chart with Mrs A of the influences on her smoking helped to lessen her guilt, e.g. no health warnings in 1940s, positive role models smoked, husband had always smoked and she was unsupported in her attempts to stop. Also Mrs A hated having chemotherapy; with reconceptualisation, she saw it as positive – it was slowing the disease process down and she wanted that. She learnt simple visualisation and relaxation techniques to help the process of having chemotherapy (J Wickings 2007, personal communication). Cognitive–behavioural therapy is often short term, skills oriented and focused on the present. Mental health practitioners who offer this option are often much appreciated by terminally ill people, because their only agenda is to talk and help with psychological pain (Turk and Feldman 2000).

Recently a trial has been conducted looking at the effectiveness of brief training in cognitive–behavioural therapy techniques for palliative care practitioners. The trial was deemed successful and it was concluded that palliative care practitioners could be trained in cognitive–behavioural therapy techniques by a simple and brief training course. However, supervision is necessary to ensure maintenance of skills and confidence in their use (Mannix et al. 2006). A review of the literature on the nature of depression in Parkinson's disease concluded that it was a promising option for depressed patients coping with Parkinson's disease; however, more research is recommended (Cole and Vaughan 2005).

Hypnosis and related therapies

Hypnosis for symptom support including anxiety (evidence level A)

A hypnotic trance is described as a state of heightened and focused concentration and thus it can be used to manipulate the perception of pain (Breitbart et al. 2005b) and other symptoms. It is well established that hypnosis can be used as an adjunct to the management of cancer pain (Spiegel 1985; Douglas 1999). Hypnotherapy can also be used effectively in the management of invasive procedures that cause discomfort and pain (Montgomery et al. 2002). There have been a number of studies that demonstrate that the use of hypnosis and self-hypnosis can be useful in chemotherapy-related nausea and vomiting (Burish et al. 1983; Walker et al. 1999).

A review of 22 studies looking at behavioural interventions and hypnosis demonstrated these interventions as being effective with respect to specific symptoms such as anxiety, pain, nausea and vomiting (Trijsburg et al. 1992).

There is also mounting evidence that it is useful as an adjunct to more conventional psychotherapy treatments. A meta-analysis of 18 studies in which cognitive–behavioural therapy was compared with the same therapy supplemented by hypnosis was carried out by Kirsch et al. (1995). They concluded that hypnosis did substantially enhance treatment outcome. Thus, the average client receiving cognitive–behavioural hypnotherapy showed greater improvement than at least 70% of clients receiving non-hypnotic treatment.

Hypnosis for quality of life (evidence level B)

Liossi and White (2001) evaluated the efficacy of clinical hypnosis in the enhancement of quality of life in patients with advanced cancer in a randomised controlled clinical trail. Fifty terminally ill patients received either standard medical and psychological palliative care or standard care with the addition of hypnosis. The patients in the hypnosis group had weekly hypnosis sessions with a therapist for 4 weeks. The quality-of-life outcome measures used were: Hospice Anxiety and Depression Scale (Zigmond and Snaith 1983) and the Rotterdam Symptom Checklist (de Haes et al. 1990). The results demonstrated that the people in the hypnosis group had a significantly better overall quality of life and lower levels of anxiety and depression when compared with the standard care group. Studies also demonstrate that hypnosis can enhance coping abilities (Walker 1992; Walker et al. 1999) and help to reduce anxiety and depression (Burish et al. 1983; Trijsburg et al. 1992). There is in fact a large body of evidence to support the use of clinical hypnosis (Prince of Wales's Foundation of Integrated Health 2003). A more detailed look at some of these studies is included in Chapter 7.

There are contraindications for hypnosis, perhaps the most important one being where there is a pre-existing psychiatric condition or in depressed patients. It is also important to be aware of inexpert use. Clinicians should not work outside their own areas of expertise and training.

Relaxation and visualisation – quality of life (evidence level A)

Relaxation is a core skill for mental health practitioners, occupational therapists and physiotherapists. Relaxation is commonly achieved by focusing attention systematically on one's breathing, on sensations of warmth in the body and on the release of muscular tension in body parts. Verbal suggestion and imagery can be used to help promote this process. Increasingly doctors, nurses, complementary therapists and other allied professions are using relaxation and guided imagery techniques in supportive and palliative care. The question that arises is: are these conventional health-care practitioners in effect using hypnosis? Health-care professionals using hypnotic techniques such as relaxation, visualisation and guided imagery perhaps need to reflect on this and reappraise how well prepared and trained they are for this role (Prince of Wales's Foundation of Integrated Health 2003).

Relaxation and imagery were researched in the treatment of breast cancer by Bridge et al. (1988): 154 women with breast cancer stage I or II were included in the study; 15 dropped out before the end of the study. Researchers spent time with patients once a week. Control individuals were encouraged to talk about themselves. A relaxation group was taught concentration on individual muscle groups. A third group was taught relaxation and imagery – the imagery was a peaceful scene of their own choice. Relaxation and relaxation+imagery groups were given a tape-recording repeating instructions and told to practise for 15 minutes each day. Initial scores for the profile of mood states (Curran et al. 1995) and the Leeds general scales for depression and anxiety (Snaith et al. 1976) were the same in all groups. At 6 weeks total mood disturbance scores were significantly less in the intervention groups. Women in the combined intervention group were more relaxed than those receiving just relaxation training. Mood in the control group was worse. Women aged 55 and over benefited more.

Walker et al. (1999) looked at the effect of relaxation combined with guided imagery on quality of life and response to chemotherapy in 96 women with newly diagnosed breast cancer. Patients were randomised to control (standard care) and experimental (standard care plus relaxation training and imagery) groups. The imagery was to visualise host defences destroying tumour cells. Psychometric testing to evaluate mood and quality of life were carried out, before each of the six cycles of chemotherapy and 3 weeks after cycle 6: tests of personality and coping strategy were carried out before cycles 1 and 6. Clinical response to chemotherapy was evaluated after six cycles of chemotherapy using the UICC (Union International Contre le Cancer) criteria and pathological response was assessed from the tissue removed at the time. As hypothesised the experimental participants were more relaxed and easy going during the study. Quality of life was better in the experimental group (Global Self Assessment and Rotterdam Symptom Checklist – de Haes et al. 1990). The intervention also reduced emotional suppression (Courtauld Emotional Control Scale – Watson and Greer 1983). The incidence of clinically significant mood disturbance was very low and the incidences in the two groups were similar. Although the groups did not differ in clinical or pathological response to chemotherapy, imagery ratings were correlated with clinical response. Walker et al. (1999) suggest that these simple, inexpensive and beneficial interventions should be offered to patients wishing to improve quality of life during treatments.

General approach

Much has already been written in this book about the importance of an empathic approach, with the aim of health professionals having a mutual understanding with the patient of their predicament. This approach can help to reduce anxiety and less anxious patients may feel less pain. Beecher (1959) first reported this connection between perception of pain and anxiety when he was attending to soldiers badly wounded in combat. When removed to a field hospital, these soldiers often reported far less pain than would be expected. We also know from classic nursing research that patients who are kept well informed of routine events around hospital stays and methods of pain relief employed will perceive less pain than those who are not (Hayward 1975; Boore 1978). The Hope studies (Herth 1990a; Buckley 1998) demonstrated that maintaining independence and control can lessen psychological pain. As in the Hope Studies, Kirk (1992) found in her study that professionals showing an interest in an individual gave the patient confidence in self-worth and personal coping ability. It is important, therefore, that when approaching people in pain an accurate and thorough assessment is carried out (see Chapter 12). All procedures regarding therapeutic approaches to pain should be agreed with and, if necessary, carefully explained to the patient. The patient taking an active role in their pain control will, in most instances, get the maximum benefit from the intervention and have a greater sense of well-being. There will be times, however, when patients do not want, or perhaps are too ill for, active involvement. As usual the professional needs to respond to this accordingly. I have heard this referred to as dancing with our patients.

Religion and prayer (evidence level C)

The concept that facing death often brings the individual's spirituality into sharp focus is discussed in Chapter 6. Although spirituality is considered to be broader than religion, for many religion is a big part of their spirituality. In both Chapter 6, on hope and spirituality, and Chapter 8, on bereavement, discussions on religious customs as death nears have been included. Failure to recognise and observe the religious beliefs and customs of individuals can lead to considerable existential pain. When patients were asked if they would welcome enquiry about their religious/ spiritual lives if they became gravely ill, two-thirds said that they would and only 16 per cent said that they would not. Interestingly only 15% reported that a doctor had made a spiritual enquiry (Ehman et al. 1999).

It is argued that making sense is central to all shades of spirituality and crucial to the code of making the most of living with dying (Kellehear 2000). For many people, making sense is achieved within a religious context. Therefore, the role of a religious representative can be central in helping with that process.

In a study of 457 cancer patients, 271 (59%) used prayer and in a terminally ill sub-group 25 (52%) used prayer. The primary reasons for using prayers were described as anxiety reduction and to influence the course of the disease (Vachon et al. 1995).

In a randomised, double-blind study on prayer in a coronary care unit, patients in the group prayed for did better by having fewer deaths, were less likely to require endotracheal intubation and ventilatory support, fewer potent drugs were administered, there was a lower incidence of pulmonary oedema and less cardiopulmonary resuscitation was needed (Byrd 1988).

Singh (1998) describes a period of surrender into transcendence as being a time when a person may see visions of spiritual figures – family members or friends – who have died, and they can rest in the 'natural great peace'.

PHYSICAL APPROACHES

Application of heat

There are many technical ways of applying thermal therapy for the relief of pain, e.g. short wave diathermy, infrared radiation, and the reader is referred to specialist texts for these; these interventions need the expertise of a physiotherapist. This text confines itself to the use of electrical heat pads – which are in fact usually the shape and size of a hot water bottle. A hot water bottle used safely, i.e. do not use boiling water and ensure that it will not leak, has the same effect. Heat therapy is particularly soothing for deep aching pains and muscle pain. It is thought to be useful for the following reasons:

- By stimulating the thermoreceptors of the skin and possibly those in the deeper tissue, it closes the spinal cord pain gates, thus reducing intensity of pain transmission (Charman 1995). Psychologically warmth is nurturing.
- Raising the temperature accelerates metabolic processes, so vasodilatation may assist in the removal of oedema and metabolic waste products. It may also increase phagocyte and other white cell efficiency in, for example, combating local infection and removing dead cell debris (Charman 1995).

Application of cold

Ice has been used instinctively for many years to cool pain caused by inflamed tissue, whether resulting from burns, infection or allergic conditions. Recent acute trauma injury and burns benefit from prompt application of cold to reduce further damage and limit the inflammatory response (Charman 1995). The application of cold reduces metabolism and nerve conduction. The skin thermoreceptors are activated and this may divert the brain's attention from the nociceptors. Cold therapy is usually applied using ice cubes wrapped in 'terry towelling', or commercially available cold packs that are gel filled and stored in the refrigerator. Packets of frozen peas can, similar to gel packs, easily shape themselves to the part that needs relief, but they need to be wrapped in 'terry towelling'. However, freezing temperatures or near freezing temperatures should not be directly applied to the skin, because there is a real danger of tissue damage as a result of excess chilling and vasoconstriction (Charman 1995).

Transelectrical nerve stimulation (evidence level C)

A simple transelectrical nerve stimulation (TENS) system consists of a small battery-operated electrical pulse generator and electrodes. The electrodes are applied to the skin, usually close to the painful areas. The electrical stimulations can be pulsed or continuous and their intensity increased.

The first use of electricity to help in pain control goes back to about 2500 BC. In Ancient Egypt stone carvings in tombs from the Fifth Dynasty depict fish, *Malapterusus electricus* (a species of cat fish found in the river Nile), used in the treatment of painful conditions.

Theoretically, the percutaneous electrical stimulation provided by TENS helps to close the gate of the dorsal horn to incoming nociceptive stimulation. Clinical evidence to support this theory was provided by Wall and Sweet (1967) in their report on the use of high-frequency percutaneous electrical nerve stimulation for the relief of chronic neurogenic pain. Further interest was generated by Dr Norman Shealy in 1974. Shealy (1974) helped to develop a dorsal column stimulator. This involved the surgical implant of electrodes in the dorsal column of the spinal cord, which are operated by an external battery-operated device. Initially, patients were given a trial of electrical percutaneous stimulation. If they responded favourably then they were offered the dorsal column implant. Interestingly, some patients in Shealy's work responded better to TENS than they did to dorsal column stimulation (DCS). However, the efficacy of TENS is controversial and clinical trials to date are inconclusive.

Essentially, people should want to use the TENS method and believe in its efficacy. It is often a modality that will appeal to people who prefer to reduce oral medications. It has a great advantage of giving the patient control over time of use, frequency of use and intensity of sensation. TENS has minimal side effects. Documented contraindications include (Bercovitch and Waller 2005):

- Severe allodynia
- Incompetent patients
- Cardiac pacemakers
- Allergy to electrodes
- People suffering from epilepsy
- When driving or operating machinery
- During pregnancy
- Electrode placement on the anterior aspect of the neck, over the carotid sinuses and eyes
- Use of microwave with TENS.

TENS is non-invasive and cheap. Anecdotally problems exist with its use because health-care professionals are inexperienced and therefore under-confident in supervising it. It is of course far better if it is supervised by an expert; usually a physiotherapist can provide this expertise. In the absence of specialist expertise, health professionals should work in partnership with the patient and together they follow the instructions and help find the best way of using it, thus building the confidence of both patient and professional. When talking about TENS in the classroom, students have frequently commented that they experienced its use during labour pains in childbirth and it is a very effective method of pain control.

Palliative radiotherapy (evidence level A)

Radiotherapy is treatment with ionising radiation that causes damage to cellular DNA. Commonly, in clinical practice X-rays are used, produced from an X-ray machine or linear accelerator and gamma rays produced from a radioactive source (Hoskins 2005). Radical radiotherapy aims to cure a local tumour by complete eradication of the cancer cells. The aim of palliative radiotherapy is, however, to control local symptoms with minimum associated acute radiation reactions. During radical radiotherapy, the aim is also to minimise associated long-term tissue damage, which is achieved by first giving small doses of radiotherapy and building them up over a period of time; thus patients require radiotherapy on a daily basis over a period of time, e.g. 6 weeks. However, this timescale is not appropriate in palliative care where a treatment period of 6–8 weeks could be a major proportion of the patient's remaining time (Hoskins 2005).

The main reason for palliative radiotherapy is to achieve pain relief and the overall effect is to shrink the tumour. This approach is useful where solid tumours are pushing on nociceptors and also where tumours are occluding a small space. Palliative treatments can be delivered in one or two treatments. This will not kill all cancer cells (between 60 and 80% of the total are killed in the first one or two radiation treatments). It is rarely necessary to extend palliative radiotherapy over more than 1 week, i.e. two treatments. This results in less troublesome side effects (Hoskins 2005).

Sometimes, immediately after a treatment of radiotherapy, a tumour, because of the irritation of cells, becomes slightly enlarged before the shrinking process begins. Therefore, symptoms can seem temporarily worse. This should settle down after a few days.

Combining the responses of 16 surveys that detailed almost 2500 treatments for bone pain, gave a mean complete response rate of 52% and a mean overall response rate of 86% (only four of the studies included data on duration of response). However, 1 year after treatment 65–90% of the patients included in the studies were still pain free (Gilbert et al. 1977; Garmatis and Chu 1978).

As most bony metastases are the result of vascular spread isolated deposits are not uncommon. For these people, hemibody radiotherapy is a treatment option and it provides relief in about 75% of patients (Twycross 1995).

Palliative radiotherapy is usually well tolerated. The patients may feel tired – more tired than usual. Sometimes the patient is nauseated, particularly if the radiotherapy treatment involves the abdomen (Watson et al. 2006).

Acupuncture

The word acupuncture is derived from the Latin *acus* – needle – and *pungere* – to pierce. This therapeutic technique, which involves the insertion of fine needles into the skin and the underlying tissues at specific points, has its origins at least 2000 years ago in China (Ma 1992). Qi (pronounced chee) is a fundamental concept in traditional Chinese medicine. Qi is usually translated as energy, and is associated with the image of a warm heart, a full stomach and a sense of well-being in health (Birch and Felt 1999). A person's qi is present at birth and circulates throughout the body, thus maintaining its physiological functions. When qi is fully dissipated death occurs. Maintaining qi to some extent depends on balancing the two opposites. Qi circulates in the body along meridians, which are deep channels joining a series of acupuncture points on the surface of the body. There are 12 paired, 2 unpaired and several extra meridians. Traditionally, to make a diagnosis after taking a history, a complex tongue and pulse diagnosis at both radial arteries can subtly diagnose disease in 12 distant organs (Filshie and Thompson 2005).

A current proposed mechanism for acupuncture analgesia is that, by stimulating peripheral nerves in the muscles, messages are sent to the central nervous system (CNS). In the CNS the spinal cord, hypothalamus/pituitary and midbrain are activated to release endorphins and enkephalins, which block pain perception (Pomeranz 2000).

For chronic pain management (evidence level C)

There is extensive anecdotal evidence to support the use of acupuncture for chronic pain. Numerous publications describe the use of acupuncture analgesia (White 1998). In China 6% of surgical operations are performed with acupuncture as the only analgesia (Filshie and Thompson 2005). However, in a systematic review of 10 randomised controlled studies evaluating the effectiveness of acupuncture for chronic pain, some were described as being of poor quality and overall the evidence provided was described as conflicting (NICE 2001). There are many difficulties inherent in conducting a randomised controlled study to assess the effectiveness of acupuncture and it is outside the scope of this book to examine them. That said, the anecdotal evidence from our patients should not be dismissed. In palliative care the failure of pharmacological measures to control pain has led to using treatments without drugs, such as acupuncture. In a summary of two extensive audits, acupuncture helped patients who were excessively sensitive to normal doses of analgesia and also those who still had pain when on recommended doses (Filshie and Redman 1985; Filshie 1990). Filshie and Thompson (2005) also note that acupuncture can be helpful and relaxing for people who are having difficulties coming to terms with their illness or who are distressed by anger or denial.

Acupuncture is currently performed in over 84% of pain clinics (Woollam and Jackson 1998; Clinical Standards Advisory Group 2003). Twenty-one per cent of GP practices offer access to acupuncture (Thomas et al. 2001). It would seem that acupuncture is established as a standard complementary form of treatment in addition to orthodox treatment methods.

For nausea and vomiting (evidence level A)

The P6 acupressure point is found just above the wrist, i.e. three finger-breadths above the distal skinfold of the wrist joint, between the tendons of the palmaris longus and carpi radialis muscles (Roscoe et al. 2002).

Many randomised controlled studies have been conducted, mainly using the traditional P6 point with a variety of stimuli to reduce chemotherapy-induced nausea and vomiting. Acupuncture, electroacupuncture, acupressure and TENS were all compared with a control treatment. Seven of eight studies reviewed were positive. Being proactive in preventing nausea and vomiting by use of the P6 point is more successful than treating nausea and vomiting once it has occurred (Dundee et al. 1987; Stannard 1989; Dibble et al. 2000; Shen et al. 2000; Macmillan Cancer Relief 2002).

Vickers (1996) concluded, in a systematic review of the research, that although not all studies were methodologically perfect P6 acupuncture seemed to be an effective antiemetic technique. It is worth noting that this review was based on 33 controlled trials published worldwide. Vickers identified 12 of the trials as being high-quality, randomised, placebo-controlled trials in which P6 acupuncture point stimulation was not administered under anaesthesia. Eleven of these trials involving 2000 patients showed an effect of P6. The reviewed papers showed consistent results across different groups of patients and different forms of acupuncture point stimulation (Vickers 1996).

Research looking at the efficacy of acustimulation wristbands for chemotherapy-induced nausea yielded positive, but not conclusive, results (Roscoe et al. 2002).

For breathlessness (evidence level D)

There is a paucity of trials in the use of looking at the use of acupuncture/acupressure in breathless patients. In spite of this, Ernst (2001) when reviewing the evidence felt that the data supported the use of acupressure to relieve breathlessness for patients with severe chronic obstructive pulmonary disease.

As a result of observations that acupuncture gave subjective improvement in breathless patients, Filshie et al. (1996) conducted a pilot study on 20 patients to look at the effect of acupuncture on the symptom of cancer-related breathlessness at rest. Outcome measures showed significant improvement, on a visual analogue scale (VAS), of subjective scores of breathlessness, relaxation and anxiety at 90 minutes. There was also an objectively significant reduction in respiratory rate that was sustained for the treatment period. Seventy per cent (14/20) reported symptomatic benefit from the treatment. Eight of these patients agreed to have indwelling studs into the sternal point, aiming to prolong the response. Patients could then massage the studs during periods of breathlessness and panic, or before trivial exercise. This gave more control to the patients. All reported varying degrees of benefit lasting up to 2 weeks.

The two sternal semipermanent needles are now available and can be used in palliative care units. They are called ASAD – short for **a**nxiety, **s**ickness and **d**yspnoea – points. They can remain in place for up to 4 weeks covered by a clear plastic dressing (Filshie and Thompson 2005).

COMPLEMENTARY THERAPIES

Massage and aromatherapy massage (evidence level for anxiety reduction A; to reduce pain, nausea and improve sleep pattern level D)

Massage and aromatherapy massage are popular complementary therapies in the palliative care world and have been subjected to well-designed research studies.

Corner et al.'s (1995) study compared back massage in 52 patients. Patients were assigned to three different groups: a control group of patients who were unable to attend a course of massage, a group receiving massage with a plain carrier oil and another receiving massage with a blend of essential oils. Participants completed the Hospital Anxiety and Depression (HAD) scale (Zigmond and Snaith 1983) and Quality of Life Symptom of Distress scale (Holmes and Dickerson 1987), providing quantitative data. Pre- and post-massage interviews gave qualitative data. The study concluded that massage has a significant effect on anxiety and that this effect is greater when essential oils are used.

In Wilkinson et al.'s (1999a) study, a consecutive series of 103 patients were randomly allocated to one of two groups: those receiving a full body massage with carrier oil only and those receiving a full body massage with carrier oil and 1% Roman Camomile essential oil. Members of both groups showed a statistically significant reduction in anxiety after each massage on the State–Trait Anxiety Inventory (STAI) (Spielberger et al. 1983). Wilkinson et al. (1999a) concluded that 'massage with or without essential oils appears to reduce levels of anxiety. The addition of essential oils seems to enhance the effect of the massage and improve physical and psychological symptoms as well as overall quality of life'.

A larger study by Cassileth and Vickers (2004) involving 1290 patients over a 3-year period used 0–10 rating scales for pain, fatigue, stress/anxiety, nausea, depression and 'other'. After the massage, symptoms were reduced by 50%, even for patients reporting high baseline scores. Outpatients improved about 10% more than inpatients. Benefits persisted, with patients experiencing no return to baseline scores through a duration of a 48-hour follow-up; 48 hours may not sound very long, but it may be a sizeable time at the end of life.

These are three well-conducted research studies among many. A Cochrane systematic review conducted by Fellowes et al. (2004) concluded that there was insufficient evidence to form firm conclusions about the benefits of massage and aromatherapy massage for cancer patients. It did conclude that massage alone and massage with aromatherapy oils might reduce anxiety in cancer patients in the short term. More evidence is needed to assess its effectiveness on physical symptoms. However, we must wonder at the wisdom of applying hard science in this way to complementary therapies, particularly complementary therapies in end-of-life care.

The application of rigorous statistical analysis diminishes the individual story. However, it is the individual story that can be extremely powerful in demonstrating the value of a given intervention. I have often used one-off hand and foot massage intuitively. I call this first aid complementary therapy.

Here are two examples of its use.

Case study 1

Mr A was an 86 year old. His prognosis was expressed in terms of weeks. He was determined to remain independent and required minimal help with hygiene needs. I went to his room routinely to find that he had been incontinent of faeces. He had clearly sought to find a lavatory and faeces were spread around the room as well as on his body. It took a long time to clean Mr A and his room. An empathic approach and efforts to preserve his self-esteem centred around conversation of how to reduce the chance of a recurrence. His shame and embarrassment were palpable. Returning with a cup of tea for him, intuitively I offered to massage his feet, to which he readily consented. The massage lasted about 15 minutes. He seemed to relax and we chatted quietly about his family, making no reference to the previous episode. His visitors arrived just as I was finishing. He smiled and greeted them warmly; his son remarked on how rested he looked. Mr A said he felt like 'a cat that had been given cream'.

Buckley (2002b)

Case study 2

Niki was an 18 year old dying of cancer. She lived with her parents and younger sister. She had accepted her prognosis in an almost matter-of-fact way and had supported her family and fiancé as they battled to accept the thought of losing her so early. Niki had been overweight before her illness and her weight loss as a result actually suited and pleased her. She wore beautiful clothes and looked very good in them. About 3 weeks before her death, her mother phoned me to request an urgent visit. Niki, she said, had 'lost it' and was hysterical. She was indeed very upset when I arrived. Almost overnight her legs had both become very swollen with oedema and she was becoming jaundiced. The newly acquired pride in her body image was crumbling fast. I talked about support tights, keeping legs up and con-tacting her GP, possibly for diuretics. After that there was little I could offer from my 'nurse's toolbox', so I suggested massage – she accepted. I spent about 30 minutes massaging both feet. She was calm and sleepy when I finished. I visited again later in the day and taught her mother how to do it. Massage was performed three or four times a day until she died. She enjoyed the sensation of the massage and felt calm and sleepy afterwards. Her mother was very comforted at being able to help her daughter in this tangible way.

Palliative care is about the individual and the individual's experience. 'You matter because you are you and you matter until the last moment of your life.' This is a famous quote from Dame Cicely Saunders.

Buckley (2002b)

Reflexology (evidence level D)

Reflexology like acupuncture has its roots in ancient times. Paintings from a physician's tomb provide evidence of treatments being carried out in India in 5000 BC. The Chinese may have used it since 4000 BC and foot treatment is documented by the Yellow Emperor who died in 2598 BC.

Reflexology is described as a sophisticated system of touch, usually on the feet, but sometimes on the hands, ears, face, tongue and back. The theory is that work on specific areas of the feet can influence other areas of the body (Tiran 2002). According to Lett (2000) it is a means of maintaining homeostasis, aiding relaxation and also triggering the body's innate self-healing capacity.

There is a good deal of anecdotal evidence to support the use of reflexology in cancer care. Good effects are reported for relaxation, well-being and stress relief (Gillard 1988; Stephenson 1996; Botting 1997; Joyce and Richardson 1997.

Modern medicine speculates on how it works. It may be that the pressure of reflexology stimulates larger peripheral nerves, thus closing the gate to stimulation of the smaller peripheral nociceptors, hence relieving pain. Another theory is that reflexology may release endorphins and enkephalins by CNS stimulation. Enkephalins and endorphins are frequently referred to as the body's natural pain relievers and mood enhancers.

A Cochrane systematic review of the use of reflexology in improving physical and psychological well-being of patients with cancer found no less than 312 references, a sign of how much interest there is in the use of reflexology. However, only three met the inclusion criteria. The review found methodological problems with both randomised controlled trials in the three studies selected (Fellows et al. 2004). The two most robust studies were conducted by Grealish et al. (2000) and Hodgson (2000).

Grealish et al. used a nursing intervention of foot massage on 87 patients hospitalised with cancer. Patients were randomly allocated to one of three factor control groups. Using visual analogue scales to measure self-reports of pain, nausea and vomiting and relaxation, their findings supported foot massage having a significant immediate effect on pain, nausea and relaxation.

Hodgson's (2000) study of 11 patients with cancer compared the effects of a course of real or placebo reflexology treatments on quality of life, using Holmes and Dickerson's (1987) scale. All the patients in the reflexology group reported an improvement in their quality of life. However, improvement in breathing was the only individual system with a statistically significant result. Both groups said that the treatments were relaxing, calming and comforting.

Various audits of services have concluded that relaxation, relief from tension and anxiety, and improved well-being are the primary benefits of reflexology in palliative care (Hills and Taylor 2001; Milligan et al. 2002; Gambles et al. 2002).

Aromatherapy (evidence level D)

According to Buckle (2003) aromatherapy is the fastest growing of all complementary therapies. Some of the evidence base has been reviewed in the earlier section on aromatherapy massage.

Aromatherapy is described as the systematic use of essential oils in treatments to improve physical and emotional well-being (National Occupation Standards for Aromatherapy 2002). Essential oils can be used in a variety of ways; as well as massage, oils can be used in vaporisers, baths, creams, lotions and compresses, and are absorbed via the skin as well as being inhaled.

The therapeutic effect of oils has been described as working in the following way by Kohn (1999). The fragrance of the oils stimulates the sense of smell, which elicits certain emotions. The limbic system of the midbrain, which is concerned with emotion as well as visceral functions, may be involved in the release of hormones that influence mood. If essential oils are used in health care, they should be used and mixed by a trained aromatherapist who is registered with a professional body. Local policy may be designed for the safe use of a range of

Table 10.2 Examples of properties of some essential oils

Specific essential oils with antiemetic properties (Buckle 2003)

- Cardamon
- Ginger
- Lavender
- Peppermint: this has been used for the treatment of nausea for hundreds of years. However, too much can cause nausea

Essential oils recommended for use in chronic pain (Buckle 2003)

- Black pepper
- Clove bud
- Frankincense
- Ginger
- Juniper
- Lavender (spike)
- Lavender (true)
- Lemongrass
- Marjoram (sweet)
- Myrrh
- Peppermint
- Rose
- Verbena
- Ylang Ylang

essential oils by other members of the health-care team, e.g. in vaporisers. Aromatic oils in vaporisers, baths or added to a carrier oil can be used in symptom control as an adjunctive therapy or sometimes tried as an alternative to an orthodox therapy (see Table 10.2).

Many studies have been done in an effort to provide an evidence base for the practice of aromatherapy. Jane Buckle's book, *Clinical Aromatherapy* (listed at the end of this chapter), provides an indepth look at the use of aromatic oils in health care. As with many complementary therapies, in spite of strenuous efforts, there is a poorly defined evidence base for aromatherapy. However, it was one of the most widely used complementary therapies in supportive and palliative care in a survey carried out in the late 1990s. Service evaluations and audits highlight that patients perceive it as effective and beneficial (Dunwoody et al. 2002).

Energy therapies

The use of energy therapies is perhaps the least understood and acceptable to western orthodox practitioners. As in all therapies, complementary or orthodox, patients will feel easier and more enthusiastic about some than others. In an ideal world patients should make their own choices. The health-care professional, it could be argued, has an ethical duty to try to ensure that patient choices are well informed, as discussed at the start of this chapter.

Reiki, spiritual healing and therapeutic touch

Although these therapies have separate trainings and slightly different approaches they also have strong similarities.

Reiki

Reiki is defined from two words: *rei* meaning higher intelligence that guides the creation and functioning of the universe and *ki* referring to the life force energy that flows through every living thing, including plants, animals and human beings (Quest 1999). Reiki was rediscovered in Japan as a method of healing in the 1800s. The main aim of reiki is to bring about balance in mind, body and spirit to improve well-being. There are no religious connotations and therefore no particular belief system is necessary to give or receive reiki.

During a reiki treatment the recipient remains fully clothed and may sit or stand. The practitioner holds his or her hands on or just above certain parts of the body. Reiki energy is channelled for the 'greatest and highest good' of the recipient and is understood to flow in response to need from the recipient (Prince of Wales's Foundation of Integrated Health 2003).

A study by Wardell and Engebretson (2001) looked at biological correlates of reiki healing. After receiving reiki for 30 minutes, 23 healthy individuals were measured by biological markers after the test and these were compared with before the test. The markers included respiratory rate, pulse rate, blood pressure and salivary immunoglobulin tends. Significant biochemical and physiological charges in the direction of relaxation were found. There is a lack of scientific evidence to support reiki in supportive and palliative care. However, there is mounting anecdotal evidence that, through its profound relaxation effect, reiki alleviates anxiety, stress and perception of pain, and promotes a feeling of well-being, particularly relating to psychospiritual well-being (Mansour et al. 1999).

Patients' voices are considered central to informing service development within the modern NHS (DH 1997). As Burden et al. (2005) state, this being so, research into how patients experience reiki should acknowledge the value of how they feel. This would emphasise the importance of the patient's voice underpinning services at all levels from policy development to service delivery.

Spiritual healing (evidence level C1)

Healing has been practised over the centuries and has been documented in all major civilisations and cultures. Healing in this context is not to be confused with providing a cure; rather it is concerned with any positive action directed by one person to another with the intention of helping. A caring touch, a kind word, attentive listening and a smile are all healing (Brown 1998). In this context, healing links closely to research looking at hope, in which patients frequently stated that the small things that people did, e.g. being friendly and interested in them, gave them a feeling of hopefulness (Herth 1990a; Buckley and Herth 2004).

A healing session usually lasts about 20 minutes. A spiritual healer prepares for a session by atunement. This means that they still themselves to find their inner core of peace. They will focus their attention on the highest source of peace and love in the universe that they can imagine. The healer then consciously directs this experience of union with the universal source through themselves to their patients. This is called channelling. This type of healing may be called 'laying on of hands', although the hands are normally held a short distance from the body (Brown 1998).

Brown (1998), a GP, established a healing clinic in his practice some 20 years ago. Patients referred to the healing clinic tend to be those with long-standing chronic conditions. Using a quality-of-life questionnaire as a measure of outcome, he was able to demonstrate consistently patients showing changes of statistical significance after eight weekly sessions and at follow-up of 26 weeks. Healers do not usually relate to the disease entities of conventional medicine, but aim to help the person in more general terms, e.g. by increasing well-being (Ernst 2001).

There is an enormous amount of contemporary interest in healing. Benor (2001) did a meta-analysis of 191 controlled studies across a broad range of conditions and organisms. Fifty per cent of the trials were described as having significant outcomes in favour of healing. Abbot describes Benor's interpretation of data as unconventional. A further meta-analysis of 59 randomised clinical trials, comparing healing with a control on human participants, found no firm conclusions about the efficacy or inefficacy of healing (Abbot 2000).

Spiritual healing is a popular therapy in supportive and palliative care (Macmillan Cancer Relief 2002). 'The process of healing, either in the general sense or specifically spiritual healing, is to be compassionate and caring. The goal of healing is to facilitate spirituality. Patients are encouraged to understand their illness and find meaning and purpose' (Brown 1998, p 380).

Therapeutic touch

This is emerging as one of the most popular energy healing methods. In spite of its name, it involves no direct contact. Healers hold their hands a few inches above the patient's body and sweep away blockages in the patient's energy field (Cassileth and Schulman 2005). Therapeutic touch is not regarded as involving channelling of energy, but more as a mutual process, a healing meditation. It has been described as an attempt to focus completely on the well-being of the patient in an act of unconditional love and compassion (Quinn and Strelkaukas 1993).

In a group of 60 people, participants in a control group were treated with mimic touch and an experimental group received therapeutic touch. The results supported the hypothesis that the therapeutic touch group would experience greater relief from headache and indeed this persisted for 4 hours after treatment.

Probably as important as the research are audits and evaluation of services – in other words patients' voices support therapeutic touch. In an audit by Hallett (1996) with oncology patients, she found the following response to therapeutic touch:

- 75% said that they were coping better
- 70% reported feeling less anxious
- 47.5% felt happier
- 75% felt more peaceful and calm.

Other responses included coping better with chemotherapy and radiotherapy (32.5%); 40% reported feeling in more control and 37.5% felt that therapeutic touch had helped them to adjust to their diagnosis. A later audit by Hallett produced very similar findings.

CREATIVE THERAPIES

Rosetta Life

The value of creative therapies at the end of life have been brought into focus in recent years by the activities of the charity Rosetta Life (www.rosettalife.org). This charitable organisation is now working across 25 hospices in the UK and abroad, and it represents the voice of hospice users and their families and carers. Working in collaboration with artists in residence in hospices, it devises national projects that celebrate creativity for people receiving end-of-life care.

Rosetta Life was conceived by Lucinda Jarrett while she was working as a volunteer at St Joseph's Hospice in London. The original project was called Life Stories. It was specifically set up to enable people facing death to tell their stories and share experiences that matter to them and their families. Lucinda's talent meant that the narratives were not confined to the written word – for some, a very precious medium, for others less attainable – but included video recording, theatrical productions, as well as music and painting and other media. Individuals can narrate their unique story in a style and medium of their choice and patients in groups can present a collective narrative. The Rosetta website is a rich and steep learning curve in what people can achieve and contribute at the end of life. Examples of their current works can be seen on the website at www.rosettalife.org.

Rosetta requiem (an example of one project) enables people to express themselves through art at a time when words fail. The collection of films and songs includes collaboration between Roots Manuva and a teenager from Great Ormond Street Hospital, and Maxine Edgington's song, 'We Laughed', which she wrote for her daughter as a legacy. The song was put to music by Billy Bragg and became a top 20 hit. It is available for purchase from Rosetta Life's website (www.rosettalife.org).

There are many other examples of different projects using a great variety of artistic media on their website. They are now widening their website access and developing partnerships with regional Motor Neurone Disease Associations, the Multiple Sclerosis Society and the Stroke Association, aiming to help people living with chronic illness to participate online in the arts projects that are run regionally and nationally.

Art therapy

Art therapy is not an occupational or diversional therapy. It provides a supportive environment in which a person can make a connection with a qualified art therapist and explore personal issues. It provides an opportunity to express emotions that may feel unacceptable to the patient, e.g. in art therapy, pounding clay, scribbling violently on paper gives permission to express strong feelings. Art therapy also allows for the development and expression of more positive feelings, e.g. tenderness, hope or beauty (Wood 2005).

Developing research methodology that can evaluate the effectiveness of art therapy is a considerable challenge. A review of art therapy literature suggests that it can positively contribute to patients' well-being and, in some cases, be more effective than other interventions (Reynolds et al. 2000).

Note that it is not intended in any way here to devalue the arts and crafts sessions that take place in many health-care settings. As an onlooker to these sessions, the degree of involvement and enjoyment that they can bring are very obvious. Being creative at the end of life creates a juxtaposition that can bring enormous satisfaction as, for example, an unexpected legacy is created. I believe that this can be a positive adjunct in supporting patients in existential pain.

Music therapy

Music therapy, with its ability to offer an experience of time that is qualitatively rich and not solely chronologically determined, is a valuable intervention in palliative care. It has the power to calm and stir us, and it is this potential that a music therapist can bring to the palliative care setting. Music therapy is suitable for patients and those closest to them who want to explore whether different musical experiences can help them to encounter the illness experience. People do not have to have a musical background to gain from music therapy, any more than they have to be an artist to enjoy and gain from art therapy (Aldridge 1999).

Music for pain (evidence level A)

A Cochrane review was carried out to evaluate the effect of music on acute and chronic cancer pain intensity, pain relief and analgesic requirements. Randomised controlled trials that evaluated the effect of music on any type of pain in children or adults were included. Trials that reported on concurrent non-pharmacological therapies were excluded. Fifty-one studies involving 1867 individuals exposed to music and 1796 control individuals met the inclusion criteria.

It was concluded that music should not be considered a first-line treatment for pain. Listening to music for treatment offers low cost, ease of provision and a safe approach to supporting people in pain. The review authors felt that music reduced pain, increased the number of patients who reported at least 50% pain relief and reduced requirements for morphine-like analgesia. They noted that the magnitude of their positive effects is small and the clinical relevance of music for pain relief unclear (Capeda et al. 2006).

Music for nausea and vomiting (evidence level D)

A randomised study with 33 patients undergoing bone marrow transplantation found less nausea and fewer instances of vomiting in the group who received music therapy (Ezzone et al. 1998). A case–control study involving patients receiving a bone marrow transplant also demonstrated decreased nausea with music therapy (Sahler et al. 2003).

CONCLUSION

There are many approaches to pain and symptom control cited here that are under-utilised, even when there is evidence to support their use. It is hoped that, in the future, we will see this changing and that patients will be offered more choice at the end of life.

MAIN IMPLICATIONS FOR PRACTICE

- It is important to keep an open mind to different ways of supporting patients experiencing pain and difficult symptoms.
- Although collecting an evidence base is valued, in the pursuit of this we should not close our minds to the collective voices of patients.
- Health-care professionals have a responsibility to ensure that they are well informed about what services exist locally to them.
- When introducing new services, e.g. complementary therapies, it is important that robust policies are in place to support the implementation and protect the patient.

SUGGESTED FURTHER READING

Brown CK (1998) The integration of healing and spirituality into health care. *J Interprof Care* **12**: 373–8.

Buckle J (2003) *Clinical Aromatherapy: Essential oils in practice*, 2nd edn. Edinburgh: Churchill Livingstone.

Carroll D, Bowsher D (1995) *Pain Management in Nursing Care*. Oxford: Butterworth Heinemann.

Douglas DB (1999) Hypnosis: Useful, neglected, available. *Am J Hospice Palliative Care* **16**: 665–70.

Moorey S, Greer S (2002) *Cognitive Behaviour Therapy for People with Cancer*. Oxford: Oxford University Press.

Prince of Wales's Foundation of Integrated Health (2003) *National Guidelines for the use of Complementary Therapies in Supportive and Palliative Care*. Available at: ww.fihealth.org.uk.

Websites

www.fihealth.org.uk
www.rosettalife.org.uk

Chapter 11
The history of the use of strong opioids for cancer pain

KEY POINTS

- **Narratives of pain**: patient narratives in the post-war years of the twentieth century highlight that cancer patients often suffered unremitting intractable pain.

    Neurosurgical techniques for the relief of pain were favoured. Morphine was seen as a last resort for doctors and they feared patients becoming addicted.

- **Studies of pain and the use of morphine**: studies by Dame Cicely Saunders, Robert Twycross, John Bonica and Raymound Houde all demonstrated the value of individually titrated morphine for patients with cancer pain. This culminated in the World Health Organization's analgesic ladder.

    The International Association for the Study of Pain constructed the WHO ladder; its use is explained.

- **Re-education**: patients and health-care staff needed re-education. Morphine seldom causes severe psychological dependence (as seen in abuse) when used for pain relief.

    Patients need reassurance that morphine is no longer used as a last resort in cancer care.

- **Adjuvant approaches**: adjuvant approaches and analgesics for specific pains are highlighted.

- **Different routes of administration**: a strong opioid is a term used to describe all morphine-type drugs.

    Different routes of administration are highlighted with reference to use of a syringe driver.

    Syringe drivers: The rationale for the dose of drugs that are prescribed for syringe drivers is explained. The dose is the equivelent to the oral dose being taken by the patient.

It would be an impossibility ever to fully assess the impact that the two world wars of the first half of the twentieth century have had on our society. Within health care, scientists, doctors and surgeons were stimulated to develop new drugs, new approaches, and more advanced and radical surgery, in the effort to prevent death and, where possible, to cure and restore. Although perhaps not felt consciously by many, it is almost certain that the tremendous increases and advances made in medical science were the result of man's love of his fellow man – a feeling of responsibility to give the very best care to those who suffered injury and disease as a direct result of war.

The poor health of conscripts for World War II reflected the plight of the health of our nation. Many potential conscripts were underweight and malnourished, and so failed the medical to join the fighting. Immediately after the war, the National Health Service was born and so the progress in medical science continued. With regard to pain relief, the dominant approach developed at this time was the neurosurgical one. Much work went into developing methods of destroying peripheral nerves and central pathways. Nerves can be exposed by open surgery, but with the development of techniques to inject substances into nerves, less drastic operations were possible (Melzack and Wall 1996). This new-found optimism in health care in newly developed hospitals and research centres worldwide led to the idea that cancer could be cured or contained (Seymour et al. 2005).

However, many patients with cancer in the early post-war period presented very late. Only terminal care was available in these situations and, as such, admission to hospital was rare. Probably as a result of this, the pain of advanced cancer was initially neglected as a worthwhile object of study (Seymour et al. 2005).

Beecher (1959) is among the first to relate perception of pain to the state of the mind. During World War II he worked on the battlefields. He was astonished that injured soldiers carried into combat hospitals complained of so little pain. Most of the soldiers denied having pain from their extensive wounds or had so little that they did not request medication. Beecher (1959) highlighted that these men were not in a state of shock and nor were they unable to feel pain; they would complain about inept venepuncture, for example! He attributed their failure to feel pain to a sense of relief at having escaped alive from the battlefield.

STUDIES AND NARRATIVES

Commonly studies in the post-war period highlighted that dying people at home were suffering many intolerable symptoms, including pain. One such major study in this country by Cartwright et al. (1973) was undertaken in 12 registration districts in England and Wales; 960 deaths in all were explored with bereaved relatives; 66% of patients suffered pain. Narratives about painful death were occurring outside medicine. As early as 1959 in Linda Caven's book, *Twice a Victim*, she describes herself being smitten with the most agonising pain, due to cancer, and she feared that her groans would wake other patients. In the 1970s Victor and Rosemary Zorza's account of the story of their 25-year-old daughter dying from skin cancer made the national press and touched the heart of the nation. This statement sums up perhaps how she felt: 'If I am going to spend a large part of the rest of my life in pain and in hospital, I think I would prefer to die quickly' (Zorza and Zorza 1980).

Bonica (1979, p 12) describes the narratives of cancer patients to that date as 'pathetically soul-stirring sights of dying patients in pain, in need of relief that frequently does not come'.

Pain relief

It was not until towards the end of the twentieth century that a consensus about the use of opioids for intractable pain was agreed. Radical neurosurgical procedures were seen by some as the first method of choice (White 1950), and the predominant philosophy in the 1950s and 1960s was that all avenues, both non-pharmacological and pharmacological, should be pursued before turning to opioids as a 'last resort' (Seymour et al. 2005). Indeed I remember as a student nurse in the early 1970s, caring for patients with enormously distressing pain and the reluctance of doctors to prescribe opioids, and nurses to give them.

Fear of addiction, tolerance and euphoria related to opioids were evident in major medical textbooks of the time (Seymour et al. 2005). There was a fear among the medical profession of *confining patients to a prison of addiction and mind-altering euphoria* and also of hastening death (Cole 1956). Simone de Beauvoir's (1965) account of her mother's death graphically illustrates these fears of medics. A physician warned her dying mother: 'You are going to become a real drug addict.' Patient narratives in the second half of the twentieth century frequently highlighted the agony of cancer pain. The patient's voice in print had little impact on the medical approach to pain control. However, the publishing of works with patients by doctors did effect a change in some medical areas (Winslow et al. 2005) – notably the early published works of Dame Cicely Saunders.

Pain is what the patient says it is

> Pain is what the patient says it is and exists when the patient says it does.
>
> McCaffery and Beebe (1994)

This much quoted definition probably endures because it epitomises what has become the dominant approach to pain control, in particular pain control in cancer care. Dame Cicely Saunders' concept of total pain originally emerged after a conversation with a patient, Louie, who said 'It began in my back, but now it seems that all of me is wrong' (Saunders in Clark 2006, p 87). Hence she then regarded pain not only as a physical feeling, but also as incorporating psychological, spiritual and social factors. Saunders comments that Louie (the name of the patient) could not, in her own words, and nor can we in our approach and treatment, deal with the elements of total pain separately.

Pioneering the new approach

As with all innovations there is no sudden change and there are always unsung heroes who have pioneered and believed in successful approaches long before they become established. In the 1930s Alfred Worcester is quoted as saying 'it matters much that we give ourselves with our pills' (Worcester 1935).

John Bonica

John Bonica had been an anaesthetist in an army hospital during World War II. Bonica, like his colleague Beecher, was convinced of the importance of emotion on the impact of the felt component of pain. He argued that the contemporary approaches to pain, i.e. neurosurgical or opioids given too late in too little doses, excluded the influence of the mind and were inadequate. In 1953 he published the first modern textbook on pain management. In it there was a section devoted to cancer pain. In this section he unfolded a 'masterly' thesis that represented officially a new approach to pain that is not merely physiological. He presented pain as a dual phenomenon and argued that what the patient thinks, feels and does about the pain he perceives is important. Doctors, he said, should base their clinical approach on patients' accounts of their intractable pain (Bonica 1953).

Dame Cicely Saunders

As highlighted in Chapter 1, Dame Cicely Saunders read medicine in order to fulfil her vocation to study pain relief among dying patients, and to develop techniques for the control of cancer pain that could be used in all clinical settings (Seymour et al. 2005). She qualified in 1957, 4 years after Bonica's book was published. In the year that she qualified she published her first paper, and within this she laid out the fundamental elements of a new philosophy on the care of those who are dying, in which she stated that the role of the doctor was to stay with the dying patient to enhance the patient's inner resources, and continue to apply their knowledge to bring relief and comfort during suffering (Seymour et al. 2005).

Seymour et al. (2005) identify Saunders' address, 'The management of intractable pain' at the Royal Society of Medicine in 1962, as one of the most critical presentations that she gave. Here she showed doctors and surgeons that what they had been taught and what they teach and practice were wrong. The paper was based on her systematic observation of 900 dying patients. She interviewed and tape-recorded her conversations with these patients. On the basis of her observations, she recommended that patients with cancer pain should have opioids administered on a regular basis. She argued that in their circumstances opioids were not addictive, that tolerance was not a problem and that giving morphine orally worked by relieving pain and not masking it. By the time she left St Joseph's in 1965 Saunders had collected detailed descriptions of 1100 patient experiences (Seymour et al. 2005).

One of Cicely Saunders' great strengths was her networking and sharing of ideas and expertise with others. She liaised with Bonica in the USA and also with Raymond Houde, Ada Rogers and Kathleen Foley.

Raymond Houde

The work of Raymond Houde and his colleagues was sponsored by grants from, among other organisations, the Committee of Problems of Drug Dependency. In their study each patient was his or her 'own control'. This was a crossover study design in which patients received a series of graded doses of test medications randomised against known medications. They were asked to self-report on pain level and degree of relief from pain. Ada Rogers, a research nurse, was involved in these studies for over 20 years. She talks of the importance of having a good rapport with the patients. It was essential, she reports, to engage and listen to the patients, as well as administer and evaluate the effects of the medication. Originally the work of Houde et al. was aimed at eventually finding a drug that was superior to morphine for pain relief. However, by 1970 they were persuaded that the many substitutes tested did not compare with morphine. Morphine, they concluded, was the best drug available (Meldrum 2005).

Robert Twycross

Dame Cicely was aware that there was a need to provide the maximum evidence possible. In 1971 she appointed Robert Twycross as a research fellow who did a series of clinical studies to provide further evidence for the use of strong opioids (morphine) in cancer pain. He did a series of studies that provided this evidence and published four papers in 2 years on this subject (Seymour et al. 2005).

In parallel with this Candace Pert, in 1972, isolated, for the first time, an endorphin – a naturally occurring morphine-like substance in the brain (Pert 1997). In addition, in 1965 Melzack and Wall published their 'gate control' theory of pain. The gate control theory complements the approach that pain is multifactorial and not just a physical sensation. This contributed to leading the way to new research and new approaches to the concept of pain (Melzack and Wall 1996).

International Association for the Study of Pain

In the main, the founding of the International Association for the Study of Pain (IASP) has been attributed to John Bonica, who had campaigned for better pain management for over 20 years. The IASP was founded in 1973. Other members of the group were Robert Twycross and Kathleen Foley, who had been working with Raymond Houde, and Vittorio Ventafridda, an equally zealous Italian campaigner for improvement in pain management. Bonica invited over 350 researchers and clinicians from 13 countries around the world to take part and launch the IASP. Currently, the IASP has over 6900 members from 106 countries. Its mission is to bring together scientists, clinicians, health-care providers and policy-makers to stimulate and support the study of pain, and to translate that knowledge into improved pain relief worldwide. It is a non-government organisation affiliated to the World Health Organization (WHO), its secretariat being based in Seattle, Washington. It publishes the journal *Pain* (www.iasp-pain.org.2006).

WHO ANALGESIA LADDER

At a meeting of the IASP in Venice in 1978, Twycross presented a chart that defined progressive stages of analgesia: aspirin, codeine and morphine. As the patient reached the limits of each stage of relief the doctor should move the patient on to the next step. At the third stage (strong opioid e.g. morphine), the dose should be tailored to the individual until the patient was pain free (Twycross 1997).

Twycross recommended that analgesia should be given by the clock, i.e. regularly as opposed to an as-needed regimen, which was used by Houde at Sloan Kettering. The Sloan Kettering as-needed regime, as opposed to 'by the clock', was supported by regular visits from Ada Rogers, the nurse assistant researcher, and this ensured that patients were not forced to wait for pain relief. Houde argued that regular dosing for every patient might lead to over-medication and that a new pain indicative of a new complication may not be felt and reported. Twycross did not dispute this; however, he emphasised the need for constant monitoring and review of the patient. However, he insisted that *continuous pain required regular preventive therapy* (Twycross 1997).

Twycross has taken the concept of regular giving of strong opioids as a golden rule in cancer care. He challenged the idea that tolerance in these circumstances was unavoidable. He prospectively charted the medications of 115 patients over a period of 7 years. Patients who died soon after the study began often required higher doses in their last days. Those who survived longer periods were often able to reach a stable plateau level in which their dosage remained stable for months. Some were able to reduce their dose and even stop taking the drug altogether. These findings, reported at a Florence meeting of the IASP, were received with enthusiasm by British colleagues and incredulity by American colleagues (Twycross 1999). After the meeting in Milan the WHO published as *Cancer Pain Relief* guide in 1986. The WHO three-step analgesia ladder was also launched (Figure 11.1).

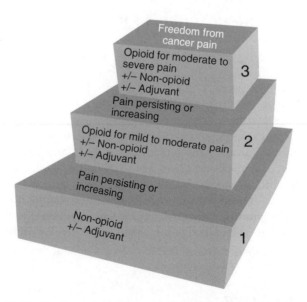

Figure 11.1 World Health Organization's analgesic ladder for cancer pain. The WHO has developed a three-step 'ladder' for cancer pain. If pain occurs, there should be prompt oral administration of drugs in the following order: non-opioids (aspirin and paracetamol); then, as necessary, mild opioids (codeine); then strong opioids such as morphine, until the patient is free of pain. (Reproduced with the permission of the WHO.)

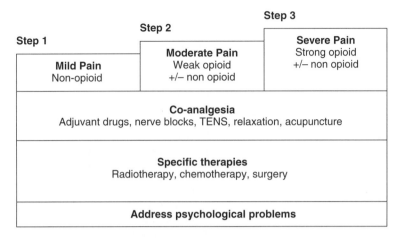

Figure 11.2 Adapted WHO analgesic ladder. (Reproduced with the permission of Western Palliative Physicians.) The steps are as follows:

Step 1 Non-opioids, e.g.
Paracetamol: oral or rectal
Non-steroidal anti-inflammatory drugs (NSAIDS): useful for any pain aggravated by movement; risk–benefit balance must always be considered; renal impairment is common with NSAIDs; relatively contraindicated in heart failure; gastric protection with misoprostol or proton pump inhibitors (PPIs) is advisable; choice of NSAID is largely dictated by local preference, e.g. ibuprofen, diclofenac, naproxen

Step 2 Weak opioids, e.g.
Codeine with paracetamol (co-codamol)
Tramadol
Dihydrocodeine

Step 3 Strong opioids, e.g.
Morphine
Diamorphine
Oxycodone
Hydromorphone
Fentanyl

The WHO analgesic ladder has been widely disseminated throughout the world. However, opioid analgesics are insufficiently available, especially in developing countries, and prescription of morphine is limited to a small number of doctors and is unavailable in many countries of the world (De Lima 2006).

A modified version – the Wessex palliative care physicians' analgesic ladder – is shown in Figure 11.2. I like this local adaptation. It quite clearly demonstrates the value of non-pharmacological approaches.

The WHO analgesia ladder is, in effect, a statement of principles that can be used with a varying degree of interpretation as opposed to a rigid framework. Studies to validate the WHO analgesic ladder show that, by using this approach, pain relief can be achieved for between 77% and 100% of patients with advanced cancer who have pain (Foley 2006). At the heart of this approach is patient involvement and understanding of their medication. This has always been so. In many situations a

Table 11.1 Adjuvant approaches for specific pains[a]

Pain	Possible approaches
Neuropathic pain This pain is associated with sensory changes. It is aching in nature. Sometimes 'burning' and 'shooting' sensations are described	• Refer to specialist palliative care team earlier rather than later • Approaches include trials of antidepressant and or anticonvulsant drugs • Steroids may be trialled • Acupuncture, TENS, neural blockage
Bone pain	• Early referral for radiotherapy • NSAIDs • Intravenous infusions of bisphosphonates – oral bisphosphonates • Consider referral to orthopaedics for patients at risk of pathological fracture
Muscle pain	• Muscle relaxant drug therapy • Physiotherapy • Aromatherapy • Relaxation • Heat pads
Abdominal pain	• Check for constipation • For colic use an anticholinergic drug • For liver capsule pain consider dexamethasone in combination with opioids ± NSAIDs
Bladder spasm	• Anti-spasmodic, e.g. oxybutynin • NSAIDs • If catheterised, may be intravesicle bupivacaine
Acute pain in short, e.g. changing a painful dressing	• Immediate-relief morphine one-sixth of total oral morphine daily dose • Nitrous oxide – as Entonox • Seek advice of specialist palliative care unit for alternative suggestions

[a]These are considered in cases where the pain is only partially opioid responsive or neurological in nature.
NSAID, non-steroidal anti-inflammatory drug; TENS, transcutaneous electrical nerve stimulation.
Adapted from Wessex Specialist Palliative Care Units (2007).

multidisciplinary approach is needed to acquire pain relief. Table 11.1 shows adjuvant approaches for specific pain.

Main general principles of WHO analgesic ladder

• Pain assessment and continuous reassessment are vital.
• Patients should enter the step of the ladder corresponding to the intensity of their pain. If a patient has severe pain, he or she should be entered at step 2 or 3 and not started on step 1.

- If analgesics that are given regularly (by the clock) on step 1 or 2 of the ladder are ineffective, the patient should be moved to the next step and *not* given another drug in the step that they are already on.
- Adjuvant drugs (e.g. non-steroidal anti-inflammatory drugs for bone pain), to complement opioids and/or control side effects (antiemetics for nausea), are important.
- Adjuvant approaches, e.g. use of complementary therapies, are an important part of the approach to the ladder.
- Wherever possible drugs should be given by mouth.
- Analgesics should be given by the clock as opposed to as needed.
- Opioid doses should be titrated to the individual.
- Attention to detail and constant reappraisal are necessary.

Titrating strong opioids

- To gain control of pain it is important to titrate the dose of opioid to the individual.
- If using a normal release opioid, either elixir or tablets, give it every 4 hours.
- Give as-needed doses that are equal to the 4-hourly dose.
- Morphine is still the drug of choice
- A starting dose of 2.5–5 mg morphine is recommended for elderly or frail people or those with poor renal function, e.g. creatinine >200 µmol/1 (Regnard and Hockley 2004).
- Dose increments of 4-hourly immediate-release morphine can be increased in 30–50% increments. In general titration should not be more than 30–50% in 24 hours (Watson et al. 2006).
- In practice this is as follows:
  2.5 mg → 5 mg → 10 mg → 15 mg → 20 mg
  30 mg → 40 mg → 60 mg → 90 mg
  120 mg → 150 mg → 200 mg
  There is no maximum dose if the pain is morphine sensitive (Watson et al. 2006). However, only a minority will need more than 30 mg 4 hourly.
  Note that in frail and elderly people and those with impaired renal function, the time interval may need to be lengthened to reduce side effects (National Council for Palliative Care 2003; Regnard and Hockley 2004).
  Note that it is custom and practice not to wake the patient for a 02:00 dose. However, it is probably wise to rouse the patient gently for the 06:00 dose.
- Review doses regularly and make an increase if using two or more breakthrough doses in 24 hours.
- Once pain has been controlled it is usual to change from 4-hourly immediate relief morphine to a modified-release morphine. The 12-hourly dose will be half the dose given in 24 hours, e.g. if giving 60 mg in 24 hours the modified release will be 30 mg every 12 hours.
- The as-needed dose for breakthrough pain will remain a 4-hourly dose, e.g. in the case of 60 mg in 24 hours, as-needed dose is 10 mg.
- If 30 minutes after an as-needed dose for breakthrough pain the pain is not relieved, the patient requires a full reassessment (Wessex Specialist Palliative Care Units 2007).

Commencing with modified-release morphine

It is not always possible to manage a 4-hourly regimen on normal release morphine. At home patients will sometimes find it difficult to measure elixirs and, indeed, to remember to take them. Lack of qualified staff to check morphine 4-hourly in care homes is problematic. *It is advisable to seek the guidance of a specialist palliative care physician when titrating morphine in these circumstances.*

Information for patients

- Patients and their relatives will often need to be reassured that use of morphine for pain is very different from abusive morphine use. Psychological dependence (addiction) does not occur if morphine is used correctly for pain (Twycross 1997).
- As a result of the early history of the use of morphine, i.e. 'it was a last resort' and 'held over until the patient was very near death', patients may also need to be reassured about the contemporary approach that introduces morphine at a much earlier stage. They may be reassured to know that patients can take morphine for some years for pain and they may have their dose reduced and even stopped with no ill effects.
- It is important that patients understand the need for regular 'by the clock' administration.
- It is important that patients understand as-needed medication and that, if it does not work in 30 minutes, this needs to be reported to their clinical nurse specialist or GP if at home.
- Educate the patient about potential side effects and how to manage them.
- Patients may be reluctant to start on morphine because they fear there will be nothing left to alleviate their pain if it escalates. They need to be reassured that unlike step 1 and 2 drugs, morphine has no ceiling amount.

Note that the WHO three-step ladder has been developed for use in patients with *cancer pain*. Its transferability to treat patients with other illnesses is, in the main, under-researched. However, transferability of this method to people with other illnesses is discussed in Chapters 13 and 14.

SIDE EFFECTS

Constipation

Many patients requiring opioids are not able to take a high-fibre diet and drink plenty of fluids. Exercise is often limited. Constipation is virtually inevitable. The prophylactic use of aperients is usually recommended: a stool softener for hard stools and stimulants if stool is difficult to expel. Patients on regular opioids will almost certainly need both.

Nausea and vomiting

Nausea, on its own or with vomiting, is a fairly common side effect of opioids. It is wise to inform the patient who is opioid naïve that vomiting and/or nausea may occur. It is not recommended now that antiemetics be given prophylactically; however, an appropriate antiemetic, e.g. low-dose haloperidol or prochlorperazine, should be at hand, just in case (Hanks et al. 2005). The nausea and vomiting may disappear after a week, but may recur if the opioid dose is increased.

Sedation

Initiation of opioid therapy may induce sedation and it is wise to forewarn patients about this. It is usual for patients to develop a tolerance to this effect. If this symptom persists, a reduction in dose can be tried and/or another analgesic option considered. However, there is also a precedent for using dextroamphetamine or methylphenidate for treatment of opioid-induced sedation (Portenoy 1994). This approach is, however, contraindicated in patients with cardiac arrhythmias, agitated delirium, paranoid personality and past amphetamine abuse (Hanks et al. 2005).

Hallucinations, confusion and delirium

Some mild cognitive impairment may well occur after commencing an opioid, or increasing the dose of one. Pure opioid-induced confusion, similar to drowsiness, tends to be transient in nature. If the confusion/delirium persists, although it may be caused by the opioid alone, it could be associated with moderate-to-severe renal impairment, dehydration, hypoxaemia, hypercalcoemia or neoplastic involvement of the CNS. Clearly, these potential underlying causes need investigating by the medical team. If pain is controlled, a reduction of the opioid by 25% may help. Changing to another opioid drug or reducing the dose of opioid by using the intraspinal route is a potential option (Hanks et al. 2005).

Multifocal myoclonus

Mild myoclonus as a side effect of opioids is not unusual. Occasionally, myoclonus can be severe and distressing and contribute to breakthrough pain. If the dose of opioid cannot be reduced, switching to another opioid should be considered. Sometimes treatment with a benzodiazepine or an anticonvulsant may be considered (Hanks et al. 2005).

Allergy

Opioids can cause histamine release and result in pruritis. This occurrence is rare. However, patients will say that they are allergic to opioids. This often means, when a history is taken, that the patient has had a bad experience with an opioid side effect. This underlines the importance of patient education about side effects (Hanks et al. 2005).

Respiratory depression

When opioids are titrated in the way described in this book, clinically important respiratory depression is rarely seen. Pain antagonises the central depressant effects of opioids (Twycross 1997). However, opioid-induced respiratory depression could be a problem if the pain is suddenly eliminated, e.g. as in nerve blockade, and the opioid is not reduced. It is important, as stated previously, to reassess the opioid regimen regularly.

Opioid toxicity

Occasionally patients will be sensitive to the effects of opioids or the dose prescribed may be more than they need (see above). Characteristics of opioid toxicity are pin-point pupils, decreased level of consciousness and respiratory depression. Clearly the patient needs an urgent medical examination. It may be enough to omit a dose and then reduce the dose. The patient may need naloxone, which is a potent opioid antagonist.

Opioid rotation (or switch)

Anecdotal evidence supports that patients who develop adverse side effects to morphine may benefit by switching to an alternative opioid. By use of this approach improvements in cognitive impairment, sedation, hallucinations, nausea and vomiting and myoclonus have been commonly reported (Hanks et al. 2005). This approach requires a good knowledge of equianalgesic tables and, even with this, patients are at risk of over- and under-dosing because of individual sensitivities (Hanks et al. 2005). *Prescribers are advised to seek the advice of a specialist palliative care consultant.*

Alternative opioids include the following:

- Methadone: however, dangerous accumulation can occur and it is best restricted to those with extensive experience (Wessex Specialist Palliative Care Unit 2007).
- Hydromorphone has been used in countries where diamorphine is unavailable for many years. It is about seven times as strong as morphine, so expertise and great care are needed in titrating doses – need specialist palliative care expertise.
- Oxycodone has been used for many years in the USA and has been available in the UK only for 5 years. There is evidence that it is useful for neuropathic pain. Again, seek the advice of local specialist palliative care experts.

ALTERNATIVE ROUTES FOR ADMINISTRATION OF STRONG OPIOIDS

Transdermal

In recent years self-adhesive skin patches have been developed for the administration of strong opioids. They are useful when the oral route is difficult, e.g. dysphagia, repeated vomiting or tablet phobia. They help to increase compliance because after application their effect will last for some days, e.g. fentanyl lasts for

72 hours. Opioids delivered in this way lay claim to being less constipative than orally administered opioids.

Guidelines for use

- The transdermal route is really only suitable for those patients already established on a steady dose of morphine.
- The patch should be applied to dry, non-irradiated, hairless skin on the upper arm or trunk. Body hair may be clipped but not shaved. Some patients may need Micropore around the edges of the patch.
- Peak plasma concentrations of, for example, fentanyl are reached only 12–24 hours after applying the patch. Therefore, in view of this:
  - patients converting from 4-hourly normal release must continue regular normal relief morphine for the first 12 hours and then review
  - patients converting from 12-hourly modified-release morphine should apply the first patch at the same time as taking the final 12-hourly dose and then review after 12 hours.
- If converting from a syringe driver, maintain the syringe driver for 12 hours after applying the first patch.
- Normal-release morphine should be prescribed for breakthrough pain – this should be equivalent to a 4-hourly dose, i.e. one-third of a 12-hourly dose if previously taking slow-release morphine twice daily.
- After 48 hours if the patient has needed two or more as-needed doses of morphine the patch strength should be increased.
- Remove patch, e.g. fentanyl, after 3 days and change the position of the new patch to rest the skin.
- A reservoir of fentanyl accumulates in the skin under the patch and significant blood levels persist for some 24 hours or more. This is significant only if fentanyl is discontinued.
- About 10% of patients may experience opioid withdrawal symptoms when changing from morphine to transdermal fentanyl. As-needed doses of morphine can be used for these symptoms, which are described as 'gastric flu-like'.
- In febrile patients the rate of absorption of fentanyl may increase. Patients should be warned to avoid any external heat source over the patch, e.g. hot water bottle, electric blankets. Patients may shower with a fentanyl patch, but should not soak in a hot bath.
- *Prescribers are advised to seek the guidance of a palliative care specialist in managing the introduction of strong opioid patches in patients with a history of taking oral opioids.*

Always remember to take the old patch off before putting on the new one.

Spinal route (epidural and intrathecal)

The discovery of opioid receptors in the dorsal horn led to the development of intraspinal opioid delivery techniques. There are no trials comparing the intrathecal and epidural routes. However, the epidural route is generally preferred because the technique to accomplish long vein administration is simpler (Hanks et al. 2005). The general indications for use of spinal analgesics in palliative care are when the pain is not controlled by systemic analgesics, or when pain control is adequate with systemic administration, but there are unacceptable adverse effects (Swarm et al. 2005).

An approximate dose calculation from subcutaneous diamorphine is:

- Epidural 1/10th of systemic dose
- Intrathecal 1/10th of epidural dose: ie 1/100th of systemic dose.

Thus, if a patient was on 100 mg subcutaneous diamorphine a day, the equivalent epidural dose would be 10 mg in 24 hours and the equivalent intrathecal dose would be 1 mg/24 hours (Fallon and Hanks 2006). The addition of a local anaesthetic, e.g. bupivacaine, to an epidural or intrathecal opioid has been demonstrated to improve analgesia while avoiding increased toxicity.

Insertion of an intraspinal catheter requires the expertise of an anaesthetist or expert pain consultant. With the improvements in catheter and pump technology, the use of spinal analgesia is becoming more common. The use of lines tunnelled subcutaneously can reduce the risk of infections (Fallon and Hanks 2006). On-site education of staff is needed to reduce potential complications. The management of these systems of delivery is complicated by the variety of different pumps available.

Subcutaneous route via a syringe driver

The syringe driver is a small portable battery-powered pump that delivers drugs via a syringe subcutaneously as a continuous infusion. The syringe driver has now become commonly used in palliative care. It can be used when the oral route is difficult because of nausea and vomiting and dysphagia. It can also be useful in severe oral tumours or when the mouth is very sore and infected, and is used towards the end of life when patients can no longer swallow. It is a way of maintaining a steady plasma level of drugs. The use of the syringe driver in palliative care was pioneered by Dr Patrick Wright at the Michael Sobell House in Oxford. He was convinced of its place in palliative care when a young woman with two young children was dying of ovarian cancer. She and her husband had organised a family holiday at Butlins in Bognor Regis. However, her pain had been difficult to control and was achieved only by using a syringe driver. Wright contacted the local health centre in Bognor and they agreed to change the syringe driver every 24 hours. The family enjoyed their holiday in spite of the patient being quite close to death. The diamorphine had to be kept at the police station. It was this experience that convinced Wright that the syringe driver had a big place in palliative care (Graham and Clark 2005).

Syringe driver myths

My experience dictates that it is fairly common for relatives, friends and sometimes colleagues to think that larger doses of strong opioids are added to the syringe driver and that this will hasten death. It is important to dispel this myth and explain to patients, relatives and friends that the dose of strong opioid is equivalent to what the patient would have taken orally. It is useful to explain that, because of more efficient absorption from the subcutaneous site, actually only a third of the total daily oral dose of strong opioid is added to the driver. A pre-prepared leaflet also emphasising this may well be useful. If the patient has been on an antiemetic it is good practice also to add this.

Local experience dictates that the use of drugs for anxiety and terminal agitation should be added only if the patient has been taking these orally or if agitation becomes apparent and communication is difficult because of the patient's deteriorating level of consciousness. This needs to be explained carefully to relatives and friends. Advance care planning with the patient can address the potential for this. A colleague related to me how comforted her dying father was to be able to have a conversation about how to address his needs if he became agitated as he was dying. He gave instructions for drugs to be used if no physical cause of any potential agitation could be indentified.

Cautionary note

Many different syringe drivers are on the market. Some deliver drugs in 1 hour, some in 24. Always check that you have the correct driver for the individual prescription. It is important to have a clear and concise syringe driver policy available to health professionals to avoid delays and mistakes in practice.

The doctrine of double effect

The doctrine of double effect is established in English law. An 81-year-old widow who had suffered a stroke was prescribed morphine by Dr Bodkin Adams in 1957 – she later died. The judge commented that, although there was no defence for mercy killing, the doctor was entitled to do all that was proper and necessary to relieve the patient's suffering even if those measures incidentally shortened life (McHale and Tingle 2002). Dr Moor was acquitted of murder in 1999. He had been accused of administering a lethal dose of morphine. However, he confessed that he had done so to relieve pain, not to kill. This verdict established that doctors who administer drugs to relieve pain are acting within the law, whether or not the patient dies as a result (McHale and Tingle 2002).

However, the important point to make here is that strong opioids titrated in the way suggested in this book do not result in the patient dying prematurely provided that, in the relatively rare event of opioid toxicity, it is diagnosed and treated appropriately. This use of opioids bears no relationship to the doctrine of double effect.

CONCLUSION

The titrated use of opioids in palliative care has meant that thousands of people have been relieved of intractable pain in their dying period, freeing them to reflect on their lives and spend relatively pain-free precious time with their friends and relatives. Understanding the history of the use of opioids against the backdrop of patient and relative narratives of dying in intractable pain is helpful to put its use in context, when perhaps faced with health professionals who query its use in specialist palliative care. The individual titration of an opioid is imperative to its safe and correct use for pain control. The development of the syringe driver means that, when patients can no longer swallow, they can still have their pain relieved.

MAIN IMPLICATIONS FOR PRACTICE

- Historically cancer pain was dreaded. Patient narratives are an enduring reminder of this.
- The WHO analgesic ladder used in cancer pain can provide relief for 77–100% of patients. Unfortunately access to strong opioids is not possible in many countries for a variety of reasons.
- Adjuvant analgesia and approaches are an important part of the WHO analgesic ladder.
- Transferability of the WHO analgesic ladder to patients with other illnesses is under-researched and unclear.
- Titrating strong opioids for the individual patient takes confidence and skill, and advice should be sought from a specialist palliative care practitioner.
- Patients need to be educated about the correct use of strong opioids for pain. It does not result in the severe psychological dependence seen in morphine abuse.
- Strong opioids are no longer seen as a last resort.
- Patients and health carers need to be proactive in minimising side effects of strong opioids.
- The syringe driver is a useful method of managing symptoms when the oral route is not possible.

SUGGESTED FURTHER READING

Dickman A, Schneider J, Varga J (2005) *The Syringe Driver*, 2nd edn. Oxford: Oxford University Press.

Chapter 12
Concordance and advance care planning

KEY POINTS

- **Focus on a patient-centred approach**: there is a risk that, in the palliative arena, we could lose the focus on psychosocial and spiritual aspects of care. Ironically this may in part result from the success of using opioids to help with cancer pain, which has stimulated a hidden curriculum promoting the biomedical ethic at the expense of the holistic one.

  There is a multidisciplinary spontaneous call for a patient-centred reflective approach to care encouraging concordance.
- **Advance care planning**: this can be a statement of wishes and preferences that must be considered carefully by health-care and social-care professionals when assessing a person's best interests. It is not legally binding.
- **Advance decisions to refuse treatment**: this must relate to specific circumstances. Valid advance decisions that are refusals of treatments are legally binding. Careful assessment of the validity and applicability of an advance decision is vital before being used in clinical practice.
- **Key times for advance planning needs to be written into policies**: advance care planning should be written into operational policies and given protected time. Professionals should instigate opportunities for advance planning at key points in the patient's illness trajectory. These key points should be identified in advance care planning policies.
- **The Mental Capacity Act**: the implications of the Mental Capacity Act should be understood by all professional disciplines. A person should be presumed to have capacity unless lack of capacity is clearly demonstrated. The person is not to be treated as if he or she has a blanket lack of capacity, and this must be determined on a decision-by-decision basis.
- **Self-care and clinical supervision**: good communication skills, self-care and clinical supervision will enhance the professional's ability and confidence to lead on advance care planning.

In many ways palliative care can be seen as the forerunner to a reflective/patient-centred approach model. Dame Cicely Saunders' vision was to achieve a radical new approach to care with attention not only to physical needs, but also to emotional, social and spiritual problems. That said, Corner (2004) highlights that good pain and symptom control has become the raison d'être of palliative care. Perhaps a natural consequence of this and the medical influence of palliative care is that, over time, the radical new approach has become embedded within the traditions and discourses of health care, particularly the biomedical ethic. Symptom management is often seen as the focus for palliative care. The success of using opioid drugs to help with cancer pain has led to the search for new and better drugs for management of other symptoms. Frequently, drug treatment is the first, and perhaps the only, approach to problems reported by patients (Corner 2004). It can be argued that other aspects of the experience of symptoms, such as suffering, distress, the ability to function and even personal autonomy, have been relegated to secondary importance (Corner 2004).

No one would deny the importance of good pain and symptom management. In the Hope Study 10 of the 16 patients could remember times when a pain or symptom had been so bad that they 'wanted to die'. One man said 'I was in so much pain at the time that it really would have been a relief to slip away, then the next day you feel better and wonder, why did I feel like that' (Buckley and Herth 2004). However, I think that we need now to be mindful in palliative nursing of continuing to be proactive in nurturing a patient-centred, reflective approach to our care.

PATIENT-CENTRED CARE: CONCORDANCE

Reflective narrative

There is a spontaneous call from the multiprofessional arena for a more patient-centred, partnership-reflective approach to care (aspects of this are dealt with in more detail in Chapters 3, 4 and 5). The calls are in many ways uncoordinated and passionate. The last time such a passionate call was made was in the late 1970s and this resulted in the nursing process approach – the tool for delivering individual care – and I think most professionals of my generation would agree that the aim then was good, but the mark was missed.

The fact is that health-care professionals can deliver an efficient and health-promoting service on a daily basis, without it necessarily being patient centred or reflective. It takes passion and enthusiasm to shape and mould oneself to each individual patient, in order that they can make a choice as to the role they want in their own health care; it does, however, reap enormous personal rewards in terms of self-esteem and professional job satisfaction.

Christopher Johns: nurse and complementary therapist

Christopher Johns (2006b) replaced the nursing process model of care, based on the 12 activities of daily living (Roper et al. 1980), with a reflective model for clinical practice at Burford Community Hospital. Central to this is that the core therapeutic of nursing practice is 'the practitioner being available – working – with relationship focused to enable the other to find meaning in their health–illness experience, to make best decisions and help take appropriate action to ease suffering and meet their life needs' (Johns 2006b, p 120). The information gained from patients about their illness experience is written as an unfolding narrative; in other words each 'difficulty or symptom' expressed by the patient should be recorded in terms of how it impacts on their life and how they cope with this. Fundamental to the unfolding narrative is 'turning into the person in each unfolding moment'. To be able to do this Johns (2006b) uses nine reflective cues:

1. Who is this person?
2. What meaning does this illness/meaning have for the person?
3. How is this person feeling?
4. How has this event affected their usual life pattern and roles?
5. How do I feel about this person?
6. How can I help this person?
7. What is important to this person to make their stay with us comfortable?
8. What support does this person have in life?
9. How does this person view the future for themselves and others?

Multidisciplinary: patient-centred communication

Johns' (2006b) concept of the unfolding narrative is not dissimilar to the guidance given on assessment by the Cancer Action Team NHS (2007). They state that, when taking a history of a person's illness experience at each key event, the following should be ascertained:

- Facts: what was found, what happened?
- Perceptions: what was understood, what the person thought was happening, what sense the patient was making of things – any links being made?
- Feelings: how does the person feel about what is happening or what they are experiencing?
- Coping: how does the person feel that they are coping with events, symptoms and feelings?
- Previous experiences: has the person related previous experiences and if so how did they cope and from where did they gain support?

Doctors: patient-centred care

Similarly, these two approaches are echoed in the patient-centred clinical method, advocated by Stewart et al. (2003). Stewart (2001) maintains that, in order for a consultation to be patient centred, it should have the following core elements:

- Exploration of the patient's concerns and need for information.
- Seeking understanding of the patient's world in terms of integration of life issues and emotional issues.
- Finding common ground on what the issues are and reaching a mutual agreement on management.
- Enhancing prevention and health promotion.
- Enhancing the continuity of a relationship between patient and professional.

Pharmacists: concordance

Within the world of pharmacology a new way of looking at medicine taking has been articulated that promotes patients' beliefs and rights, giving them equal weight to those of health-care professionals. In 1995 a small group of pharmacists met with a common interest, the effective use of medicines – in other words to discuss reasons why patients do not take their medicines as directed by the prescriber (Bond 2004). Incidentally, it is estimated that 30% of prescribed medication is not taken as directed. In a model of compliance, if a patient does not take a medicine as prescribed, it is seen as misunderstanding or wilful disobedience of the prescriber's wishes. Out of the 1995 meeting the concept of concordance was highlighted. The model of concordance overtly recognises that it is the patient who makes the final decisions whether or not to take medications. The aim in concordance is to promote a discourse that makes explicit any differences between patients and professionals and to promote a decision-making approach that respects these differences (Britten and Weiss 2004).

ADVANCE CARE PLANNING

In the past it was not uncommon for major decisions about care to be made in a reactive mode and sometimes without reference to the patient. In an unexpected acute event this will inevitably still happen. However, in the twenty-first century an operational policy should exist that dictates that protected time must be given after the unexpected event for advance care planning in the light of a similar event occurring again. This should be done with the patient, and/or relatives or someone with lasting power of attorney for the patient.

An advance care planning discussion should ideally begin with establishment with the patient of a mutual understanding of the diagnosis and prognosis (see assessment in Chapter 3 on communication skills). It would be difficult to proceed without this. However, in practice sometimes communication is difficult perhaps because the patient may be confused, demented or in denial. Advance planning may involve the patient appointing a person who will have lasting power of attorney for them. This is a new statutory form of power. Anyone with mental capacity can appoint someone to make decisions on their behalf if or when they lose mental capacity (Mental Capacity Act 2005).

It is important to note that advance care planning, statements of wishes and preferences, and advance decisions also occur as a process of discussion with the patient and care providers, irrespective of discipline. Everyone has responsibility here so education of all staff disciplines is important. Communicating spontaneous and informal discussions about wishes and preferences, to case managers, clinical nurse specialists and medical consultants, i.e. key workers, is a vital commitment, as is ensuring that conversations are carefully and fully documented. All care organisations would do well to provide a specific document on which of these conversations could be recorded. In-house training should encourage staff of all disciplines to familiarise themselves with updates by checking this document each time before giving care at the end of life.

However, it is important that the health professional has the core competence to support the type of decision made. Although being able to explain the concept of advance care planning and guidance is the remit of all involved in the direct care of patients, advance decisions to refuse treatment, for example, will need the support of consultant clinical staff and GPs. Complex legal and ethical issues will need input from legal and medical consultants (see www.endoflifecare.nhs.uk2007).

Statement of wishes and preferences

A statement of wishes and preferences embraces a range of written and/or recorded words from the patient in which wishes and preferences in relationship to future treatment and care are stated (see www.endoflifecare.nhs.uk2007). This may include details of feelings, beliefs and values that govern the person's decision-making in both medical and non-medical matters. Wishes and preferences may be related to all aspects of care from thoughts about life-prolonging treatments to preferences about bathing versus showering. Statements of wishes and preferences must be considered carefully by health-care and social-care staff when assessing a person's best interests, but they are not legally binding in the same way that an advance decision is (see www.endoflifecare.nhs.uk).

Advance decisions to refuse treatment

Advance decisions must be specific, i.e. the decision must relate to the refusal of a named specific treatment in a particular set of circumstances. Valid advance decisions are legally binding. It is imperative that the validity and applicability of an advance decision are carefully assessed in clinical practice before it is applied.

Advance decisions to refuse treatment should be fully and carefully documented with the patient's agreement (see www.endoflifecare.nhs.uk2007). They need to be regularly discussed with the patient and efficiently communicated to the key people involved in the patient's care. *Regularly* needs to be defined in practice areas. Policies for advance planning should specify this. The multidisciplinary team, in its widest sense, should share documentation and procedures for this central and vital function. Documentation should include the rationale for decision-making, and it should seek to demonstrate that the patient has been supported in making an informed decision. Ideally the documentation should be signed and dated by both the patient and the health-care professional who is key in supporting the patient in making the decision. Record keeping is pivotal in ensuring that advance planning is effective. Many organisations are now working to produce appropriate paperwork on which to make advance decisions. Advance decisions to refuse treatment should be regularly updated.

Best interests

The Mental Capacity Act stipulates that anyone making a decision for another who lacks capacity will be required to take any statement of wishes and preferences into account when assessing best interests. Part of assessing best interests is making reasonable efforts to ascertain what wishes and preferences may be (see www. endoflifecare.nhs.uk2007). This is important because an objective account of best interests will hold that there is always an action (or inaction) that is in the individual's best interest. The objective account is defined as maximising the individual's well-being. However, when considering best interests there is a vital distinction to be made between need and want – what an individual might need and what they might want may not coincide.

The subjective account of best interests is defined in terms of what the individual would be expected to choose if they were competent. This of course means that strong personal beliefs and commitments may play a decisive role in the best interests of an incompetent person (National Council for Hospice and Specialist Palliative Care Services 2002). The Mental Capacity Act sets out a specific process that must be applied when assessing best interests (National Council for Palliative Care 2005c).

Key ethical principles often quoted in palliative care suggest that, in demonstrating sound decision-making, the professional needs to be able to demonstrate:

- Respect for the autonomy of the person, i.e. the right of self government.
- Beneficence, i.e. active goodness and kindness.
- Non-maleficence, i.e. that there should be no wrong doing or evil intent.
- Justice, i.e. social justice being mindful of resources.

National Council for Hospice and Palliative Care Services (1993)

Initiating advance care-planning conversations

All too often advance care planning does not take place. Reactive decisions are made about care that can have profound consequences for quality of life. Advance planning conversations can be difficult to open. However, it is important that health-care professionals take the initiative in this. People only die once and, although they are the experts on themselves in terms of preferences, values and personal goals, they are not the experts on dying – as far as the patient is concerned you are. Health professionals may not feel like the experts but they will, in the main, have seen death before. It is also important for professionals to remember that patients may not necessarily understand the extent of their role. Although professionals have philosophies of care that are very familiar to them, the patient may have neither read nor understood them. Part of our role should be interacting with the patient in a way that educates them on what help and support we can extend to them.

When piloting the Preferred Place of Care document, which prompts conversations on future care in the face of deterioration, Pemberton et al. (2003) were surprised at the reactions of staff and the extent of their needs. Many found these conversations difficult/impossible to have. They concluded that health professionals need a good deal of education on communication skills to prepare for advance planning conversations, and also a supportive working environment where they can debrief. The national advanced communication skills programme can help to address these needs. The reader is referred again to Chapter 3 which discusses communication skills and Chapter 4 which addresses self-care and awareness.

It is important to highlight again that one of the main aims of communication in health care is to seek permission from the patient to have a conversation about their future and to proceed at a rate and depth determined by them. Some patients may never want conversations about advance planning and this should be respected. Health professionals nevertheless have a responsibility to instigate opportunities for these discussions.

There is evidence that sensitive advance planning can strengthen coping mechanisms and hope. Also evidence supports that in advance planning there will be fewer emergency decisions or crisis admissions to hospitals (Gold Standards Framework 2007).

Shah et al. (2006) did a feasibility study to estimate the views of patients about discussing their life-threatening illness. They used vignettes to instigate discussions on prognosis, seriousness of their illness and needs for supportive care. The participants were 20 patients with advanced cancer and 20 patients with advanced non-malignant disease (heart failure, chronic obstructive pulmonary disease and renal failure). This study concluded that these patients did not object to questions about end-of-life care and were able to judge their own health status and life expectancy.

Timing and policies

Advance care planning needs protected time. It should no longer be the case that 'if it comes up we discuss it'. Although no pressure should be put on patients to discuss things for which they are not ready, health professionals should provide opportunities for discussion. The end-of-life care document (see www. endoflifecare2007) suggests that the following events may trigger advance care planning discussions:

- life-changing event, e.g. death of spouse, close relative or friend
- following a new diagnosis of a life-limiting condition
- when assessing an individual's needs
- in conjunction with prognostic indicators (see www.goldstandardsframework. nhs.uk/non_cancer.php)
- multiple hospital admissions
- admission to care home.

Discussion about introduction and cessation of treatments to assist quality of life in palliative care also needs to address advance planning. These treatments may include:

- non-invasive positive pressure ventilation
- percutaneous endoscopic gastrostomy
- deactivation of implanted cardioverter devices.

Resuscitation and artificial hydration are also issues that patients may want to discuss. It should be part of written policies that these discussions take place. It would be useful for all health-care settings to devise designated documentation for this.

THE MENTAL CAPACITY ACT 2005

The Mental Capacity Act is concerned with decision-making in situations where individuals lack the capacity to make their own decisions. It has implications for all health settings and, like advance planning, and in conjunction with it, requires that policies be drawn up to incorporate its implementations into everyday practice. One of the important parts of the Mental Capacity Act is the new statutory power for anyone with capacity to choose a person (an attorney) to make decisions on their behalf if they lose capacity (see www.endoflifecare2007).

The Mental Capacity Act is underpinned by five key principles and they are:

1. A presumption of capacity: everyone has a right to make their own decisions and so should be presumed to have capacity unless lack of capacity is clearly established.
2. Individuals should be supported to make their own decisions. A person must not be treated or assumed not to be able to make their own decisions unless all practicable steps have been taken to help him or her do so, without success.
3. People have the right to make decisions that seem eccentric or unwise.
4. Best interests: decisions made on behalf of a person who lacks capacity must be demonstrated as working in that person's best interest.
5. The patient's rights and freedoms must be restricted as little as possible.

Before making a decision on behalf of the patient, regard has to be given to whether the purpose underlying the act or decision can be achieved in a way that is less restrictive to his or her right to freedom of action (NCPC 2005c).

It is also important to recognise that capacity might fluctuate and a person is not to be treated as if they have a blanket lack of capacity. Capacity must be determined on a decision-by-decision basis. It is outside the scope of this chapter to provide fully comprehensive information on both advance care planning and mental capacity. It is important that all health-care professionals have a thorough understanding of the two important initiatives. Further reading is suggested at the end of this chapter.

This short chapter comes before Chapter 13 which looks at 11 prevalent symptoms in patients with a variety of illnesses, e.g. cancer, AIDS, heart failure, COPD and renal failure. The onus is on helping the patient to make choices about treatments and approaches, and not for the professional to assume 'ownership' of the symptoms. The aim is a reflective approach that promotes patient-centred care, resulting in concordance as opposed to prescribing a plan of care with which the patient is expected to comply. Clearly, advance care planning can help to increase patients' sense of coping and control. Advance planning discussions may be difficult to initiate but are likely to result in a strengthening of patient/professional relationships.

MAIN IMPLICATIONS FOR PRACTICE

- Contemporary health-care professionals need to be able to take a reflective patient-centred approach to care (see Chapter 5).
- Health-care professionals should take responsibility for instigating conversations about advance care planning.

- Permission to address issues of advance care planning needs to be gained from the patient. The rate and depth of the planning should be decided by them.
- Clear policies should exist in all health-care settings for the recording of spontaneous discussions expressing wishes and preferences about future care.
- Time for advance care planning should be built into organisational policies and given protected time.
- Documentation forms for recording all conversations concerning advance care planning should be designed and referred to routinely at the start of each shift.
- Advance refusals of treatments should be regularly reviewed. It is imperative to define regularly in terms of specific timing.
- Staff of all disciplines should be educated about and know their responsibilities with regard to advance care planning and the Mental Capacity Act, in terms of both statutory requirements and local policies.
- Further training in advanced communication skills and self-care should be a priority, as should provision for clinical supervision.

SUGGESTED FURTHER READING

Downie RS, Randall F (2006) *The Philosophy of Palliative Care*. Oxford: Oxford University Press.

Johns C (2006) *Engaging Reflection in Practice – A narrative approach*. Oxford: Blackwell Publishing.

Munroe B, Oliviere D (2003) *Patient Participation in Palliative Care: A voice for the voiceless*. Oxford: Oxford University Press.

National Council for Hospice and Specialist Palliative Care Services (1993) *Key Ethical Issues in Palliative Care*. London: NCHSPCS.

National Council for Hospice and Specialist Palliative Care Services (2002) *Vital Judgements*. London: NCHSPCS.

National Council for Palliative Care (2005) *Guidance on the Mental Capacity Act*. London: NCPC.

Websites

www.endoflifecare.nhs.uk
Advance Care Planning: A guide for health and social care staff
www.dca.gov.uk/legal-policy/mentalcapacity/publication.htm
Making Decisions: A guide for people who work in health and social care
www.goldstandardsframework.nhs.uk/_advance_care.php

Chapter 13
Eleven prevalent symptoms

KEY POINTS

- **History**: the history of symptom support and management lies in cancer care. It is important to develop methods of best practice across all diseases.
- **Prevalent symptoms**: 11 prevalent symptoms for patients with cancer, acquired immune deficiency syndrome (AIDS), end stage heart disease, chronic obstructive pulmonary disease (COPD) and renal disease are looked at in this chapter, and ways of supporting patients with them explored with the emphasis on a patient-centred approach.

  With concordance in mind the symptoms of pain and nausea are accompanied by a patient contract that provides the patient with choices about treatment approaches. These have not been used in practice but are included as a possibility for future practice.
- **Psychosocial care**: this chapter focuses on the impact of a given symptom and addresses specific interventions to support the patient with that symptom. This is done against the backdrop of the earlier chapters in this book, which address psychosocial care in some detail.

HISTORY

The history of palliative symptom management lies in the management of patients with cancer. Little attention has been paid to patients with other life-threatening diseases (Gibbs et al. 1998). How much of the knowledge and expertise developed in cancer care can be applied to other illnesses is in the process of being explored. Each disease has its own trajectory and anecdotally there is an anxiety of professionals in palliative care around being able to cope with a series of acute episodes that may occur in patients dying of heart failure and COPD, for example, as opposed to the steady decline often associated with cancer. Although research continues to find what is best practice, the world does not stand still.

Solano et al. (2006) aimed to determine to what extent patients with chronic diseases have similar symptom profiles. After a systematic search of medical databases and textbooks they identified 64 original studies reporting on 11 common symptoms among end-stage patients with cancer, AIDS, heart disease, COPD and renal disease.

In this chapter these 11 common symptoms are looked at and ways of supporting patients with them suggested, based on current evidence and examples of best practice. The symptoms are:

- Pain
- Nausea and vomiting
- Constipation
- Diarrhoea
- Anorexia
- Fatigue
- Breathlessness
- Confusion
- Insomnia
- Anxiety (adjustment disorder)
- Depression.

Table 1.1 (see page 7) details the prevalence of these symptoms in advanced disease.

PAIN

Assessment

There has been a good deal of activity in producing pain-rating scales that help people to describe the nature and intensity of their physical pain. The Brief Pain Inventory (BPI) and BPI Short Form are validated pain instruments. The instrument is available in many different languages and contains a body diagram, numerical rating scale for pain severity, relief and interference with function (Daut et al. 1983). For BPI see Box 13.1.

Numerical rating scales of 0–10 can be used. In a multinational sample, an analysis of pain severity suggests that 1–4 may be mild pain, 5–6 moderate pain and 7–10 severe pain (Serline et al. 1995). Perhaps the most well known is the McGill Short Form. This is an adaptation of the McGill Pain Questionnaire, which was devised for use in pain research. It has 17 items: present pain intensity, pain severity, visual analogue scale and ratings of 15 descriptors (Melzack 1987). It is available in several different languages. *The McGill Short Form* is available for viewing: community.ocr.org.uk/core/community/public_download.

The literature suggests that the diagnosis of pain in certain groups of elderly patients was improved by using assessment instruments, rather than simply asking 'Do you have pain?'. Routine use of assessment tools in cognitively intact and mild-to-moderately cognitively impaired palliative care patients increases the diagnosis of pain; however, people often need help in completing assessment instruments as opposed to self-reporting. This is particularly true for elderly people (Portenoy et al. 2005).

The assessment of pain in people with moderate-to-severe cognitive impairment remains a challenge (Portenoy et al. 2005). There is evidence to support that pain is both underestimated and under-managed when people are severely cognitively impaired (Sengstaken and King 1993; Morrison and Siu 2000). It is important to trust

Box 13.1   Brief Pain Inventory (reproduced with permission of Professor Charles S Cleeland)

1903

Date: ☐☐ / ☐☐ / ☐☐
(month)   (day)   (year)

Subject's Initials: ------------------

PLEASE USE   Study Subject #: ☐☐☐☐
BLACK INK PEN

Study Name: ------------------------------

Protocol #: -------------------------------
PI: ---
Revision: 07/01/05

Brief Pain Inventory (Short Form)

1. Throughout our lives, most of us have had pain from time to time (such as minor headaches, sprains, and toothaches). Have you had pain other than these everyday kinds of pain today?

☐ Yes   ☐ No

2. On the diagram, shade in the areas where you feel pain. Put an X on the area that hurts the most.

Front

Right   Left

Back

Left   Right

3. Please rate your pain by marking the box beside the number that best describes your pain at its worst in the last 24 hours.

☐ 0   ☐ 1   ☐ 2   ☐ 3   ☐ 4   ☐ 5   ☐ 6   ☐ 7   ☐ 8   ☐ 9   ☐ 10
No   Pain As Bad As
Pain   You Can Imagine

4. Please rate your pain by marking the box beside the number that best describes your pain at its least in the last 24 hours.

☐ 0   ☐ 1   ☐ 2   ☐ 3   ☐ 4   ☐ 5   ☐ 6   ☐ 7   ☐ 8   ☐ 9   ☐ 10
No   Pain As Bad As
Pain   You Can Imagine

5. Please rate your pain by marking the box beside the number that best describes your pain on the average.

☐ 0   ☐ 1   ☐ 2   ☐ 3   ☐ 4   ☐ 5   ☐ 6   ☐ 7   ☐ 8   ☐ 9   ☐ 10
No   Pain As Bad As
Pain   You Can Imagine

6. Please rate your pain by marking the box beside the number that tells how much pain you have right now.

☐ 0   ☐ 1   ☐ 2   ☐ 3   ☐ 4   ☐ 5   ☐ 6   ☐ 7   ☐ 8   ☐ 9   ☐ 10
No   Pain As Bad As
Pain   You Can Imagine

Box 13.1   (*cont'd*)

1903

Date: ☐☐ / ☐☐ / ☐☐
(month)   (day)   (year)

Subject's Initials: ----------------
PLEASE USE BLACK INK PEN   Study Subject #: ☐☐☐☐

Study Name: ----------------------------------

Protocol #: ------------------------------------
PI: ---
Revision: 07/01/05

7. What treatments or medications are you receiving for your pain?

[grid of empty boxes]

8. In the last 24 hours, how much relief have pain treatments or medications provided? Please mark the box below the percentage that most shows how much relief you have received.

0%	10%	20%	30%	40%	50%	60%	70%	80%	90%	100%
☐	☐	☐	☐	☐	☐	☐	☐	☐	☐	☐

No Relief   Complete Relief

9. Mark the box beside the number that describes how, during the past 24 hours, pain has interfered with your:

A. General Activity

☐ 0   ☐ 1   ☐ 2   ☐ 3   ☐ 4   ☐ 5   ☐ 6   ☐ 7   ☐ 8   ☐ 9   ☐ 10
Does Not Interfere   Completely Interferes

B. Mood

☐ 0   ☐ 1   ☐ 2   ☐ 3   ☐ 4   ☐ 5   ☐ 6   ☐ 7   ☐ 8   ☐ 9   ☐ 10
Does Not Interfere   Completely Interferes

C. Walking ability

☐ 0   ☐ 1   ☐ 2   ☐ 3   ☐ 4   ☐ 5   ☐ 6   ☐ 7   ☐ 8   ☐ 9   ☐ 10
Does Not Interfere   Completely Interferes

D. Normal Work (includes both work outside the home and housework)

☐ 0   ☐ 1   ☐ 2   ☐ 3   ☐ 4   ☐ 5   ☐ 6   ☐ 7   ☐ 8   ☐ 9   ☐ 10
Does Not Interfere   Completely Interferes

E. Relations with other people

☐ 0   ☐ 1   ☐ 2   ☐ 3   ☐ 4   ☐ 5   ☐ 6   ☐ 7   ☐ 8   ☐ 9   ☐ 10
Does Not Interfere   Completely Interferes

F. Sleep

☐ 0   ☐ 1   ☐ 2   ☐ 3   ☐ 4   ☐ 5   ☐ 6   ☐ 7   ☐ 8   ☐ 9   ☐ 10
Does Not Interfere   Completely Interferes

G. Enjoyment of life

☐ 0   ☐ 1   ☐ 2   ☐ 3   ☐ 4   ☐ 5   ☐ 6   ☐ 7   ☐ 8   ☐ 9   ☐ 10
Does Not Interfere   Completely Interferes

and follow up on the intuition of the carer that something is wrong when people are cognitively impaired, even if the carer finds it difficult to be specific. An assessment tool that has been found to be reliable in the cognitively impaired who cannot speak is the Pain Assessment in Advanced Dementia Scale (PAINAD: Warden et al. 2003). The scoring system asks the scorer to rate the patient's status in the following areas: breathing, negative vocalisation, facial expression, body language and consolability. The tool comes with detailed information about criteria for scoring the patient's status – 0, 1 or 2 in each area, 0 being a generally relaxed and peaceful state and 2 indicating difficulty in the area and distress.

PAINAD is available to download at www.lumetra.com/uploadedfiles/resource-center/tools/pain/pain-assessment-advanced-dementia-definitions.pdf.

Doloplus 2 Scale

The Doloplus 2 Scale was put forward by Wary et al. (1993) as a heteroevaluation of pain in elderly people and patients who are unable to communicate. They draw their inspiration from the Douleur Enfant Gustave Roussy (DEGR) scale for young children and have adapted it for use in elderly people (Lefebvre-Chapiro and Sebag-Lanoë 1996). It is based on the observations of patients in 10 different situations that could potentially reveal pain. These behaviours are classified into three groups: somatic reactions, psychomotor reactions and psychosocial reactions. For the Doloplus 2 Scale see the Addendum at the end of the chapter.

The Doloplus 2 was developed in France. The Doloplus group continues to work on evaluating the tool and it has been extensively tested in Europe. It is described as a comprehensive tool for assessing pain in non-verbal elderly people. However, it is felt that translation issues are evident and further study or description regarding the use of the Doloplus 2 Scale in English-speaking populations is needed (Herr et al. 2004).

Assessment of total pain

Total pain is defined as physical, psychological, social and spiritual. Although the pain-rating scales featured here do include a social and psychological component, others not cited do not. It would be good practice therefore to accompany the use of a pain-rating scale assessment with an interview with the patient, where the patient's cognitive state permits.

Seek the patient's permission to talk with them about what is happening and how things are going. You might say something like, 'I just wonder if there is any more we can help you with'. It might be useful to prearrange this so that the patient can organise for someone to be with them if they choose.

> I have read your notes and am aware of the history of your illness and it is recorded medically, but I wonder just what you are making of all of this – what effect does it have on you and your life?

Some key questions as the patient unfolds their story may be:

- How is all this making you feel?
- What is uppermost in your mind at the moment?

- In all of this, what is the worst thing for you?
- How are you managing to cope with all of this?
- In the past, when things have been difficult, how have you coped? Who has helped you?
- How are you feeling in your spirits?
- Do you have a religious or other spiritual conviction? Is there anyone we could contact to support you in this?
- Are there any worries financially or socially that we may be able to help you with?

After listening and empathising with the patient, you might suggest:

Clearly we cannot fix all of this for you – I wish we could. However, there is a range of different approaches that we can offer that may help with your coping. Are any of these something that you feel may help? (For approaches to patients who are in denial, angry, finding it difficult to talk, etc., please see Chapters 2 and 3.)

With concordance in mind, rather than being overly prescriptive in treatments and approaches offer the patient choices about their care (Box 13.2). Some people may find making choices at this time difficult or impossible and of course this should be respected.

Physical pain and approaches in different diseases

The WHO analgesic ladder, including the titration of opioids, as described in Chapter 10, was conceived and designed for patients with pain associated with cancer. The evidence base lies there. The following includes reference to how these principles have been applied since palliative care has increased its horizons to encompass people dying of other illnesses.

AIDS

Of patients with AIDS 63–80% reportedly have pain (Solano et al. 2006). A recent study suggests that 50% of pain syndromes are directly related to HIV infection and 30% to the therapy for HIV disease (Breitbart and Patt 1994). There are many different causes of pain in AIDS patients; however, neuropathic pain with peripheral neuropathy is a frequent one (Lipton 1994). AIDS-related pain has many similarities to cancer pain, in particular the increasing incidence with advancing disease and the impact on quality of life (Woodruff and Glare 2005). Assessment and diagnosis of pain in AIDS are as for cancer. Where an underlying pathology can be determined, it should be treated as clinically appropriate, e.g. as in opportunistic infection.

The neuropathic pain that occurs with AIDS has been subject to a number of treatment trials with no conclusive results. Gabapentin has been reported to be effective (Hirschtick and Von Roenn 2006). The WHO analgesic ladder applies equally well to patients with AIDS (Woodruff and Glare 2005). That said, several important drug interactions may occur between opioids and other medications taken by patients with AIDS (Piscitelli and Gallicano 2001), and therefore titration would need specialist input and careful monitoring. Where possible the oral route

---

Box 13.2   Some approaches available to help you. Which approach(es) do you think will best suit you?

Patient contract for pain care
Your professional carer will be able to explain some of these options to you. Please tick the ones that you think might suit you best

Psychological
Meet with psychologist/psychiatrist who may suggest a variety of approaches as well as listening and talking:
cognitive–behavioural therapy (help you to take control of your thoughts)
hypnosis
relaxation and visualisation

Physical approaches
Meet with doctor to review your medication for pain
Meet with physiotherapist who may suggest:
use of heat
use of cold
transelectrical nerve stimulation (non-invasive – easy to use)
acupuncture

Complementary therapies
Meet with complementary therapies' coordinator, who might suggest:
massage and aromatherapy massage
reflexology

Spiritual approaches
Meet with a minister of your religion
Meet with complementary therapies' coordinator who may suggest:
reiki
spiritual healing   } These are all completely non-denominational
therapeutic touch

Patient signature   Professional signature
Review date

Note that health professionals should be knowledgeable about these different treatments in order that they can be explained clearly to patients. These approaches are discussed in some detail in Chapter 11.

---

should be used. However, sometimes severe associated gastrointestinal disease makes this difficult (Woodruff and Glare 2005). Patients will then require either parenteral treatment or the transdermal route (Newshan and Lefkowitz 2001).

End-stage heart failure

Between 41 and 77% of patients in end-stage heart failure suffer pain (Solano et al. 2006). Coronary artery bypass and transplantation are treatment for refractory angina. However, towards the end of life, surgery is often not an option.

External pneumatic counter-pulsation devices

The external pneumatic counter-pulsation device is experimental. Recent studies suggest that it may be useful in severe angina (Arora et al. 1999). The device consists of inflatable bands for the limbs. The bands inflate in diastole, improving diastolic blood flow to the coronary arteries.

Implantable spinal cord stimulators

These were first developed by Shealy in 1974 and are discussed briefly in Chapter 10. The device is inserted into the epidural space and it provides paraesthetic stimuli over the area where anginal symptoms are present. As with transelectrical nerve stimulations (TENS) devices, patients control how much stimulus is given (McGavigan and Dunn 2005).

Pharmacology

As well as angina people with end-stage heart failure often have generalised aches and pains in muscles and joints. The use of non-steroidal anti-inflammatory drugs (NSAIDs) should be avoided, because of their adverse effect on renal functions and the tendency to increase fluid retention (McGavigan and Dunn 2005).

Opioids are of irrefutable value in treating acute left ventricular failure by helping with associated breathlessness, although the mechanism for this is poorly understood. There is anecdotal evidence to support the use of opioids in chronic heart failure and Duncan et al. (2006) identify this as an area for research. However, McGavigan and Dunn (2005) state that the need for short- and long-acting opioids should be assessed regularly in end-stage heart failure. They highlight that, as opioids are helpful for both breathlessness and pain, they are a useful addition in end-stage heart failures (McGavigan and Dunn 2005).

In the symptom control guidelines for patients with end-stage heart failure, the Working Party of the Merseyside and Cheshire Specialist Palliative Care and Cardiac Clinical Networks (2005) recommends the use of the WHO three-step analgesic ladder.

Pain in COPD

In spite of between 34% and 77% of patients with COPD experiencing pain, there is a paucity of literature about pain relief in this area. Chest pain is a feature of COPD and this can be a result of a variety of causes, e.g. chest infections and chest traumas caused by coughing. Intercostal nerve blocks may be helpful. Breathlessness with its associated anxiety and restlessness is within the concept of total pain. There is a consensus that the use of opioids is justified for the relief of these symptoms in the terminal phase (NICE 2004c; Leach 2005; Randall-Curtis and Rocker 2006). Randall-Curtis and Rocker (2006) state that opioid therapy should be considered not only at the end of life but also in stable patients with COPD when breathlessness is severe in spite of maximum bronchodilator therapy.

End-stage renal failure

Pain is a problem in 47–50% of patients with end-stage renal failure (Solano et al. 2006). Barakzoy and Moss (2006) trialled the use of the WHO analgesic ladder in 45 patients with end-stage renal failure. They concluded that the WHO ladder did lead to effective pain relief in haemodialysed patients. However, more work in terms of a larger and more diverse dialysis population is necessary.

Neurological disorders

Pain occurs in around 50% of people with multiple sclerosis (MS) (Moulin 1989) and up to 75% with motor neurone disease (MND) (O'Brien et al. 1992). The most common pain problems are associated with dysaesthesia (impaired touch sensation) and muscle spasms, and unfortunately there is evidence that pain is often under-treated in these circumstances (Archibald et al. 1994). There are tremendous benefits to patients in terms of pain prevention when the early expertise of physiotherapy and occupational therapy is introduced. Later physical therapies including application of cold, heat and TENS among other modalities may be helpful. These are discussed in more detail in Chapter 11. NSAIDs and antispasmodic drugs also may help.

Neuropathic pain may well respond to neuropathic agents such as amitriptyline and gabapentin (Burman 2006). A recent paper reported that the use of gabapentin in combination with an opioid is more effective then either drug on its own (Gilron et al. 2005).

Successive studies have shown that pain is a problem in end-stage MND (O'Brien et al. 1992; Hicks and Corcoran 1993). A retrospective study of 32 patients showed that 72% received both oral and parenteral opioids and 94% received parenteral opioids. The median oral dose was 60 mg in 24 hours with a median duration of 51 days, and the median parenteral dose 180 mg in 24 hours, with a median duration of 3 days. It was felt that these results demonstrated that strong opioids can be used safely and effectively for patients with MND (Oliver 1998). In conclusion, Oliver wrote that strong opioids can be used to reduce a patient's distress in end-stage MND and should not be withheld.

NAUSEA AND VOMITING

Definitions

Nausea is described as an unpleasant feeling of the need to vomit. It is often accompanied by autonomic symptoms, e.g. salivation, cold sweat, pallor, tachycardia and fear. Retching is defined as rhythmic, laboured, spasmodic movements of the diaphragm and abdominal muscles, occurring in the presence of nausea and possibly culminating in vomiting – but not always. Vomiting is forceful expulsion of gastric contents through the mouth (Twycross and Wilcock 2001).

Early research indicates that, in cancer patients, nausea is a symptom for 50–60%. However, vomiting is less common, occurring in about 30% of these patients (Dunlop 1989). Solano et al. (2006) identified nausea as being a problem for patients: with cancer 6–68%, AIDS 43–49%, heart disease 17–48% and renal disease 30–43%. However, vomiting was not listed among the 11 prevalent symptoms, which is

---

Box 13.3   Vomiting scale

Grade
0 No nausea or vomiting
1 Nausea
2 Transient vomiting
3 Vomiting requiring therapy
4 Intractable vomiting

---

based on a systematic review of 64 studies. This has implications for supportive management of nausea. In a busy environment, nausea as a symptom can be easily overlooked; vomiting is usually not. For this reason, the routine use of the vomiting scale can be a useful tool to incorporate into the documentation of patients being cared for in all health-care settings. This could be a useful adjunct to routine documentation and would immediately identify patients suffering nausea with no vomiting, as well as patterns of vomiting (Box 13.3).

The neural pathways that mediate nausea are unclear; however, evidence suggests that they are the same pathways that mediate vomiting (Allan 1993). It therefore follows that the treatment for nausea and retching is the same as that for nausea with retching and vomiting. It may be that a lesser activation of the neural pathways leads to nausea without vomiting. Research in recent years has identified different stimuli that can cause vomiting and, although the research has been done mainly in cancer patients, it transfers well to patients with other illnesses.

Neural pathways and vomiting

Lying within the fourth ventricle of the brain is the area postrema and this also includes an area called the chemoreceptor trigger zone. These areas are outside the blood–brain barrier and are bathed in systemic blood. In the area postrema, dopamine receptors are sensitive to high concentrations of toxins, e.g. opioids, calcium and urea. Input from the vestibular apparatus and vagus nerve is also received in the area postrema. The emetic pattern generator is close to the area postrema; however, it lies fully within the blood–brain barrier. It contains the greatest concentration of 5-hydroxytryptamine or serotonin (5HT) receptors in the brain stem in its deeper layers (Twycross and Wilcock 2001). It is therefore important to assess the patient with nausea and/or vomiting carefully, in order to identify the cause. Different causes of vomiting will involve a slightly different set of neural pathways. Much work has been done to develop antiemetics that block different neural pathways (Table 13.1).

Stimuli that cause vomiting can occur from:

- The vagus nerve
- Other visceral nerves
- The vestibular apparatus
- Blood borne toxins
- Higher centres, e.g. cortex of brain.

Table 13.1   Medications used in nausea and vomiting

Gastric stasis	Domperidone
	Metoclopramide
Motion sickness (positional)	Cyclizine
	Hyoscine hydrobromide patch
Toxic	Haloperidol
	Prochlorperazine
	Levomepromazine
(Chemotherapy)	(Consult oncology colleague)
Raised intracranial pressure	Dexamethasone
	Cyclizine
Anxiety	Diazepam
	Lorazepam
	Propranolol
Infection	Antibiotics

The drugs are matched to the neural pathways that they are reputed to block, so accurate assessment for causes of nausea and vomiting is essential.

Reasons for nausea and vomiting, highlighting assessment points

Reflux vomiting

This occurs when there is a 'mechanical' reason for the vomiting, e.g. as in hiatus hernia, or from an abdominal tumour or ascites which causes pressure.

Assessment points

Vomiting occurs when not expected and often nausea is absent, e.g. it may occur when bringing up wind, eating or changing posture, e.g. stooping or sitting up in bed.

Gastric stasis

Gastric stasis can occur as the result of severe constipation (often opioid induced), or when a new drug is introduced, which slows down the gut's natural movement.

Assessment points

Often there is a large amount of vomit and patients may also complain of epigastric pain, which is oesophageal reflux. Patients may feel very full and have no appetite. Sometimes hiccups are a feature.

Gastrointestinal obstruction

This can occur when people have colon cancer or other abdominal cancers that press on their intestines. It may occasionally result from severe constipation.

Assessment points

Vomiting is forceful and in large amounts, and there is an offensive smell caused by faecal material.

Motion sickness

Movement-associated nausea and vomiting can occur as a side effect of opioids, increasing vestibular sensitivity. It is suggested that this may also occur when internal organs are distended and distorted, which in turn increases traction on the mesentery during movement (Mannix 2005).

Assessment points

Vomiting may occur suddenly on movement, e.g. lifting up the bed or getting out of bed. Nausea may well be absent.

Toxic sickness

Patients may vomit as a result of imbalance in blood chemistry, e.g. high blood urea and high calcium levels (hypercalcaemia is regarded as a palliative emergency and will be dealt with in Chapter 15). Some drugs can also cause nausea and vomiting, e.g. opioids and digoxin.

Assessment points

Pallor and a brown-coated tongue can indicate urea. Nausea, accompanied by confusion or drowsiness, may indicate uraemia and hypercalcaemia. Check treatment card for any new drugs written. The doctor will want to check the patient's blood chemistry.

Raised intracranial pressure

Often regular vomiting, perhaps with little nausea, will occur with someone who has a brain tumour and rising intracranial pressure. Patients may have either primary or secondary brain tumours.

Assessment points

Symptoms other than vomiting may include severe headache, blurred vision and a change in conscious level.

Higher centres – psychological factors

People can vomit because of fear, excitement, seeing revolting sights or smelling revolting smells.

Assessment points

Careful history taking encourages expression of anxiety and fear. Be observant for smells and sights.

Infection

Any infection can cause nausea and vomiting; in particular it is not unusual for urinary tract infections to manifest in this way.

Assessment points

Look for signs of fever, record temperature and take a midstream specimen of urine (MSU) and blood for blood cultures. If the patient history suggests a gastrointestinal infection then *isolation care* should be implemented *immediately*. Recent outbreaks of norovirus have been problematic in patient units. This virus can survive in the environment for several days and is easily transmitted. The illness usually starts with a sudden onset of nausea, often with projectile vomiting and watery diarrhoea.

Assessment in general

It is important to take a detailed history to try to establish, with the patient, why nausea or vomiting is occurring. For a nursing history use of the assessment points cited in the text would be a good starting point. The patient will need a full medical examination by the doctor. It is important to invite patients to tell their story to get a picture of how these symptoms are impacting on their quality of life. For the purpose of research, nausea is measured using a visual analogue scale and vomiting is quantified as the number of episodes in a 24-hour period (Hesketh et al. 1998).

With concordance in mind there is scope for patients who want to make choices about the approach for helping with nausea and vomiting (Box 13.4).

General approach

- Isolation care if gastrointestinal infection is suspected.
- Correct what is correctable, e.g. relieve constipation, change drug regimen if possible.
- Environment: many people will want to be cared for in a well-ventilated and possibly a quiet environment, although it is important not to assume this. It may be, for some, that the distraction of a busier area is welcome, particularly if the feeling of nausea is fearful for them.
- Good quality music of the patient's choice, using a Walkman or MP3 player, for example, may be helpful and calming.
- An aromatherapy burner with lemon, ginger, peppermint or spearmint in the room may be helpful.
- People usually have clear ideas about how much support they want while vomiting – some people want to be alone, others find another being present supportive. It is important to ascertain the patient's preference here.

Box 13.4   Feeling sick and being sick

Name _____ Date _____

Here are some approaches available to help you. Which approach or combination of approaches do you think would suit you best?

Physical
Medication – discuss with your doctor or clinical nurse specialist
Meet with physiotherapist to discuss use of acupuncture or acupressure, e.g. 'sea bands'

Psychological
Meet with psychologist/therapist to discuss, using hypnosis or relaxation and visualisation or other therapies

Complementary therapies
Meet with complementary therapist to discuss use of aromatherapy, e.g. an aromatherapy oil burner or an aroma therapy 'sniff stick'*

Music therapy
This can be discussed with the complementary therapist.

Signature_____ Review date _____

*Sniff sticks are being introduced in this country (Harris 2004). An aromatherapy sniff stick is made up by an aromatherapist for individual patients. An anti-nausea sniff stick would consist of a blend of lemon, geranium, ginger and spearmint.

- For those people whose consciousness level is impaired, the availability of suction apparatus and the use of the recovery position are important for airway protection during vomiting; clearly these patients should not be left alone when vomiting.
- It is not usual practice to use a nasogastric tube in palliative care; however, flexibility is the key and, if the patient asks and sometimes they do, then this could be tried.
- Most people will want to freshen up after vomiting – a quick wash of face and hands may be welcome.
- People may want a mouthwash or a few sips of fluid. Some favourite mouth washes or sips after vomiting are: ginger beer, flat Coca-Cola, flat lemonade, soda water, diluted peppermint water.
- Present food chosen by the patient attractively and, in the first instance, in small portions.

Intractable vomiting

For intractable vomiting or intractable nausea it may be necessary to deliver antiemetics subcutaneously, via a syringe driver. It is best to seek the advice of a specialist palliative care physician or clinical nurse specialist (CNS) in this event (see Table 13.1).

CONSTIPATION

Constipation is a common problem in palliative care. It is frequently stated that 50% of patients admitted to hospice care are constipated. Solano et al. (2006) report a prevalence of 23–65% in cancer patients and 34–35% in patients with AIDS, and 38–42%, 27–44% and 29–70% in heart disease, COPD and adrenal disease, respectively. It can cause great distress and has been quoted as rivalling or exceeding pain in the amount of distress that it incurs (Sykes 2005). During the illness trajectory of many patients, there will be episodes of chronic constipation brought on by opioid medications, autonomic failure, immobility and decreased fluid intake. Severe constipation can result in abdominal pain, intestinal obstruction and urinary retention. Symptoms may also include anorexia, malaise and mental confusion.

The Rome Criteria are frequently used for diagnosing constipation in research (Derby and Portenoy 1997). According to the Rome Criteria, constipation is present when two or more of the following symptoms have existed for a period of at least 3 months:

- Straining at stool at least 25% of the time
- Hard stools at last 25% of the time
- Incomplete evacuation at least 25% of the time
- Two or fewer bowel movements per week.

Common causes of constipation

- Dehydration, as a result of poor fluid intake, diuretic therapy, vomiting, fever or polyuria
- Immobility and weakness
- Low-fibre diet
- Loss of muscle tone
- Drugs, in particular opioids, antispasmodics and tricyclic antidepressants
- Lack of privacy
- Spinal lesions.

It is important that palliative care professionals understand and emphasise to patients that stool content consists mainly of sloughed intestinal endothelial cells and micro-organisms, and not only digested food (Bruera and Fadul 2006). Thus, patients who are hardly eating anything at all can and do become constipated.

Assessment

- As in many areas in health care, this can be embarrassing for the patient to address. The health professional usually needs to take the lead in establishing an easy rapport, making this an open and frank discussion, in order to get a comprehensive picture of the patient's bowel movements or lack of. Many patients will be extremely relieved to be able to discuss this very intimate and troublesome problem. Patients with cognitive impairment may not be able to fully cooperate with the assessment as described here, and information may need to be gained from a carer or trusted relative.

- When assessing a person's bowel function, it is important to know what a usual pattern is for them. *Bowels opened* is a meaningless statement unless accompanied by a description of the faecal material and the opinion of the patient as to whether this was a full bowel movement or not. The Bristol Stool Chart can help enormously in this. It may cause embarrassment when shown to the patient – and, hopefully, mirth. However, it is essential to get a good description and history of recent bowel movements. Patients may be passing a liquid stool and still be very constipated. This is called constipation with overflow. The *Bristol Stool Chart* can be viewed on: http://en.wikipedia.org/wiki/Bristol_Stool_Scale.
- The doctor may perform an abdominal examination, which may reveal the presence of distension, tenderness or faecal mass in the large intestine. A plain abdominal radiograph can be extremely useful in determining the extent of the problem.
- Digital rectal examination can reveal stenosis, tissue scarring, rectal tumour, haemorrhoids or rectal mass, as well as impacted faeces. An empty rectal vault can suggest proximal impaction or obstruction. Digital rectal examination is an invasive procedure and should not be considered as a primary investigation in the assessment of constipation. It should be performed only by either a doctor or a nurse who is deemed competent to do so (RCN 2003).

Management

Prevention is always better than cure

- Weak patients, e.g. patients with advanced cancer, will almost certainly need laxatives when being prescribed weak or strong opioid drugs; often a stool softener and stimulant is needed. Patients can be educated to titrate the dose, until a good evacuation is achieved. Ascertain whether the patient has a preference for a particular aperient.
- A review of a patient's predisposition to constipation should be carried out when prescribing any drug with constipation as a side effect, e.g. tricyclic antidepressants, antispasmodics, ondansetron. Where appropriate add an aperient.
- As patients get weaker and less able physically, review their exercise regimen with them. Patients may often want to keep active, but fear falling. The physiotherapist and occupational therapist can be invaluable here, in helping to work out individual exercise and activity plans. Indeed constipation may, in part, be caused by an inability to walk to the toilet. Help with this may need to be organised. Again the occupational therapist and/or physiotherapist can often provide invaluable help here. Aids such as a walking frame and raised toilet seat can make a big difference.
- Self-esteem: consider with the patient whether they feel that their privacy is protected when using the toilet, e.g. they may be using a commode. If only curtains are providing a screen for a patient using a commode, this alone is a good reason why they might be constipated. Organise for the patient to have easy access to a toilet or to be in a private room.
- As patients weaken, their desire for food and drink may fade. It is helpful to discuss this with the patient and look at ways of maximising fibre and fluid intake without it feeling a burden to the patient. The dietitian may help here.

- It is really important to emphasise to the patient that, although they are not eating very much, they can still became constipated. This is a result of the accumulation of faecal matter, formed from gut secretions, cells and bacteria (Wessex Specialist Palliative Units 2007).

This health promotional approach provides opportunity for patients to reflect on their thoughts and feelings about their predicament with the professionals. Here the responsibility for preventing constipation is shared – an example of partnership working. This is infinitely preferable to simply assuming that the patient will be too weak to consider an exercise programme or maintaining fibre in their diet – a paternalistic approach.

Rectal agents

About a third of patients receiving opioid therapy need suppositories or enemas for established constipation (Twycross and Wilcock 2001). Clearly, it is very important to explain rectal procedures carefully to the patient and seek consent to proceed. Some suppositories work by softening the stool, while others work as a rectal stimulant. Careful assessment will indicate which is needed. It is important that the patient understands the procedure and is encouraged to 'hold on' to the suppositories for as long as possible, e.g. 20–30 minutes is good. Ensure that a toilet or commode is ready for the patient and that they can summon help to reach it when they are ready. Often one stool-softening suppository and one bowel-stimulating suppository are inserted at the same time. It is important that the bowel-stimulating suppository is placed in contact with the bowel wall.

Enemas

Enemas are usually reserved as a second-line approach to rectal agents and are indicated when the rectum is loaded with hard stool. Again a combination of stool softening and bowel stimulation can be used. A pattern that is often used and can be very successful is as follows:

- Administer an oil-based enema last thing before sleep. If there are no contraindications and the patient finds it reasonably comfortable, tip the foot of the bed, so that gravity can aid retention. Some oil-based enemas may contain nut oil, so do enquire about allergy before proceeding
- The following morning offer a stimulant enema, e.g. phosphate. The patient may have already had their bowels open. Discuss with them if the stimulant enema is necessary; often it can produce a further result. Again, it is important to discuss the procedure with the patient so that the importance of retaining the enema for as long as possible can be appreciated.

Manual evacuation

Manual removal of faeces may sometimes be necessary. It is used as a last resort and should be discussed with the multidisciplinary team before proceeding. Clearly, it is important that the patient understands what this procedure entails, before consenting to it. Usually, nurses will be expected to have undergone specific training for this. It is important that the person carrying out this procedure is competent to do so (RCN 2003). It is advisable to use a local anaesthetic gel. It is also advisable that this procedure be accompanied by some form of sedation or analgesia.

Particular caution is needed in:

- Patients with inflammatory bowel disease
- Patients with a tendency to bleed and/or on anticoagulant therapy
- Patients with an anal fissure (can be a complication of constipation) and/or haemorrhoids
- Patients with spinal cord injury. There is evidence to demonstrate that failing to support people with a spinal cord injury, who need a manual evacuation, can place them at risk of developing autonomic dysreflexia. This is a syndrome characterised by hypertension, bradycardia, severe headache and pallor below, and flushing above, the cord lesion, and perhaps convulsions. This syndrome is unique to people with spinal cord lesions and can lead to damaging outcomes, such as cerebral haemorrhage or myocardial infarctions (RCN 2003).

Complementary therapy – massage

A well-trained and experienced masseur will be able to massage over the area of the ascending, transverse and descending large intestine. Anecdotal accounts support that people undergoing such an abdominal massage do find it helpful for constipation. A small study by Preece (2002), with 15 patients attending a hospice day-care unit, involved teaching patients abdominal massage. The technique consisted of a daily massage, using two specific strokes, repeated six times for 10 minutes or until the patient's, carer's or masseur's hands got tired! Patients in the study reported less discomfort and pain from constipation, following a period of self-administered abdominal massage. Although the study did not prove the efficacy of relieving constipation, the individual comments of some of the participants are very illuminating:

- Patient W 'I use the massage twice a day and it has meant that I no longer get tummy cramps or an awful wind, I am able to go to the toilet once a day, instead of feeling that I need to go several times.'
- Patient G 'Using abdominal massage has meant that I no longer need to take my opening medicine. When I feel that my colostomy is not working properly, I massage myself and it works every time.'
- Patient X 'When I do abdominal massage, I feel that I am doing something to help myself and I don't have to ask anyone else to do it for me. I like the soothing feeling the massage gives, as well as the nice smell of the lotion.'

Preece (2002, p 104)

A systematic review of several studies looking at abdominal massage for constipation suggested that none of the trials was free from methodological flaws. However, the reviewer, Professor Edzard Ernst, medical director of the Department of Complementary Medicine at the University of Exeter, states that abdominal massage is a promising, although unproven, treatment option for chronic constipation and further investigation is needed (Ernst 1999).

Constipation can be a distressing and demoralising symptom. It is hard to imagine the experience of receiving suppositories, enemas and manual evacuations. Patients need a high level of expertise and kindness from professionals to make these experiences bearable. Attention to the dependent patient's hygiene and great care with local pathology, e.g. haemorrhoids, fissures and soreness, is very important. Offering a 'first aid complementary therapy session', e.g. hand and foot massage, after completion of a bowel intervention, may go some way to helping to maintain self-esteem and dignity.

DIARRHOEA

Diarrhoea is defined as the urgency to pass stools frequently. A single loose stool is not defined as diarrhoea. Sykes (2005) states that three unformed stools in 24 hours can be termed diarrhoea and that, if it persists over 3 weeks, it is defined as chronic. Most diarrhoea in the general population is caused by a gastrointestinal infection and lasts only a few days. Clearly, if this occurs in a hospital or hospice, isolation nursing is required to reduce risk of spread. The *Clostridium difficile* micro-organism is probably the most common cause of infectious diarrhoea.

When considering diarrhoea as a problem in the traditional palliative cancer setting, it is estimated that about 7–10% of patients when admitted to a hospice have diarrhoea. However, perhaps the reason that it is among the prevalent symptoms in palliative care, as reported by Solano et al. (2006), is because diarrhoea affects up to 90% of patients with HIV infection and AIDS (Woodruff and Glare 2005). It is estimated that there are 40 million people in the world living with AIDS (UN AIDS 2001). Developments in antiretroviral therapy have had a profound effect on the clinical course of HIV infection and AIDS. The combinations of antiviral therapy are known as highly active antiretroviral therapy (HAART) and progressive work is ongoing. HAART is very expensive and not available to most of the world's population who have HIV infection and AIDS (Woodruff and Glare 2005). In fact 95% of the world's HIV-infected people live in less developed countries. Often these people not only do not receive antiretroviral therapy, but also do not receive antibiotics for opportunistic infections that include causes of diarrhoea (Woodruff and Glare 2005). The reported prevalence of diarrhoea in other illnesses is 3–29% in cancer, about 12% in heart failure and 21% in renal disease (Solano et al. 2006).

Causes of diarrhoea/fluid stool

- Iatrogenic: this may be because of an accidental overdose of an aperient. Other drugs that may be responsible include NSAIDs, chemotherapy agents, antibiotics, iron preparations and elixirs that contain a disaccharide, and also antiretroviral therapy in patients receiving treatment for HIV.
- Faecal impaction: patients who are grossly constipated may suffer an overflow of liquid faecal material. This can be profuse and often a source of incontinence.

Sometimes the impaction can be the source of an intestinal obstruction or partial obstruction.

- A recent history of radiotherapy in the abdominal area.
- Malabsorption syndrome: failure of pancreatic secretion, as in carcinoma of the pancreas, can lead to steatorrhoea. Gastric surgery can also lead to this, e.g. gastrectomy, partial or total colectomy.
- Tumours in the colon or rectal area can alter bowel movements, sometimes resulting in diarrhoea.
- Dietary factors: an excess of fibre or fruit may cause diarrhoea on occasions. Sometimes, enteric supplements can cause diarrhoea.
- Anxiety: extreme anxiety may cause gastrointestinal disturbances.
- Infective: this is a particular problem with HIV and AIDS, where, in most cases, it will be caused by opportunistic infection, often with more than one organism at a time.

Assessment

It is important to gain a detailed history, which includes:

- Frequency of episodes of liquid stool
- Amount and description of stools:
  - watery stools, with or without lower abdominal cramps, can indicate large bowel colitis, which may be due to gastrointestinal infection; watery diarrhoea is a feature of *C. difficile* and the norovirus
  - mucus in stools (slippery stools) with specks of blood and altered colour, e.g. yellowish or greenish, can also indicate infection
  - fatty offensive stools (float in toilet), i.e. steatorrhoea, can indicate malabsorption, indicating problems in the small intestine
  - a sudden change from constipation to liquid stools, which are the 'usual colour' and smell offensive, could indicate faecal impaction and/or partial intestinal obstruction
- Review drug regimens with patients, looking for a likely cause
- Check for signs of infection; take temperature and send off stool for culture and sensitivity three times on subsequent days.

Management

- **Potential cross-infection**: patients should be nursed in isolation until the cause of the diarrhoea has been established. This is to avoid spread of infection.
- Antibiotics for any infective causes. Note that, if the cause is *C. difficile*, this presents a particular problem because it is resistant to most antibiotics.
- In the case of AIDS, diarrhoea may be a result of a wide variety of infections and it is advisable to seek advice from an AIDS specialist and bacteriologist.
- Correct whatever else is correctable.
- **Symptomatic treatment** with anti-motility, anti-diarrhoeal drugs, comprising the opioid and non-analgesic opioid derivatives, e.g. loperamide, codeine,

phosphate. In AIDS-related diarrhoea, morphine orally or diamorphine/morphine by continuous subcutaneous controlled injection (syringe driver) may be necessary (Twycross et al. 2002).

- **Independence**: assess with the patient their proximity to, and ability to reach, a toilet – at least until a diagnosis is made the patient should have their own toilet if this is possible; it also can help allay the patient's anxiety about potential smell, splashing, etc. in the toilet. If a commode is necessary, organise managing this with the patient. Creative care may be needed to ensure that the patient has absolute privacy when on the toilet.
- **Smell**: the patient's room/area should be kept well ventilated and the smell from diarrhoea well managed. The aromatherapist may well be able to help here.
- **Skin care**: skin around the anus may become sore and excoriated, adding to the patient's distress. Soft absorbent toilet paper should be used. This issue should be sensitively discussed with the patient. Keeping the skin clean and dry after each bowel action is important. The patient may well need help with this. Sometimes a small amount of barrier cream, after washing, around the anal and peri-anal area can be helpful, particularly if the patient is very hot or to some degree incontinent.
- **Hygiene**: meticulous hand washing by patient and professionals is a priority.
- **Food and drink**: this should be discussed and addressed on an individual basis with the patient. A small attractive meal, when the patient feels like it, is often a guiding rule. The dietitian may help here.
- **Dehydration**: if diarrhoea is persistent and oral intake poor look for signs of dehydration. The doctor might want to check urea and electrolytes. It may be that intravenous rehydration is required.
- **Rehabilitation**: palliative patients may be severely exhausted by an acute episode of diarrhoea. It is very important to help the patient regain their maximum level of independence following such an episode. The physiotherapist and occupational therapist can make a valuable contribution here.
- **AIDS patients** with severe or prolonged diarrhoea may require enteral nutrition, by either nasogastric tube or percutaneous gastrostomy. AIDS patients with continuing diarrhoea and malabsorption benefit from total parenteral nutrition (Corcoran and Grinspoon 1999).
- **Self-esteem and anxiety**: some 'first aid' hand and/or foot massage for patients who are receptive can help with feelings of self-esteem at this distressing time. A caring touch in this way can help people to feel better about what is happening to them. An intensive course of complementary therapy, over several days, may also be helpful. Not only will complementary therapies help restore self-esteem, but the time spent with the therapist may also encourage expression of fears and anxieties and reflection on their predicament.

ANOREXIA

Anorexia is the loss or a complete absence of an appetite for food. The anorexia weight loss syndrome can be very distressing for patients and their families. In a survey of 1000 patients with advanced cancer, anorexia was superseded only by pain and fatigue as being one of the most distressing symptoms (Walsh et al. 2000). The anorexia weight loss syndrome is associated with an unfavourable prognosis in cancer patients (Dewys et al. 1980). A worse prognosis has also been demonstrated in patients with congestive heart failure in those who had lost weight, compared with those who maintained their weight (Anker et al. 1997). Also in HIV-infected patients, weight loss has been associated with disease progress (Wheeler et al. 1998) and increased mortality (Palenicek et al. 1995; Suttmann et al. 1995). The Gold Standards Framework (2007) prognostic indicator guidance includes weight loss of greater than 10% in 6 months as one of the multiple comorbidities that signals the palliative period.

The pathophysiology of the anorexia weight loss syndrome is not clearly understood, particularly in cancer patients. However, it is deemed a complex metabolic derangement that includes anorexia, early satiety weakness and anaemia, as well as weight loss (Bondly and Jatoi 2006). Although patients are experiencing inadequate energy intake, it may possibly be that they have increased energy expenditure at rest (Capra et al. 2001). Also in the anorexia weight loss scenario, unlike in starvation, loss of skeletal muscle in relation to adipose tissue is accelerated (Bondly and Jatoi 2006).

The anorexia weight loss syndrome has been less well studied in patients with cardiopulmonary disease and AIDS than in cancer patients. In patients with advanced metastatic cancer, the consensus is that no benefit is gained from parenteral or enteral nutrition (Bondly and Jatoi 2006). This phenomenon continues to be researched and is not fully understood. The reader is referred to texts referenced in this chapter for more detail.

There have been no large controlled studies in the anorexia weight loss syndrome in patients with heart failure. However, in patients with heart failure, who are clinically stable, nutritional support alone does not demonstrate a significant effect on clinical status (Broqvist et al. 1994). There is evidence that total parenteral nutrition in HIV-infected patients, with severe wasting, has shown significant improvement in weight (Kotler et al. 1990).

Assessment

There can be many reasons why someone's appetite is reduced and it is important to try to identify these and correct what is correctable, where possible. Some reasons are:

- Unappetising food and too much of it!
- Altered taste sensation – common in cancer patients
- Nausea, and nausea with vomiting
- Sore mouth, e.g. oral thrush
- Constipation
- Anxiety
- Depression
- Some drugs
- A malodorous environment
- Patients with neurodegenerative disease may also have problems swallowing as well as anorexia. Often because of their illness they find that any physical activity is a challenge and a poor state of nutrition will aggravate this. It is important

that a full assessment is carried out by the speech and language therapist and the dietitian. Enteral feeding is an option that can be discussed with the patient and they should be supported in making an informed choice about this. This is discussed in more detail in Chapter 14.

This is not an exhaustive list, but perhaps covers the main potentially reversible causes. The most important part of the assessment, when illness is advanced, is to give the patient time and space to reflect on why they are not eating and how they feel about it. It is desirable, if the initial conversation reflects on this, that it takes place between the patient and professional. Hearing the patient's narrative, as opposed to the friends' or relatives', helps to achieve a mutual understanding between the professional and the patient, of what the meaning of not eating holds for them.

It is also important to assess the effect of the patient not eating on close friends and relatives. In advanced cancer there is some evidence to suggest that weight loss and anorexia may be more distressing for those who care for the patient, than for the patient him- or herself. There is anguish in food refusal for carers (Poole and Froggart 2002). Not providing or preparing food any more can sometimes feel like love or nurture is being withdrawn. Friends and relatives need help and support with this.

Management

A careful physical and psychological assessment should reveal any particular reason for anorexia. It may be that simply relieving constipation will restore a healthy appetite. Sometimes, towards the end of life, the patient is ready to stop eating – it has become a chore – and sometimes the patient is generally eager to try to recover some appetite. It is important to support the patient in whichever choice they make. In some instances, the way a patient feels about eating or not, in this situation, is a metaphor for how they feel about dying.

Body image and self-esteem

Whatever the patient's choice, attention to self-esteem and body image can have a positive impact on quality of life, particularly if weight loss is a problem. Altered body image can be associated with many disease processes and not simply related to weight loss:

- Encourage, if possible, the patient to wear clothes that fit – this may involve enlisting a family member or friend to 'take in' clothes, so as to avoid a 'baggy effect', or indeed 'let out' clothes as may be needed when limbs are swollen from oedema.
- The patient may gain comfort and advice on coping by joining a formal or informal group of patients in similar circumstances (see Chapter 7).
- Look good and feel good; pampering sessions in day centres and as part of a group may be helpful.
- Continue to compliment the patient on their clothes, hairstyle, etc.

- Encourage the family and friends to take photographs and make videos of the patient with their loved ones as they are. This will help to avoid the looking back syndrome and lamenting what is lost rather than 'love me as I am'.
- Complementary therapies, e.g. touch therapies, spiritual healing and aromatherapy, can help people with a challenging body image to feel valued and pampered. Teaching relatives and friends to massage the patient can provide a new dimension, when old recognised signs of love and bonding, e.g. sexual ones, may be lost.
- A gentle and regular exercise programme may help reduce muscle wasting and assist in a feeling of well-being. Ideally, such a programme should be individually tailored for the patient with the physiotherapist.

The patient who chooses not to make efforts to eat at the end of life

- Health professionals should respect this and the patient should be supported in their decision.
- Often, it is the relatives and close friends who need the most help to accept this. The professional may act as a mediator in this arena. It is important to have empathy with the 'food is love' feeling and the idea that relatives are 'abandoning' their responsibilities. Rather, use these conversations as an opportunity for the relative/friend to reflect on the progression of disease and the impact that this is having on feelings and relationships. Ideally, this can be done with the patient and relative together, to promote companionship at this challenging time.
- Flexibility is key. It may be a good idea to have favourite food to hand in case things change. Gently encourage the patient to keep drinking their favourite drinks.

The patient who chooses to make efforts to continue to eat

The patient and key person taking care of catering should be given advice along the following lines:

- Try not to be constrained by usual eating times. Aim for small frequent meals, when desired. Try to eat or drink something nourishing every 2 or 3 hours.
- If possible have meals prepared in advance – chilled or frozen, as appropriate – and eat when hungry. Have nourishing snacks always available.
- Substitute nourishing drinks for tea, coffee and squashes, which have little nutritional value.
- Encourage the use of a small side plate rather than a dinner plate.
- A glass of sherry or wine, before a meal, may help to stimulate appetite.
- It is advisable that the patient and key preparer of food also meet with a dietitian who can enlarge on the advice and give more creative ideas.

Pharmacology

If appetite stimulants are used, they should be closely monitored by the doctor and stopped after 1–2 weeks, if they are not helping. Drugs that may be prescribed include:

- Corticosteroids, e.g. prednisolone or dexamethasone. However, these drugs carry considerable side effects and the effects generally only last a few weeks.
- Progesterone, e.g. megestrol. The effect can last for months and is generally also associated with weight gain.

The temporary effect of these drugs can be to give the patient a feeling of well-being and a genuine appetite, facilitating some enjoyable meals with family and friends. This should not be underestimated. These may well be enjoyed and remembered by the patient's family and friends as precious moments.

Listening to the patient's story is important. This forms the cornerstone to a reflective approach, in which the patient is empowered and supported to make their own decision about eating or not. The professional needs to use their experience and knowledge of palliative care, to give the patient the confidence to make this choice and relatives and friends confidence to support it.

The last few days

In the palliative care arena the question of artificial hydration at the end of life has been much debated. Blanket policies, of course, are unacceptable and probably illegal. Medically it is important to make a distinction between patients who would benefit from hydration and those who are dying. In cancer care, for example, hypercalcaemia can cause severe dehydration that is easily reversible. There is a need therefore for careful clinical assessment before any decision is made regarding hydration.

There is concern that the dying patient may become dehydrated and feel thirsty. This is difficult to counter because we cannot gather evidence from beyond the grave and very few empirical studies have been done looking at dehydration in the dying person. However, two studies have been done that analysed blood and urine samples of terminally ill patients: Burge's (1993) study involved 51 patients and Ellershaw and Sutcliffe's (1995) 82. Both studies failed to correlate the symptoms of dry mouth and thirst with the biochemical markers of dehydration. They both concluded that giving additional fluid to imminently dying people to prevent dry mouth and thirst may well be futile. There is a consensus that impeccable mouth care is the best way to alleviate thirst.

Haas (1994) highlights potential physiological consequences of artificial hydration that may impede the patient's comfort, including increased gastric secretions that may lead to vomiting; increased urinary output that may lead to restlessness and perhaps retention, and increased pulmonary secretions that may cause dyspnoea. Additional fluids may also increase peritumoral or cerebral oedema in cancer patients, leading to pain.

However, Fainsinger (2006) writes that dehydration can lead to prerenal azotaemia and an accumulation of drug metabolites, which may cause the patient to experience delirium, myoclonus and seizures. He also maintains that hydration does not prolong the dying period and may be a comfort to anxious relatives who will feel that *something is being done.*

The decision whether to continue drinking or have artificial hydration is ultimately the patient's. However, if the patient cannot make a decision, a decision should be made by the medical consultant in discussion with relatives/friends or someone with lasting power of attorney. The decision-making process should include a full clinical examination of the patient by a doctor. Clearly, as discussed in Chapter 12, any decision made should be in the patient's best interests, taking into account any expressed wishes or preferences made when capable. If using parenteral hydration, there is a consensus that subcutaneous fluids are relatively safe and comfortable.

FATIGUE

Fatigue is one of the most common symptoms in palliative care, yet often it is unacknowledged by health professionals. It is a particular problem in AIDS, cancer, end-stage heart failure and COPD. Solano et al. (2006) report the following prevalence for fatigue: 32–90% in cancer patients and 54–85%, 69–82%, 68–80% and 73–87% in AIDS, heart disease, COPD and renal disease, respectively. The mechanism for fatigue in each disease is probably different. Fatigue in advanced cancer has received considerable attention and the reader is referred to texts referenced here for more information on this. However, no distinct neural pathway for the mechanism of fatigue has been found.

Weakness and fatigue may coexist in a large number of patients. These two overlapping components have been termed 'asthenia' by some researchers. Asthenia is defined as lack or loss of strength or energy, weakness or debility. In psychiatry, it is termed a loss of psychological dynamic force (*Mosby's Medical, Nursing and Allied Health Dictionary* – Anderson 2002). In contrast to the tiredness felt by a healthy individual, the fatigue in chronic illness is disproportionate to any activity or exertion, and can be overwhelming at all levels – physical, emotional and social. On one occasion after helping a patient with hygiene needs, I left her with a fresh cup of tea. I called in about 30 minutes later; the tea was untouched. She cried and said, 'I want it, but I can't be bothered to pick the cup up'. To me, this illustrated the profound effect that fatigue can have on the quality of life in chronic disease.

Assessment

There have been many assessment tools developed for use to assess fatigue in advanced cancer (see Loge 2006). Self-report measures seem to be preferable. Portenoy and Itri (1999) suggest the following simple method for assessing fatigue:

1. Are you experiencing fatigue?
2. If so, how severe on average has it been over the last week?
   Use 1–10 scale
   0–3 = mild
   4–6 = moderate
   7–10 = severe
3. How does fatigue interfere with your ability to function?

Here patients can express their fatigue objectively and reflectively. Health professionals can get a real sense of the impact that it is having on their quality of life. This in itself may be helpful. Sometimes, like anorexia, patients' descriptions of its impact on them can serve as a metaphor for their feelings about dying. Another tool is the Brief Fatigue Inventory (Mendoza et al. 1999) (Box 13.5).

Management

There may be an underlying contributing factor to the fatigue, in addition to the chronic illness experience, e.g.:

- Infection
- Anaemia
- Hypothyroidism
- Depression
- Unrelieved chronic pain
- Drugs for chronic illness
- Sensitivity to opioids.

It is important to correct anything that can be corrected on this list. However, in many patients, no one cause is readily identifiable and the approach to management is more general.

Education

- Patients receiving information of what symptoms to expect may well feel less stressed when they occur. Research has demonstrated that patients can interpret fatigue as a progression in their illness and/or a sign that therapies are no longer working, when this is not so (Mock et al. 2000). The benefits of patients having information about what to expect is well documented in the health-care literature (Hayward 1975; Boore 1978; Stewart 1995). Patients whom I have nursed have often been relieved to know that fatigue is a recognised symptom. By validating fatigue as a symptom, we open the door to helping the patient cope with it.
- The benefits of education of patients in groups give the added dimension of patients learning coping mechanisms from each other. See Chapter 7 for more details of this.
- The large cancer charities have developed information leaflets and audio cassettes that suggest strategies for dealing with fatigue. The advice is general and may well be helpful to patients with fatigue with illnesses other than cancer. These provide a good basis for education. Available from www.patientinfo. selcn.nhs.uk/livingwithcancer/symptomandsideeffects/fatigue.

Exercise

- We know that muscle strength decreases when people are immobile, perhaps by as much as 5% each day. The natural antidote for fatigued muscles is known to be exercising. Courneya et al. (2006) cite seven observational studies examining the association between exercise and fatigue in cancer survivors. In all studies,

Box 13.5   Brief Fatigue Inventory (reproduced with permission of Professor Charles S Cleeland)

STUDY IT no. _____   HOSPITAL no. _____

Date: ___/___/___   Time: _____

Name: Last _____ First _____ Middle initial _____

Throughout our lives, most of us have times when we feel very tired or fatigued. Have you felt unusually tired or fatigued in the last week?   Yes   No

1. Please rate your fatigue (weariness, tiredness) by circling the one number that best describes your fatigue right NOW
   0   1   2   3   4   5   6   7   8   9   10
                                                    As bad as you can imagine

2. Please rate your fatigue (weariness, tiredness) by circling the one number that best describes your USUAL level of fatigue during the past 24 hours
   0   1   2   3   4   5   6   7   8   9   10
                                                    As bad as you can imagine

3. Please rate your fatigue (weariness, tiredness) by circling the one number that best describes your WORST level of fatigue during the past 24 hours
   0   1   2   3   4   5   6   7   8   9   10
                                                    As bad as you can imagine

4. Circle the one number that describes how, during the past 24 hours, fatigue has interfered with your:

A. General activity
   0   1   2   3   4   5   6   7   8   9   10
   Does not interfere   Completely interferes

B. Mood
   0   1   2   3   4   5   6   7   8   9   10
   Does not interfere   Completely interferes

C. Walking ability
   0   1   2   3   4   5   6   7   8   9   10
   Does not interfere   Completely interferes

D. Normal work (includes both work outside the home and daily chores)
   0   1   2   3   4   5   6   7   8   9   10
   Does not interfere   Completely interferes

E. Relations with other people
   0   1   2   3   4   5   6   7   8   9   10
   Does not interfere   Completely interferes

F. Enjoyment of life
   0   1   2   3   4   5   6   7   8   9   10
   Does not interfere   Completely interferes

higher levels of exercise/fitness were associated with lower levels of fatigue. In addition, a total of 21 intervention studies have examined the effects of exercise on fatigue on cancer survivors and, with the exception of one study, all demonstrated a positive effect of exercise. Interventions consisted of supervised exercise sessions and appropriate exercise stimuli. Objective fitness indicators and validated fatigue scales were used. These studies have been described as generally being of good quality, consisting of randomised controlled trials (Courneya et al. 2006).

- As these studies have not been conducted in patients nearing end of life, and also have been done only in cancer patients, their generalisability may be limited. However, studies looking at hope in terminally ill patients identify remaining actively independent as being important to hope (Buckley and Herth 2004). Furthermore, studies looking at the relationship between hope and survival in Nazi concentration camps have been interpreted as demonstrating that having hope endows people with psychological and physical energy in adverse conditions (Frankl 1946; Korner 1970; McGee 1984).

- The best evidence available suggests that helping patients to exercise may be helpful. Ideally, each patient should have an individualised plan designed by a physiotherapist, who can take into account their individual regimen and preferences. In the interim, health-care teams will do well to devise generic regimens that can be used if there is a wait for physiotherapy.

Energy conservation

- Encouraging patients to keep a diary of the peaks and troughs of energy levels may be helpful. Patients may be able to recognise regular times when energy levels are higher. They can then plan to do their most valued activities at this time.

- Advise the patient who wants to remain independent and maintain a role in the family to speak to relatives about delegating more mundane, less enjoyable tasks.

General specific advice, e.g. housekeeping, is available from the CancerBACUP booklet and website as quoted in the education section above.

Eating and drinking

Although the role of good nutrition in cancer fatigue and heart failure is unclear, it seems wise to gently encourage patients with other illnesses to eat and drink regularly without it becoming a burden. See Anorexia earlier.

Rest and sleep

- Advise patient to sleep as long as needed to feel rested in the morning. To help ensure good-quality sleep consult the appropriate section on insomnia later in the chapter.

- Patients who try additional rest and sleep to manage fatigue do not report it to be particularly effective (Young-McCaughan et al. 2002). However, advice, such as taking a planned timed rest period lying comfortably on a bed or sofa is preferable to cat napping in the chair, is sensible. It would be advisable to rest when there is a trough in energy levels.
- Avoiding long sleeps during the day again makes sense. Planning rest with diversion can help, e.g. favourite TV programmes, videos, radio and, perhaps, time with close friends who accept a slower pace, but can stimulate with gentle conversation. Gentle creative therapies, e.g. compiling photograph albums, can be restful and stimulating at the same time.

Stress reduction

- Studies looking at decreasing stress by psychological support have also shown reductions in fatigue. Intervention here has been support groups including a focus on education and coping strategies (Speigel et al. 1981; Fawzy et al. 1990). See also Chapter 7.
- Psychological support on an individual basis could consist of hypnosis, visualisation/relaxation and one-to-one supportive care or counselling.
- Complementary therapies, e.g. massage and aromatherapy massage, can help reduce levels of anxiety (Corner et al. 1995; Wilkinson et al. 1999a).
- Fatigue can be helped by relaxation sessions.

Pharmacology

- Erythropoietin-α has demonstrated some success in cancer-related fatigue with anaemia (Ahlberg et al. 2003).
- Megestrol acetate helps alleviate anorexia and improves weight and there is some evidence that it helps in fatigue.
- Psychostimulants, e.g. dextroamphetamine, have been effective in reducing fatigue related to HIV infection, in MS and in opioid-induced sedation (Sweeney et al. 2005). Psychostimulants have also been demonstrated to be effective antidepressants (Masand and Tesar 1996; Olin and Masand 1996).

BREATHLESSNESS

The words 'breathlessness' and 'dyspnoea' are used synonymously. The word breathlessness is understood by lay people as well as health professionals and so seems a more appropriate word in a health arena, encouraging partnership care. The American Thoracic Society defines dyspnoea as 'a term used to characterize a subjective experience of breathing discomfort, that is comprised of qualitatively distinct sensations, that may vary in intensity'. The experience derives from interactions among multiple physiological, psychological, social and environmental factors, and may induce physiological and behavioural responses (American Thoracic Society 1999a). Although breathlessness is a symptom probably most frequently associated with COPD, it is also a symptom experienced in end-stage heart disease in 60–88%, cancer 10–70%, AIDS 11–62% and renal disease 11–62% (Solano et al. 2006).

Causes of breathlessness

There are many different causes of breathlessness and some are listed here:

- Pulmonary oedema
- COPD
- Chronic heart failure
- Infection
- Iatrogenic, i.e. drugs that might trigger bronchospasm or fluid retention
- Pleural effusion
- Gross ascites
- Infiltration of cancer in lungs or airways
- Lymphangitis in thorax as a result of cancer
- Pneumonitis and fibrosis resulting from chemotherapy and/or radiotherapy.

Assessment

The patient will need a full medical examination and good history to be taken, because it is important to determine the cause of breathlessness, e.g. respiratory disease, heart disease, neuromuscular disease. The patient may have multiple pathology, so the full medical assessment to determine pathophysiology is vital. This assessment may include the chest physician as well as the palliative care team.

To assess the subjective experience of breathlessness not pain, rating scales can be used. A systematic review to identify which measurement scales should be used to measure breathlessness in palliative care examined 29 existing scales. It was concluded that the NRS (Gift and Narsavage 1998), modified Borg (1970), CRQ-D (Guyatt et al. 1987) and CDS (Tanaka et al. 2000) appear to be the most suitable for use in palliative care, but further evaluation is required before adapting any scale as standard (Dorman et al. 2007).

- **NRS (Numeric Rating Scale)**: usually 0–10, labelled with verbal anchors, e.g. *nothing at all* to *maximal*.
- **Modified Borg Scale**: the modified Borg Dyspnoea Scale has verbal descriptors at each of the 10 points. Verbal descriptions range from very slight to maximal. It was conceived as a ratio scale, so that 8 signifies twice as much breathlessness as 4, for example. View at www.acbv.com/karlaz2.htm.
- **CRQ-D (Chronic Respiratory Disease Questionnaire – dyspnoea subscale)**: patient chooses the five most important activities to have made them breathless over the previous 2 weeks. There are 25 listed activities. Each activity is rated by a score where 1 is extremely short of breath and 7 is not at all short of breath.
- **CDS (Cancer Dyspnoea Scale)**: a 12-item questionnaire to assess breathing difficulty in the past 3 days. Ratings include sense of effort (five items), sense of anxiety (four items) and sense of discomfort (three items).

Breathlessness: ongoing care – an integrative model

An integrative model is built on the premise that the emotional experience of breathlessness is inseparable from the pathophysiology mechanisms and the sensory experience of breathlessness. An integrated approach is used in parallel with the conventional approach. It is a rehabilitative model of care that aims to support patients in managing their own breathlessness, rather than it being a symptom managed solely by health professionals (Bredin et al. 1999). Patients diagnosed with lung cancer participated in a multicentre randomised controlled trial, in which they either attended a nursing clinic for breathlessness or received best supportive care. Interventions carried out included:

- Detailed assessment of breathlessness and factors that ameliorate or exacerbate it.
- Advice and support for patients on ways of managing breathlessness, e.g. positioning, posture, use of devices such as wheelchairs to reduce metabolic demand.
- Exploration of the meaning of breathlessness, their disease and feelings about the future.
- Training in breathing control techniques, progressive muscle relaxation and distraction exercises.
- Goal setting to complement breathing and relaxation techniques, to help in the management of functional and social activities and to support the development and adoption of coping strategies.
- Early recognition of problems warranting pharmacological and/or medical input.

The relatives and friends of patients were also included in the programme, which was an 8-week study. Compared with controls, the patients in the intervention groups showed improvement in dyspnoea scores, performance status and emotional states. These results confirm the findings of an earlier study and show that these interventions based on psychosocial support, breathing control and coping strategies can help patients cope with breathlessness. This approach will not only help patients suffering from the distress of chronic breathlessness on a daily basis but also help them to mobilise coping mechanisms in an acute situation.

This approach is very similar to pulmonary rehabilitation clinics for patients with COPD. These are frequently led by physiotherapists and occupational therapists and have been shown to improve quality of life and function (American Thoracic Society 1999b).

Management of an acute attack of breathlessness

- Ascertain cause(s) of the current breathlessness and treat accordingly. It may be that the chest physician and palliative care team work together on this. Concurrent with this the following general measures should be employed.
- Positioning: help the patient to find the most comfortable/effective position. Patients with COPD often find that sitting up in bed or a chair and leaning

forward to rest their arms on a table – with a pillow on the table to elevate and for comfort – helps them to breathe more easily. Patients with gross oedema in the legs may find that sitting in a chair with legs down helps their breathing.

- Ventilation: it is important that the patient is in an area that is well ventilated, preferably with an open window, so that the air really feels fresh. The use of a fan directing cool air across the face may be helpful. There is a theory that the current of air from the fan may stimulate the trigeminal nerve and help to access higher neural pathways and influence the perception of discomfort positively. Individuals who were made breathless experimentally reported an improvement in symptoms when cool moving air was directed at the cheek or nasal mucosa (Liss and Grant 1988; Burgess et al. 1988).
- Oxygen therapy: this will increase the alveolar tension and therefore decrease the effort of breathing necessary to maintain a given level of O_2 in arterial blood. The concentration of O_2 given will vary with the disease process:
  - patients with asthma, pulmonary embolism and fibrosing alveolitis should receive 60%
  - patients with COPD and other causes of hypercapnic ventilatory failure require a lower concentration, e.g. 28%; this is because patients with hypercapnic ventilatory failure are dependent upon hypoxia for their respiratory drive (Twycross and Wilcock 2001)
  - a trial for oxygen therapy can be given. Usually nasal catheters are preferable to facemasks which often make people feel claustrophobic. Ideally, pulse oximetry should be used to confirm hypoxia and monitor effects of oxygen therapy. If, on review, the patient has found the oxygen useful, it can be continued; if the patient has doubts about its efficacy, it should be discontinued (Twycross and Wilcock 2001).

  Note that it may also be that oxygen therapy has the same mode of action as a fan on the face for some people – that it stimulates the trigeminal nerve.
- Reassurance: general reassurance can best be given by a kind and very confident approach. Patients need to feel that health professionals 'know what they are doing'. This can be best demonstrated by prompt attention to the patient and prompt administration of drug therapies ordered. The health professional should clearly and succinctly explain each new event, e.g. drugs given, fan, oxygen. The patient should not be left alone during the acute period. It is important to ask the patient if there is a particular intervention that they find helpful and, if so, incorporate this, which may be their usual way of coping, into the plan. Having more sense of control may help patients cope with fear and anxiety during episodes of breathlessness. A qualitative phenomenological study highlighted the themes of fear, helplessness, loss of vitality, preoccupation and legitimacy that surfaced from patients' recollections of their lived experience of breathlessness (Devito 1990). Heinzer et al. (2003) explored nursing activities that eased the intensity of symptoms with acutely breathless patients. Patients reiterated the importance of having someone with them to anticipate their needs and assist with activities. Patients talked about the need to have *someone to hold on to* and *someone to attend to their needs straight away.*

Specific reassurance should be given in response to the patient's individual expression of anxieties. They may fear suffocation and death. It is important to listen and respond empathically, gently explaining that they will not suffocate and that the therapies being offered will be helpful.

If the patient has been attending a breathlessness clinic or pulmonary rehabilitation, it may be very reassuring to see a key person from that clinic, who can remind them of their own preconceived coping mechanisms.

Drug treatments

- Nebulised saline may help if there are tenacious secretions.
- Opioids can be used for the symptomatic relief of breathlessness in palliative care. They reduce the subjective experience of breathlessness and there is no evidence that they shorten life (Wessex Specialist Palliative Care Units 2007). The opioid is titrated in the same way as described for pain in Chapter 10. If the patient already takes an opioid for pain, the dose may need to be increased by up to 50% for coexisting breathlessness (Wessex Specialist Palliative Care Units 2007) and it is advisable to seek specialist palliative care input to supervise this. During an acute episode, opioids may need to be delivered via a syringe driver. The use of nebulised opioids is not supported by scientific evidence and may induce bronchospasm (Wessex Specialist Palliative Care Units 2007).
- Benzodiazepines can be used in combination with opioids for their anxiolytic effect. Sublingual lorazepam can be used for acute crisis with perhaps diazepam as background control. Benzodiazepines can also be added to a syringe driver.

Specific treatments

Specific treatments for specific conditions should be used in parallel with the measures outlined here for supporting the patient in an acute episode of breathlessness. Examples of specific treatments are:

- Diuretics for pulmonary oedema
- Bronchodilators for COPD
- Antibiotics for infection
- Pleural aspiration for pleural effusion
- Non-invasive positive pressure ventilation (NIPPV): this method of ventilation is reliant on tight-fitting facemasks, nasal masks or helmets. Often pressure support ventilation is used with continuous positive airway pressure (CPAP). These systems are being used in neuromuscular disease and COPD, and a more detailed discussion of their use is included in Chapter 14. A Cochrane review looking at 14 good-quality randomised controlled trials concluded that non-invasive mechanical ventilation used in patients with acute exacerbation of COPD substantially improves recovery (Ram et al. 2004).

Complementary therapies

The use of complementary therapies can be introduced in pulmonary rehabilitation clinics or breathlessness classes for patients who desire this. These may give the patient extra coping strategies when faced with acute episodes of breathlessness.

- A discussion about the use of acupuncture for breathless patients is included in Chapter 10. Two sternal semipermanent acupuncture needles are now available. They are called ASAD – short for anxiety, sickness and dyspnoea points. They can remain *in situ* for 4 weeks and can be massaged by patients during periods of breathlessness and panic
- Two randomised controlled studies looked at progressive muscle relaxation to reduce anxiety associated with breathlessness. Both studies reported an improvement in dyspnoea scores in the relaxation group (Renfroe 1988; Gift et al. 1992).

Refractory breathlessness

It is relatively rare that a patient will have dyspnoea that is refractory to interventions. The patient may become exhausted and be too frightened to sleep. These patients need a prompt and urgent referral to either a specialist chest physician or a specialist palliative care medical consultant, depending where the patient is in their disease trajectory.

CONFUSION

People who are very ill, particularly those close to death, can experience confusion. The terms 'delirium' and 'acute brain syndrome' are synonymous with confusion. Sometimes the syndrome of terminal restlessness is characterised by confusion. Although patients with dementia can also experience an acute confused state, this text confines itself to an acute confused episode with no underlying mental impairment.

Solano et al. (2006) noted that confusion was prevalent in between 6% and 93% of patients with cancer, between 30% and 65% of patients with AIDS, and in up to 33% of patients with heart disease and COPD. There are many reasons why someone might become acutely confused and it is important that the multidisciplinary team works closely together to establish the cause. Many of the causes are relatively easily corrected.

Potential causes

- Drugs:
  - opioids
  - antidepressants
  - antimuscarinics
- Metabolic causes:
  - hypercalcaemia
  - uraemia
  - hyponatraemia
  - hepatic failure
  - hyper-/hypoglycaemia
  - cerebral hypoxia

- Infection:
  - in particular respiratory tract or urinary tract infection
- Severe constipation
- Urinary retention
- Intracerebral causes:
  - space-occupying lesion
  - strokes
- Environmental change:
  - in patient admissions and the accompanying unfamiliar stimuli
  - social isolation
- Alcohol and drug withdrawal.

Assessment

There are a variety of assessment tools for delirium/confusion. One of the most frequently used is the Mini-Mental State Exam (MMSE). It has been conceived as a brief tool, taking about 5–10 minutes to complete. It includes 11 simple questions, 2 of which require written answers. It has a maximum score of 30 and a cut-off score of 24, indicating cognitive impairment. It assesses orientation in time and space, instant recall, short-term memory, serial subtractions, constructional capabilities and use of language. The MMSE can be administered by lay interviewers and comes with precise instruction for administration (Breitbart and Cohen 2000). MMSE is available from www.hartfordign.org (email notification of usage to: Hartford.ign@nyu.edu).

Stedeford (1994) describes confusion as losing touch with reality. It can encompass a wide range of symptoms, including disorientation in time and space, memory failure, hallucinations and paranoia. It is often a very frightening experience, especially as the confused person may have some insight into their strange behaviour and may think at some level that they are going mad. Stedeford (1994) uses a model first employed in the study of schizophrenia to provide some insight and understanding of confusion. The model proposes that people have a filter, an automatic filter that controls the entry of stimuli into the conscious mind. The stimuli come from three main sources: the environment, the body and the unconscious. We can, for example, in a mindful state be aware of our body, our heartbeat, our breathing, the touch of our clothes; however, in 'normal' functioning much of this is 'filtered out'. In general living only the physical sensations that require action penetrate the filter, e.g. a full bladder. The level of awareness is like a volume control that is set for certain situations. Thus a mother may sleep through a massive thunderstorm, but wake if her baby cries.

We all have memories – some good, some distressing; they are part of our subconscious and may be almost forgotten. For the main part, in general we refer to recent memories. In a confused state the filter is altered and the person may be bombarded with physical stimuli and memories that were 'buried'. In addition to this the person may become extra sensitive to environmental stimuli.

Stedeford (1994) demonstrates how these components can disturb a person's experience using the following examples. A person may be deeply asleep and develop a very high temperature. Their mental state may be that of fearing death. Thus, they have a nightmare about burning to death. A person may be in a drowsy state and, as nearing death, perhaps feeling a longing to see their mother again. A person approaching may be mistaken for their mother (Stedeford 1994). Dying patients are often reviewing their lives. It is not unusual to feel guilty about certain aspects of a life. When consciousness is impaired a health professional may be mistaken for a policeman or a judge. Dying patients may relive difficult or frightening episodes in their life; likewise they can also relive the good, happy and funny moments.

As opposed to controlling the 'confused' behaviour, perhaps because it is disruptive to other patients, the aim should be to sensitively support the patient and endeavour to gain some understanding of their thoughts and feelings. While the patient is being investigated to ascertain a specific reason for the confused state, general methods should be in place that are supportive.

General support

It should be explained clearly to both patient and relatives that there is a good chance that this confused state is reversible. The steps being taken to find a specific cause should be outlined. This explanation may need to be repeated several times for the patient:

- It is probably good advice that the patient is cared for in a single room, thereby reducing the external stimuli of other patients and visitors, which could impinge on the patient's inner world and perhaps complicate it. However, this may not always be appropriate. The patient may fear being alone and it may not be possible for someone always to be with them.
- The environment should be well lit and it may well be helpful for family and friends if they could bring in objects from the patient's home to give a more familiar feel, e.g. photographs, ornaments.
- Having a visible calendar and clock may help with keeping the person orientated.
- Keep the person's routine as close as possible to what is usual for them, e.g. waking times, general hygiene habits, meal times, usual foods, usual exercise habits, TV programmes, radio programmes.
- It can be invaluable if people closest to the person can stay with them.
- Remember that simple things such as using the toilet can be a challenge to a confused person in an unfamiliar environment. So much of wandering and searching behaviour in the confused person may be a quest to find the toilet. Where possible avoid the use of commodes and urinals; they serve to confuse even more. Offer to walk with patients to the toilet at least 3 hourly.
- Each time the person is attended to, the health professional should quietly and kindly explain who they are and what they are doing.

Communication

- Sometimes patients will relive frightening episodes from their past. This is quite common in patients who have experienced armed combat. Sit quietly with the patient and encourage them to tell their story. This may be therapeutic and help them to realise that the event was in the past. Offer reassurance that they are safe now. Sometimes the person may want to tell the story over and over again. Sometimes the story may be so frightening that it may prove impossible to bring relief. In this case sedation may be required (Stedeford 1994).

- Sometimes, during a confused state, a person may feel ashamed or fearful that they are being 'judged as mad' by care staff. It is important to explain that 'there is a reason for this behaviour and we know that you, yourself, are all right'. This way the patient may learn to separate themselves from their illness. Sometimes they may even be able to laugh at their mishaps (Stedeford 1994).

- Try to respond honestly and empathically to 'strange' remarks; if a patient thinks that you are their mother, kindly explain that you are not. You may follow this with 'I expect you wish I was'. This may open a conversation about the patient's mother that could be comforting and relaxing.

- Work with the family and friends to try to make sense of what the confused person is saying, often in a jumble of words; a person can give a clue to the basis of the 'jumble'. Picking up on this clue accurately may bring some relief to the confused person and closeness in your relationship with them.

- Patients, relatives and friends may well need a good deal of support and involving them in the care plan can both help them to cope and be a source of comfort to the patient.

Medication

- Where the patient is clearly distressed and all obvious reasons have been eliminated, e.g. pain, urinary retention, and if, in spite of best supportive care, the patient remains consistently anxious, agitated or is hallucinating and/or paranoid, medication may be considered. This may be particularly appropriate in patients for whom the underlying pathology is irreversible, e.g. terminal uraemia. Specialist palliative care units will be able to advise on this and most produce a handbook with medication guidance. Prescribers can also consult the *Palliative Care Formulary* (Twycross et al. 2002). *It is important in the face of a distressed patient to pursue advice on prescribing in this situation and provide sedation that can bring peace to someone who may be suffering existential pain.*

- Medication of this sort, i.e. to sedate the person, can be considered controversial if the confused state is not agitating the patient. Towards the very end of life confusion associated with terminal restlessness is increased as a natural part of dying. In particular, hallucinations that involve dead relatives welcoming the patient to heaven can be viewed as an important transition from life to death. Where the delusions or hallucinations are pleasant and comforting, many clinicians question the appropriateness of medication (Breitbart and Cohen 2000).

Advance care planning

Talking with the patient earlier in their illness about what they would want if they become confused at a later stage is the ideal. The patient then has an opportunity to state clearly whether or not they would prefer medication that would sedate them. This may seem like a difficult conversation to have. Some patients will make it very clear that they do not want to discuss it. Others will be relieved to be able to talk this through and know that their wishes will be represented in this difficult discussion should it arise. It is important if possible to involve friends and relatives with the patient in this advance care planning.

In the absence of an advance preference here, and if the patient is in distress and it is difficult to get their permission to use drugs, the relatives/friends should be consulted. They should have the rationale for and action of any medications carefully explained to them. The final decision will be with the medical consultant who must demonstrate that actions are in the best interest of the patient. If the patient does receive medication, it is vital that the type and its action are explained. Relatives need to know that, if the medication is sedating, it is not shortening the patient's life. They also need to be able to express their fears and anxieties that they may feel, e.g. that they have already 'lost the person'. Chapter 12 discusses advance care planning in more detail. It is important that advance planning becomes routine and health-care organisations provide documentation to ease the facilitation of this.

INSOMNIA

Difficulty in sleeping is a common problem in serious illness. It is probably a symptom that is under-reported; many patients, when asked, will admit to having problems with night-time sleep for a long time. Solano et al. (2006) report sleeplessness as a symptom in up to 69% of patients with cancer, 74% for patients with AIDS and 48%, 65% and 71% for patients with heart disease, COPD and renal disease, respectively.

Some people may not be concerned that they do not sleep well at night. They may sleep during the day and rationalise why they do not sleep through the night and not mind it. Others do. Sleeplessness is a symptom not a diagnosis and so it is important that the patient and multidisciplinary team work together to establish the cause, i.e. if it is seen as a problem by the patient.

Causes

Psychological

- Anxiety: many people will report feeling wide awake when 'the world sleeps'. With no day-time distractions 'I am left alone with my thoughts – they go round and round in my head – I get frightened'.
- Depression: people who are depressed often report early waking or repeatedly waking abruptly during the night. Often this experience is accompanied by a feeling of 'doom' and despair.
- Fear: some people may report a fear of going to sleep. They may be fearful that they will die in their sleep.

Physical

- Poor symptom control: pain, discomfort or breathlessness, for example.

Drugs

- Diuretics may cause nocturia; steroids can cause patients to feel wakeful and alert. Caffeine drinks last thing at night may act as stimulants. Some drugs can cause nightmares, e.g. propranolol, fluoxetine. Withdrawal from alcohol can cause sleeplessness.

Environment

- Sleeping in a new environment may cause difficulties. Light and noise during the night can be a problem.
- Excessive sleepiness during the day can lead to sleeplessness at night. Long siestas and catnaps can be problematic.
- Periodic limb movement/restless leg syndrome can be a result of many different problems, e.g. antidepressant medication, anaemia, leukaemia, peripheral neuropathy and uraemia. Some of these conditions cannot be corrected.

The reason for sleeplessness can be multifactoral. Often, however, on assessment a probable cause can be found and adjustments made fairly easily, e.g. limit diuretics to one morning dose, ensure all steroids are taken before 14:00 and limit day-time sleeping. However, together with assessment for a specific cause, general measures to help improve sleep can be instigated.

Examine the environment in which the patient is sleeping. This can be particularly important if in a hospital or hospice. Correct what is correctable, e.g. light, room temperature, noise. However, a hospital bed at home can be a big change and make sleeping more difficult; the person may now be sleeping on their own for the first time for many years. Family, friends and professionals need to be mindful of this and hopefully creative in reducing feelings of isolation.

Day-time sleeping

For patients who are largely immobile or bedridden provide as much physical and divisional stimulation as possible for them during the day. Encourage friends and relatives to do things with the patient, e.g. put together a photograph album, play card games and watch favourite videos together.

Pre-sleep routine

Many people have a usual pre-sleep routine. It may not be something that we think about very much. As a person becomes more dependent at home as well as in hospital, they may not be able to follow their usual routine without help, e.g. it may include a warm bath, a milky drink and a good book! Help the patient to look at their current pre-sleep routine and identify if the disease progression has made it different; if so, perhaps friends, relatives or health-care professionals can aid in restoring it.

Cognitive–behavioural therapy

To help still the troubled mind, cognitive–behavioural therapy (CBT) can be helpful. Indeed, there is a good deal of evidence to support this approach (Hauri and Sateia

1985; Murtagh and Greenwood 1995). Recent research demonstrates that CBT techniques can be taught to palliative care practitioners by a simple brief training course (Mannix et al. 2006) (see Chapter 10). Jordache (S, 2007, personal communication) states that clinical nurse specialists in her organisation are fabulous behavioural therapists. They often get patients to keep diaries, set goals, work with negative thoughts and set programmes to work with fear and insomnia. CBT may involve the patient altering their night-time thoughts by listening to music or reading a book that they enjoy. It is advisable to avoid lying in bed in a wakeful state for long periods. Relaxation training can be accomplished by using tape-recorded training sessions.

Complementary therapies

An aromatherapy bath, vaporiser or massage using lavender, geranium, neroli or camomile, or a blend of these oils in an aromatherapy burner in the room, may well be very helpful. In particular, a soothing massage can aid deep relaxation.

Expressing fears and anxieties

Sometimes, at night, people find it easier to express their fears and anxieties. Maybe it is perceived that in hospital nurses have more time at night; wakeful patients should be given time and invited to talk about any concerns that they have. This, accompanied by a hand or foot massage, could be very soothing.

Medication

For some people night sedation may be the answer. Patients who are unduly anxious or depressed may be prescribed medication for these conditions that also has a sedating effect, e.g. a selective serotonin reuptake inhibitor (SSRI) to treat an underlying depression or a sedative antidepressant, e.g. amitriptyline, as a *sleeping tablet*.

ANXIETY

No health professional would be surprised that someone who has just been told, or now comes to understand, that their illness is incurable will be anxious. However, it should not be accepted as unavoidable and something patients 'have to go through'. Prevention is so much better than cure. In earlier chapters of this book are details of supportive approaches that, used skilfully, can minimise anxiety. In particular, Chapters 2 and 3, looking at facing death and communication skills, emphasise gauging information at the rate and depth dictated by the patient, and encouraging expression and support of feelings at each new event. The sick role and partnership working, in Chapter 5, examine helping patients to utilise their own coping mechanisms and the fundamentals of good information giving. Finding resilience together, in Chapter 7, looks at the potential of a variety of approaches to patient groups that are supportive and also share coping mechanisms.

Recognising anxiety

The recognition of an anxious patient can be very challenging. Patients can present with a complex mix of physical and psychological symptoms. Often the behavioural and physical manifestations of anxiety overshadow the psychological causes. Patients can become restless, jittery, hyperactive and vigilant. Symptoms of insomnia, rumination, shortness of breath, apprehension and worry can dominate (Passik and Kirsh 2006). Unfortunately, as a result of a lack of recognition of these as signs of anxiety, family, friends and health professionals can react to the symptoms of anxiety and thus often serve to aggravate them.

It can be difficult to offer support and reassurance to anxious people because they tend, like depressed people, to remember the more threatening and difficult information given, and overlook the positives and interventions that can be reassuring (Passik and Kirsh 2006). Anxiety states may often be related to fear, uncertainty and other existential issues. Loss of status, role in the family and in society, and financial worries are common stressful issues.

Assessment

If team members are finding a person challenging to manage, it is well worth reflecting on the situation, considering if anxiety may be driving 'difficult' communication. So often on the 3-day advanced communication skills course, which I am involved in running, in retrospect a difficult communication scenario fits an anxious patient template:

- Potential physical factors should be considered, e.g. steroid therapy may cause hyperactivity, thyrotoxicosis, uncontrolled pain and alcohol and/or nicotine withdrawal.
- Inviting the patient to express fears and anxieties can be valuable in finding a causative factor and can also be therapeutic. Anxiety can be helped if the patient feels heard.

Management

In many ways the management of anxiety is very similar to that of patients who are depressed and so will be dealt with generically in the next section. Medication, e.g. lorazepam sublingually as needed, is an excellent self-administered treatment for panic if other self-methods of controlling anxiety fail. Lorazepam can also be used on a regular basis twice daily if anxiety is ongoing. Sometimes a regular benzodiazepine is useful in feelings of unremitting anxiety and can help people through difficult periods in their illness.

Adjustment disorder

As the title suggests, an adjustment disorder is a person's reaction to something that is happening to them. The person may be very anxious or perhaps profoundly depressed. Professionals, friends and relatives may be hesitant to consider the person as having a 'mental' illness because the reaction is understandable and may not last for long (Stedeford 1994). Strictly speaking, for an emotional reaction to be termed an adjustment disorder, the onset must occur within 3 months of the triggering event and must not continue longer than 6 months after termination of the stressor or its consequences. However, the condition can be chronic when there is a chronic stressor (Passik and Kirsh 2006). Patients who perceive that they are given too little or too much information about their diagnosis and treatment are more likely to develop a major depressive illness, generalised anxiety disorder or an adjustment disorder than patients who feel that their informational needs were met appropriately (Fallowfield et al. 1990).

Demoralisation syndrome

In recent years the demoralisation syndrome has been discussed in the world of palliative care and perhaps this is synonymous with the term 'adjustment disorder'. People with demoralisation syndrome may not be diagnosed as being depressed because they do not usually suffer anhedonia, i.e. they can enjoy immediate pleasures; however, they are denied anticipatory pleasure because they often regard the future as hopeless (Parker 2004). At the heart of demoralisation is existential despair (Kissane et al. 2001), and the pain of this should not be underestimated. These people do need our help and support. The approach here is much the same as for depressed and anxious patients.

DEPRESSION

Paul was 28 with end-stage liver disease. He talked frankly about his impending death. He was fiercely independent and 'self-sufficient'. As he became weaker and closer to death, he developed a range of physical pains that proved impossible to diagnose and relieve. In retrospect, it seems that someone was always at his bedside examining him, discussing his physical pain and trying to find ways to help. It is only years later with more insight and experience that I feel sure that he was frightened to be alone and perhaps depressed. He could not verbalise that and we carers lacked the maturity of a reflective approach that pointed to Paul's physical pain being a metaphor for his mental anguish.

Patients with advanced disease, in particular with untreated pain, are more vulnerable to becoming depressed (Glover et al. 1995). It has been estimated that in up to 25% of patients admitted to palliative care units depression will be a significant symptom (Barraclough 1994). Some studies suggest that 80% of psychological and psychiatric morbidity in cancer patients goes unrecognised and is thus not treated (Maguire 1985).

The work of Solano et al. (2006) demonstrates depression as being prevalent in cancer (3–77%), AIDS (10–82%), heart disease (9–36%), COPD (37–71%) and renal disease (5–60%).

Although depression in cancer patients seems to be well researched, it is less so in other disease processes. However, there does seem to be a consensus that depression is under-diagnosed and under-treated in terminally ill individuals. Depression, however, significantly diminishes quality of life and complicates symptom control, resulting in more frequent admission to the inpatient care setting (Breitbart et al. 2005a).

There are many potential reasons for missing a diagnosis of depression in terminally ill people:

- The patient may not disclose their feelings. This can be because they feel a stigma attached to 'not coping' or simply that they do not appreciate that the palliative team would be interested. Patients with a physical illness will not necessarily know that we are interested in how this is making them feel unless we ask them.
- There is an expectation from health professionals that a dying person will feel sad. It is important that health professionals are able to differentiate between appropriate sadness and depression. A rough rule of thumb is that a depressed person will suffer anhedonia. This is a marked loss of interest or pleasure in activities. An appropriately sad person will still take pleasure and be interested in some activities. In other words, they can be diverted from their low feeling. That said, the appropriate sadness may be very demoralising and the patient will require an opportunity to express feelings and receive emotional support.
- Sometimes patients do not disclose a depressed mood because they may feel that they are wasting the doctor's time and that they are in some way to blame for their distress (Maguire and Howell 1992). Terminally ill people will almost always experience a functional decline and disengagement from areas of interest that may have been of secondary importance. Again, it is important to be able to distinguish between this and anhedonia.

Assessment

There is no universally agreed way of assessing for depression in the terminally ill. It is generally accepted that the criterion-based *Diagnostic and Statistical Manual of Mental Disorders*, 4th edition (DSM-IV – American Psychiatric Association 1994), which is considered to be the most widely used tool for assessing for depression in the physically healthy, is not appropriate. The DSM-IV contains two core criteria: depressed mood most of the day and anhedonia. To qualify for a diagnosis of depression, the patient should have one of the core criteria, along with four other symptoms from this criteria list: feelings of worthlessness or inappropriate guilt, diminished ability to concentrate and think, recurrent thoughts of death and suicide, fatigue, weight gain or loss, insomnia or hypersomnia. In patients with cancer or other chronic illness, weight loss, fatigue, insomnia or hypersomnia may be common and attributable to the physical illness as opposed to a psychiatric diagnosis (Wilson et al. 2000).

For the DSM-IV scale see www.jr2.0x.uk/bandolier/band99/b99-6htm/.

The Edinburgh Postnatal Depression Scale

This scale was devised by Cox et al. (1987). It is a screening tool for postnatal depression. Importantly, it has been devised so that health-care professionals, with no prior knowledge of psychiatry, can administer it (Lloyd-Williams 2006). The scale contains questions on helplessness and hopelessness, subjective low mood and thoughts of self-harm. These are considered by Casey (1994) to be particular indicators of depression in terminally ill people.

In a study of 100 patients with metastatic cancer, who were receiving palliative care, Lloyd-Williams et al. (2000) compared the 10-item Edinburgh Postnatal Depression Scale with a present state examination for depression, according to the *International Classification of Diseases* (10th revision – ICD-10 – WHO 1992) criteria. They found that using a cut-off threshold of 13 gave an optimum sensitivity of 81%, i.e. the proportion of true positives out of all positives. The specificity was 78%, i.e. the proportion of true negatives out of all negative test results. They concluded that this was a useful scale for palliative care and it has since been used in other palliative care settings, with favourable results (Lloyd-Williams et al. 2003). The Edinburgh postnatal depression screening tool can be viewed at: www.elcmht.nhs.uk/pdf/servicesandyou/Edinburgh.

More recently, Payne et al. (2007) trialled a two-question screening tool: 167 patients admitted to a specialist palliative care unit took part in the study and the screening interview took place separately from the formal psychiatric interview. The registrar asked two questions:

1. 'Are you depressed?'
2. 'Have you experienced loss of interest in things or activities that you would normally enjoy?'

Patients' responses to the two questions were documented. If a patient answered yes to one or both questions, the screening test was considered positive. The research demonstrated a sensitivity of 90.7%, but a lower specificity of 67.7%; however, the false-negative rate was low at 9.3%. It is felt that this two-question screening tool could be useful in identifying depression in palliative care patients (see also Chapter 2).

General principles of management of anxiety, demoralisation syndrome and depression

One to one

There is a consensus that the cornerstone and most important component of psychotherapeutic support for many people with serious illness is the relationship with the primary medical caregiver (Wilson et al. 2000) or the mental health practitioner (Lloyd-Williams 2006). These relationships are based on respect, mutual trust and sensitivity. It is important to see the person as a 'whole person' and respond to their own individual style and needs (Wilson et al. 2000; Lloyd-Williams 2006). It is also important, wherever possible, to ensure continuity of the primary medical caregiver (this may be a CNS) and/or the mental health practitioner.

Psychosocial interventions

- A combination of CBT techniques and supportive psychotherapy with antidepressant medication comprises an optimal approach to managing depression in terminally ill people (Maguire et al. 1985). Research on psychological approaches including CBT, hypnosis, relaxation and visualisation have been reviewed in Chapter 11. These therapies have proved valuable but are under-used. Research studies looking at the benefits of support groups and psychoeducational groups aimed at improving coping and helping with existential pain are reviewed in Chapter 7. The elements of successful groups are identified. These groups need to have clear aims and objectives and are probably best managed or supervised by a mental health practitioner.
- A survey of doctors in Canada reported that 57% had experienced requests for euthanasia. The primary reasons for these requests were persistent pain and terminal illness (Helig 1988). Pain and low levels of family support have been shown to correlate with the wish for death to come soon (Chochinov et al. 1995). The concepts of hope and spiritual pain are discussed in Chapter 7 and should be read in conjunction with this. Good supportive care can do much to help patients find hope in a seemingly hopeless situation. Clearly any request for euthanasia is an indicator of existential pain and should be dealt with empathically, and here the reader is referred to the next section dealing with suicidal thoughts for guidance in this situation.
- For patients suffering a major depression, pharmacological therapy with psychotherapy will help symptoms more quickly. The timeframe in terminal care is clearly important. Patients with a prognosis of months can perhaps afford to wait the 2–4 weeks needed for antidepressants such as SSRIs. A depressed dying patient with only 'weeks' to live may benefit from a psychostimulant. Those patients within hours to days of dying and in distress may benefit best from sedation (Lloyd-Williams 2006).

Complementary and creative therapies

These approaches can be a useful adjunct to more orthodox therapies for depression and anxiety. For some people, complementary and creative therapies can facilitate a time of special and creative peace to the experience to dying. See Chapter 11 for a review of research and current examples of good practice.

Suicidal thoughts

- Research looking at 200 terminally ill patients demonstrated that 44.5% acknowledged at least a fleeting desire to die. These periods were generally brief and did not reflect a committed desire to die (Chochinov et al. 1995). However, 8.5% (17 patients) of the 200 reported the desire for death as coming soon, consistently over time. In another study, patients with a consistent desire for death were more likely to be depressed and found to have significantly more pain and less social support than those patients without such a desire (Breitbart et al. 2000).

- Patients expressing suicidal thoughts should always be taken seriously. Asking someone gently and sensitively whether they have considered how this might be achieved, i.e. exploring intent, can give a clue to how serious this thought is. For many people, thoughts of suicide can act as a 'steam valve' and provide a forum for the patient to reflect on their feelings and how they are coping (Breit-bart et al. 1993). Spira (2000) suggests that, from an existential perspective, considering the possibility of suicide and then choosing to live will give greater value to living.
- If patients, as opposed to reflecting on the enormity of the possibility of suicide, explain how they have thought about doing it, they will need prompt follow-up, by the doctor in charge of their care or a mental health practitioner. Expressed thoughts of suicide with or without intent should always be reported promptly to a care manager.
- The support of a suicidal patient should start with a comprehensive assessment of the patient's history, thoughts and associated feeling; it should be carried out preferably by a mental health practitioner or the doctor in charge. It is imperative that the assessing person is empathic and non-judgemental, and establishes an easy rapport with the patient.
- It is also pertinent to note here that, when patients are very low and despondent, it is a myth to think that asking about suicidal thoughts will put ideas of suicide into their head (Pessin et al. 2006). If the 'suicide' question is one that you intuitively want to ask, then it is right to do so. As discussed before, it can provide a forum for reflection and be an earlier indication of the patient's extreme distress for which help can be offered.

CONCLUSION

It is intended to provide here a framework for supporting patients with the 11 prevalent symptoms that occur in a variety of diseases. Where possible the relevant evidence base has been highlighted. This chapter is designed to be comparable to an A–Z of symptoms with a little more detail. Clearly all the symptoms here have had vast amounts written about them, even if some are under-researched, and so there are bound to be omissions. I have tried to highlight the main points. The emphasis has been on recognising approaches that will be appropriate regardless of disease, as well as highlighting when different strategies may be needed because of a certain disease. The main point is that different folks require different strokes and we need to understand the symptom from the perspective of the individual as opposed to the perspective of textbooks and handbooks.

MAIN IMPLICATIONS FOR PRACTICE

- Invite the patient to tell the story of their symptom so that a clear idea of the meaning for the individual is apparent.
- Plan care in partnership with the patient unless the patient indicates otherwise.

- Aim for concordance not compliance.
- Involve friends and relatives in planning where appropriate.
- Do not make assumptions about a patient's capabilities or desires – always assess.

SUGGESTED FURTHER READING

Most specialist palliative care units produce their own handbook on symptom support. Contact your local unit and ask for a copy.

Bruera E, Higginson IJ, Ramonti C, Von Gunten C, eds (2006) *Textbook of Palliative Medicine*. London: Hodder Arnold.

Doyle D, Hanks G, Cherny N, Calman K, eds (2005) *Oxford Textbook of Palliative Medicine*. Oxford: Oxford University Press.

Lloyd-Williams M (2003) *Psychosocial Issues in Palliative Care*. Oxford: Oxford University Press.

Stedeford A (1994) *Facing Death: Patients, families and professionals*, 2nd edn. Oxford: Sobell Publications.

ADDENDUM: DOLOPLUS 2 SCALE

Reproduced with the permission of Doctor Bernard Wary.

DOLOPLUS 2 SCALE	BEHAVIOURAL PAIN ASSESSMENT IN THE ELDERLY			
Name:	First name:	Unit		Dates

SOMATIC REACTIONS

1 Somatic complaints	• no complaints	0	0	0	0
	• complaints	1	1	1	1
	• occasional involuntary complaints	2	2	2	2
	• continuous involuntary complaints	3	3	3	3
2 Protective body postures adopted at rest	• no protective body posture	0	0	0	0
	• the patient occasionally avoids certain positions	1	1	1	1
	• protective postures continuously and effectively sought	2	2	2	2
	• protective postures continuously sought, without success	3	3	3	3
3 Protection of sore areas	• no protective action taken	0	0	0	0
	• protective actions attempted without interfering against any investigation or nursing	1	1	1	1
	• protective actions against any investigation or nursing	2	2	2	2
	• protective actions taken at rest, even when not approached	3	3	3	3

SOMATIC REACTIONS

4 Expression					
	● usual expression	0	0	0	0
	● expression showing pain when approached	1	1	1	1
	● expression showing pain even without being approached	2	2	2	2
	● permanent and unusually blank look (voiceless, staring, looking blank)	3	3	3	3
5 Sleep pattern	● normal sleep	0	0	0	0
	● difficult to go to sleep	1	1	1	1
	● frequent waking (restlessness)	2	2	2	2
	● insomnia affecting waking times	3	3	3	3

PSYCHOMOTOR REACTIONS

6 Washing and/or dressing					
	● usual abilities unaffected	0	0	0	0
	● usual abilities slightly affected (careful but thorough)	1	1	1	1
	● usual abilities highly impaired, washing and/or dressing is laborious and incomplete	2	2	2	2
	● washing and/or dressing rendered impossible as the patient resists any attempt	3	3	3	3
7 Mobility	● usual abilities and creative remain unaffected	0	0	0	0
	● usual activities are reduced (the patient avoids certain movements and reduces his or her walking distance)	1	1	1	1
	● usual activities and abilities reduced (even with help, the patient cuts down on his or her movements)	2	2	2	2
	● any movement is impossible, the patient resists all persuasion	3	3	3	3

PSYCHOSOCIAL RELATIONS

8 Communication					
	● unchanged	0	0	0	0
	● heightened (the patient demands attention in an unusual manner)	1	1	1	1
	● lessened (the patient cuts him- or herself off)	2	2	2	2
	● absence or refusal of any form of communication	3	3	3	3
9 Social life	● participates normally in every activity (meals, entertainment, therapy workshop)	0	0	0	0
	● participates in activities when asked to do so only	1	1	1	1
	● sometimes refuses to participate in any activity	2	2	2	2
	● refuses to participate in anything	3	3	3	3
10 Problems of behaviour	● normal behaviour	0	0	0	0
	● problems of repetitive reactive behaviour	1	1	1	1
	● problems of permanent reactive behaviour	2	2	2	2
	● permanent behaviour problems (without any external stimulus)	3	3	3	3
	SCORE				

Doloplus 2 Scale: lexicon

Somatic complaints

The patient expresses pain by word, gesture, cries, tears or moans

Protective body posture adopted at rest

Unusual body positions intended to avoid or relieve pain

Protection of sore areas

The patient protects one or several areas of his or her body by a defensive attitude or gestures

Expression

The facial expression appears to express pain (grimaces, drawn, atonic) as does the face (fixed gaze, empty gaze, absent, tears)

Investigation

Any investigation whatsoever (approach of a caregiver, mobilisation, care procedure, etc.)

Washing/dressing

Pain assessment during washing and/or dressing, alone or with assistance

Mobility

Evaluation of pain in movement: change of position, transfer, walking alone or with assistance

Communication

Verbal or non-verbal

Social life

Meals, events, activities, therapeutic workshops, visits, etc.

Problems of behaviour

Aggressiveness, agitation, confusion, indifference, lapsing, regression, asking for euthanasia, etc.

Doloplus 2 Scale: instructions for use

1. Scale use requires learning

As is the case with any new instrument, it is judicious to test it before circulating it. Scale scoring time decreases with experience (at most a few minutes). Where possible, it is of value to appoint a reference person in a given care structure.

2. Pluridisciplinary team scoring

Irrespective of the health-care, social-care or home structure, scoring by several caregivers is preferable (doctor, nurse, nursing assistant, etc.). At home, the family and other people can contribute using a liaison notebook, telephone or even a bedside meeting. The scale should be included in the 'care' or 'liaison notebook' file.

3. Do not score if the item is inappropriate

It is not necessary to have a response for all the items on the scale, particularly given an unknown patient on whom one does not yet have all the data, especially at psychosocial level. Similarly, in the event of coma, scoring will be mainly based on the somatic items.

4. Compile score kinetics

Re-assessment should be twice daily until the pain is sedated, then at longer intervals, depending on the situation. Compile score kinetics and show the kinetics on the care chart (such as temperature or blood pressure). The scale will thus become an essential argument in the management of the symptom and in treatment initiation.

5. Do not compare scores on different patients

Pain is a subjective and personal sensation and emotion. It is therefore of no value to compare scores between patients. Only the time course of the scores in a given patient is of interest.

6. If in doubt, do not hesitate to follow a test treatment with an appropriate analgesic

It is now accepted that a score ≥5/30 is a sign of pain. However, for borderline scores, the patient should be given the benefit of the doubt. If the patient's behaviour changes after analgesic administration, pain is indeed involved.

7. The scale scores pain and not depression, dependence or cognitive functions

Numerous instruments are available for each situation. It is of primary importance to understand that the scale is used to detect changes in behaviour related to potential pain.

Thus, for items 6 and 7, we are not evaluating dependence or independence of pain.

8. Do not use the Doloplus 2 Scale systematically

When the elderly patient is communicative and cooperative, it is logical to use the self-assessment instruments. When pain is patent, it is more urgent to relieve it than to assess it. However, if there is the slightest doubt, hetero-assessment will avoid underestimation.

Chapter 14
Palliative issues in some common diseases

KEY POINTS

- **Gold standard for all**: the history of palliative care is in cancer care. The future is to achieve a gold standard approach to the care of those who are dying based on need not disease and in all care settings.
- **Doing the right thing at the right time**: explains the development and use of the Gold Standard Framework prognostic indicators.

  Identifying the palliative period in an illness is fundamental to giving good supportive and palliative care. The Gold Standard Framework prognostic indicators can be a useful aid in this process and are used to introduce each illness in this chapter.
- **Palliative issues in different diseases**: some aspects of care that are important in the palliative period for people with end stage heart failure, COPD, neurodegenerative disease, dementia, AIDS and cancer are highlighted and discussed. However, this is not a fully comprehensive text.
- **Examples of good practice**: these are highlighted. Replicating examples of good practice requires good leadership, commitment and enthusiasm.
- **Let's get real**: many dying elderly people are cared for in environments where carers are under enormous stress. In care home environments written standards of care are high; however, all too often staffing levels are low, support and training scant, and financial remuneration is small. This is not conducive to a gold standard service.

GOLD STANDARD FOR ALL

As already highlighted in this book the history of palliative care is in the care of cancer patients. We find ourselves in the twenty-first century with the challenge of formulating a palliative approach for people dying of all other diseases that will match the quality that cancer patients have had access to through the hospice movement. Furthermore, the aim is to provide a first-class palliative approach in any care setting. Patients with terminal cancer usually have a dying trajectory that is a steady decline, whereas patients with end stage heart failure and chronic obstructive pulmonary disease (COPD), for example, may have a dying trajectory that is punctuated by acute life-threatening episodes, and so those of us used to caring for people in steady decline are likely to have anxieties about our abilities in acute life-threatening episodes. The national End-of-Life Programme is a coordinated approach to achieve gold standard care for all dying people. It provides a forum for professionals to share knowledge of evidence base and best practice (see Chapter 1 for more details).

In this chapter we look at particular palliative aspects of caring for patients with end-stage heart failure, COPD, neurodegenerative diseases, dementia, HIV/AIDS and cancer. Clearly this is not a comprehensive account of care management in all of these diseases. Rather it is done against the backdrop of Chapter 13, which looks in some detail at 11 prevalent symptoms common to all of these illnesses.

Fundamental to providing best supportive and palliative care is being able to determine when it is needed! Anecdotally it is felt that the heralding of a palliative approach for cancer patients is relatively clear, i.e. those with metastatic disease not amenable to treatment, but is it so clear in other illnesses? The Gold Standards Framework (GSF) team has looked at this issue and as a result has produced prognostic indicator guidance (PIG) (Gold Standards Framework 2006). In the following section its use is explained.

DOING THE RIGHT THING AT THE RIGHT TIME

Keri Thomas and Amanda Free

Development and use of the GSF PIG paper

Difficulties identifying which patients need supportive/palliative care

One of the greatest difficulties in the area of improving care towards the end of life is identifying the right patients early enough. Once these patients have been identified and noted, specific extra support can be given according to their needs and condition, their progress can be followed more closely, inappropriate events and crises may be averted, and we can be more certain that 'the right thing happens at the right time'. This is famously more difficult with non-cancer patients than with cancer patients, whose trajectory of illness is more predictable. Patients sometimes live with chronic serious illnesses for many years before they deteriorate with advanced disease and develop 'end-stage' disease. Elderly patients may also carry the weight of several cumulative comorbid conditions, causing gradual incremental decline, 'skating on thin ice', with even less prognostic certainty. But, viewed retrospectively, it is often possible to predict that a patient was gradually or erratically deteriorating, sometimes unnoticed, sometimes with preventable suffering or unmet needs.

Why is this important? The umbrella theory

The reason that this is so vital is that we too often get this wrong, and are caught out by our lack of forward thinking and planning. Of course, we can never predict the future, and some uncertainty is inevitable, but there must be more that we as health-care providers know of the likely course of events for most of our patients, so it is our duty to light the way ahead and avoid some pot holes. Better identification and pre-planning of care must be one of the biggest levers for improvement in end-of-life care for the future. We can begin to identify who needs help using the surprise question insurance way of thinking, famously developed by Joanne Lynne from the USA, i.e. 'Would you be surprised if the patient were to die in the next year or month or week or days . . . then if you would not be surprised, what have we done to support them?'.

In a similar way, would you be surprised if it were to rain today or might you take an umbrella just in case? You might not need the umbrella, but you felt better knowing that it is there, and it might just be invaluable in a sudden shower. So, similarly, how are we protecting ourselves from the likely torrents that occur towards the end of life, many of which are predictable? If we ask ourselves the surprise question, think ahead and get prepared just in case, we feel a sense of reassurance that we have safely covered some possibilities and averted disasters, and can relax to savour the present moment. Stretching the analogy, the biggest reason for getting wet in the rain was simply that we did not read the signs of bad weather, were too rushed to think of the umbrella, did not know what you had done with it, etc. So better planning can lead to less anxiety and more organised relaxed care.

People who are most ill need most support

If we suspect that someone is nearing the final stage of life, why not anticipate – pick this patient out as having serious advanced illness and needing more intense care, assess and predict their likely needs, and ensure that the right care is provided well in advance of the time that it is required. Therefore we need a means of identifying people using possible predictors of advanced illness with the major killer diseases, and then triggering supportive care and provision before it becomes urgent. This is using prognostication not in the traditional medical way – not in answer to the question 'How long have I got, doc?' – but to be one step ahead in insurance-style thinking of what might be needed just in case: 'hope for the best but prepare for the worst.' This more proactive approach comes harder in some traditional medical thinking but is commonplace in the insurance world, or the airline business, where the mesmerising dance of air hostesses is repeated at each flight, 'just in case' we should fall into the sea and want to know where our whistle was – and we would be surprised if that should happen! Why, then, do we not ensure that we cover all eventualities with the one thing that we know happens to us all – dying.

Encouraged by work in the USA and Canada in trying to anticipate end-stage illness earlier, we developed a paper to try to help generalist clinicians to identify people with advanced illness earlier. This goes hand in hand with the development of the needs/support matrices for several patient groups (cancer, COPD, elderly people, dementia, learning disabilities, children, etc. – work that is still under way and being piloted), to act as a safety net checklist for all care staff to ensure that the right care happens at the right time for the right patient.

The PIG paper

This paper was developed after initial wide consultation with various specialist clinical bodies and special interest groups, e.g. Royal College of Physicians, Royal College of General Practitioners, national disease associations, such as Heart Improvement Programme, GPs with a special interest, standard palliative care textbooks. It was based on various prognostic indicators commonly used in the USA, which trigger referral of these non-cancer patients for hospice/palliative care. The paper is regularly reviewed and updated, and is being used in many areas across the world, as a first attempt to provide more needs-focused care, especially for those traditionally excluded from palliative care services. It is used extensively in primary care to suggest patients who might benefit from being included in the practice GSF supportive/palliative care register. It is also a core element of the GSF in Care Homes Programme, where residents' notes are colour coded according to likely stage and needs, and the needs support matrix applied. This is the first step to integrating improved identification of seriously ill patients into usual practice and giving them extra care that is appropriate to each person.

Although all prognostication is inherently inexact, the aim is to contribute to the development of nationally accepted indicators for patients in the last year of life, which will aid identification of such patients and promote excellence in end-of-life care.

Guidance on usage of the PIG paper and some needs support matrices can be found from the GSF team via www.goldstandardsframework.nhs.uk.

For examples of other prognostic indicators please see:

- Community Hospices: www.communityhospices.org/_assets/TWH_indicator_crds6.pdf
- University of Pennsylvania/Genesis Eldercare: www.mywhatever.com/cifwriter/library/41/pe6010.html
- Watson et al. (2006)
- Long-term conditions: patients at risk of hospital admissions – King's Fund: Predictive Risk Project: www.kingsfund.org.uk/health_topics/patients_at_risk/predictive_risk.html
- Further information available from the GSF central team: www.goldstandards framework.nhs.uk.

Three triggers for Supportive/Palliative Care

As suggested by the GSF (2006) these might be:

1. The surprise question: 'Would you be surprised if this patient were to die in the next 6–12 months?' An intuitive question integrating comorbidity and social and other factors.
2. Choice/need: the patient with advanced disease makes a choice for comfort care only, not 'curative' treatment, or is in special need of supportive/palliative care.
3. Clinical indicators: specific indicators of advanced disease for each of the three main end-of-life groups – cancer, organ failure, people who are elderly frail or have dementia.

General predictors of end-stage illness

Multiple comorbidities (Gold Standards Framework 2006)

- Weight loss: >10% weight loss over 6 months.
- General physical decline
- Serum albumin <25 g/l
- Reducing performance status/Karnofsky score (KPS) <50%. Dependence in most activities of daily living (ADLs).

End-stage heart failure

Heart failure is described as a common disorder affecting 1–2% of the population. There is a marked age-related increase, with up to 20% of elderly people being affected (Dargie and McMurray 1992). Therefore, with the rising number of elderly people in many countries, the incidence of heart failure will rise.

Prognosis

The mortality even in milder forms of heart failure approaches 50% in 5 years (McKee et al. 1971). In cases of severe heart failure, a 50% mortality rate in 1 year has been reported (CONSENSUS Trial Study Investigators 1987). Up to half of heart failure patients die suddenly and unexpectedly (Uretsky and Sheahan 1997). This will often be associated with an acute admission to hospital. Heart failure has been described as having the greatest negative effect on quality of life, compared with other major chronic illnesses such as diabetes, arthritis and hypertension (Stewart et al. 1989).

Staging heart failure

The New York Heart Association (NYHA) model for staging heart failure is widely used. The American Heart Association model is less used, but is described by Duncan et al. (2006) as reflecting the pathophysiology and progressive nature of the disease better (Table 14.1).

Defining the palliative period

The Gold Standards Framework (2006) and the Coronary Heart Disease (2005) Collaborative Supportive and Palliative Care for Advanced Heart Failure concur that the clinical indicators for including patients on a supportive palliative care register should be that the patient has two or more of the following indicators:

- Chronic heart failure: NYHA stage III or IV
- Patient thought to be in the last year of life, i.e. the answer is no to 'Would you be surprised if this patient died in the coming year?'

Table 14.1 New York Heart Association (NYHA) and the American Heart Association (AHA) models for staging heart failure

NYHA	Class I: patients with cardiac disease but with unlimited physical activity	Class II: patients with cardiac disease resulting in slight limitation of physical activity	Class III: patients with cardiac disease resulting in marked limitation of physical activity. Mild activity causes symptoms	Class IV: patients with cardiac disease and are unable to do any physical activity without symptoms. May be symptomatic at rest
AHA	Stage A: patients at high risk of heart failure but without cardiac dysfunction	Stage B: patients with structural heart disease *in situ* but no symptoms	Stage C: patients with structural heart disease with previous or current symptoms	Stage D: patients with refractory symptoms that require special intervention such as hospice care or positive inotropes

Reproduced from Duncan, Shah & Kearney (2006) by permission of Edward Arnold.

- Repeated hospital admissions with heart failure
- Patient has difficult physical or psychological symptoms despite optimal tolerated therapy

See also the other two triggers for palliative/supportive care and general indicators of end-stage illness at the start of the chapter.

The Cheshire and Merseyside Specialist Palliative Care and Cardiac Clinical Networks (2005) add to these criteria that the patient must know that they have a confirmed diagnosis of heart failure. Implicit in this is that someone has discussed the diagnosis with the patient.

The main symptoms for people with end-stage heart disease have been highlighted by McGavigan and Dunn (2005):

- Breathlessness
- Oedema
- Light-headedness
- Muscle wasting and fatigue
- Nausea, anorexia and disturbances of taste
- Depression and anxiety
- Pain.

These symptoms, apart from light-headedness and oedema, have been dealt with in Chapter 13. However, it is important to look at specific treatments for breathlessness. Aspects of pain in heart failure are addressed in Chapter 13.

Pharmacology for breathlessness and angina pain

On a day-to-day basis the symptoms of breathlessness and angina pain are minimised by the judicious management of drugs including diuretics, digoxin and vasodilators. Sublingual glyceryl trinitrate (GTN) can be used for acute episodes of angina. Regular quick-release oral morphine and intravenous morphine, if acutely distressed, can be used for angina and/or associated breathlessness (McGavigan and Dunn 2005). As discussed in Chapter 13 the use of non-steroidal anti-inflammatory drugs (NSAIDs) for pain should be avoided because they have an adverse effect on renal function and a tendency to increase fluid retention There is a need for specialised input to manage cardiac drugs; this can be done by a cardiologist, a heart failure nurse specialist or another doctor following drug protocols designed by the patient's cardiologist. When oedema is unstable the aim is to reduce it by adjusting diuretic therapy.

Care is focused on minimising oedema and monitoring it closely, so that increases can be detected early and diuretic therapy adjusted accordingly. The patient can be weighed each day to monitor their oedema. Clearly a reliable set of scales should be used: 1 kg of weight is equal to 1000 ml of fluid. The daily desirable weight loss is between 0 and 5 kg (McGavigan and Dunn 2005). A fluid restriction of 1.5–2 l/day is wise and no salt should be added to food at the table. Lower limb dependency can be decreased by raising the legs on a footstool when resting.

As the patient's condition continues to deteriorate, consider withdrawing drugs that have been prescribed to improve prognosis but have no symptomatic benefit (McGavigan and Dunn 2005). These drugs include angiotensin-converting enzyme (ACE) inhibitors, β blockers and spironolactone. A decision to discontinue weighing and fluid restrictions may be made will the patient.

Light-headedness

First check for postural hypotension. Reassess the need for drugs, vasodilators, β blockers and diuretics. Exclude arrhythmias as a cause of light-headedness. Ensure that the patient understands the reason for the light-headedness and explain measures taken to reduce it, i.e. management of drug therapy (McGavigan and Dunn 2005).

Implantable cardioverter device

The implantable cardioverter device detects ventricular fibrillation and delivers an electric shock in clear consciousness to prevent death. More people in the future will be coming to the end of their life with these devices in place. Patients need expert psychological support when these are placed and continuing support as their condition declines. A ceiling for its use and a time when it may be deactivated are an important part of advance care planning. It is vital that such advance planning is guided by a professional who has a full understanding of and expertise in implantable cardioverter devices. Implantable cardioverters can be programmed to provide pacemaker function only. Deactivation does not mean imminent death.

A new model of care

Traditionally, specialist palliative services in the UK are seldom involved in people with advanced heart failure, even though the need for supportive and palliative care is at least as great as for people with cancer.

Daley et al. (2006) describe a model of care that is a collaboration of three community-based heart failure nurse specialists (funded by British Heart Foundation), and existing palliative care services (this included 8 hours a week from a psychologist). In the model of care that evolved, the heart failure nurses remained the key workers throughout the illness. The model is based on the traditional Macmillan community nurse approach. The heart failure nurses provide a service that involves home visits; telephone advice and a support group run from a hospice day-care unit. The heart failure nurses use a standardised formal assessment of coping strategies, values and care preferences. They work with detailed protocols for adjustment of medication that have been agreed with the local cardiologist. The cardiologist is happy to give telephone advice to the heart failure nurses and specialist palliative care team.

In terms of experiential learning the collaboration is mutually beneficial to the heart failure nurses and the specialist palliative care team. This is very clearly and healthily acknowledged by the team. Being proactive about shared learning in a more formal sense was also an important part of the model.

Demographics

The demand on the specialist palliative care unit was relatively small. Of 491 patients referred in a 3-year period six patients had seven hospice admissions, four of which ended in death. This represented 1.1% of all hospice admissions during the period and accounted for 80 occupied bed days (0.9% of total use).

Patients' experiences

The support of the psychologist was reported as very valuable by many of the patients. One person described how the session had enabled her to swim again (in her imagination). The psychologist talked about:

> ... where would you fancy being; and at that time I must have gone out, and well, I didn't go anywhere else. I went to the swimming pool and had the time of my life. I had a good swim and a shower and I'd gone off to sleep and that's what was on my mind. I just miss the pool so much.
>
> Daley et al. (2006 p 598)

Seventeen per cent of the patients and some relatives attended the support group. Interview data from patients demonstrated that patients gained strength from being with others with heart failure and learnt coping skills. One patient's comment about the support group was:

> Well, I think it gives you a sense of continuing. That your life is still important and it's worth something. And you learn about the characters of people and how they attack it and how they make their lives worthwhile.
>
> Daley et al. (2006 p 598)

It is also important to note that this model of care is relatively cost-effective. The only additional cost to the specialist palliative care unit was the cost of running the support group, estimated at £47 per attendance (i.e. cost of general staffing, transport and hospice overheads) and the cost of 8 hours of the psychologist's list time per week, which included home visits where necessary (Daley et al. 2006).

Chronic obstructive pulmonary disease (COPD)

There is no single test for COPD. A diagnosis is made by relying on clinical judgement, based on a history and physical examination. Confirmation of the presence of airflow obstruction is made by spirometry. In the UK it is estimated that chronic respiratory diseases are responsible for about 13% of adult disability and COPD is the major cause (Royal College of Physicians 1986). Non-malignant respiratory disease has been described as the Cinderella of the many chronic diseases that require compassionate end-of-life management (Leach 2005).

Prognosis

The mortality rate for COPD is a leading cause of morbidity and mortality worldwide. The course of COPD is highlighted by Leach (2005) as being an illness characterised by a long inexorable disease, punctuated with protracted periods of disabling breathlessness, reducing exercise tolerance, causing recurrent hospital admissions and premature death.

The SUPPORT study (Study to Understand Prognosis and Preference Outcomes and Treatments 2000) enrolled seriously ill, hospitalised patients with one of six life-limiting diseases. The study found that, compared with patients with lung cancer, COPD patients were much more likely to die in the intensive care unit (ICU) on mechanical ventilation and with dyspnoea. These differences in the kind of care occurred despite the fact that most COPD patients in the study expressed a preference for an approach that focused on comfort as opposed to prolonging life (Claessens et al. 2000). Advance care planning conversations and careful documentation of these plans, as discussed in Chapter 12, are a vital part of care to avoid these discrepancies.

Staging COPD

The Medical Research Council's (MRC's) scale for grading the degree of breathlessness related to activities was developed in 1959 by Fletcher et al. Both the GSF PIG (2006) and the National Institute for Health and Clinical Excellence (NICE) guidelines (2004c) recommend that it be used as part of the criteria for assessing degree of respiratory failure (Table 14.2).

Defining the palliative period

The clinical indicators for including patients on the supportive and palliative care register of the GSF are:

- Disease assessed to be severe (forced expiratory volume in 1 second or $FEV_1 < 30\%$ predicted – with caveats about quality of testing)

Table 14.2 MRC dyspnoea scale

Grade	Degree of breathlessness related to activities
1	Not troubled by breathlessness except on strenuous exercise
2	Short of breath when hurrying or walking up a slight hill
3	Walks slower than contemporaries on ground level because of breathlessness, or has to stop for breath when walking at own pace
4	Stops for breath after walking about 100 m or after a few minutes on ground level
5	Too breathless to leave the house, or breathless when dressing and undressing

Reproduced with permission from the National Institute for Health and Clinical Excellence (NICE 2004c).

- Recurrent hospital admission (more than three admissions in 12 months for COPD exacerbations)
- Fulfils long-term oxygen therapy (LTOT) criteria
- MRC grade 4/5: shortness of breath after 100 m on the level or confined to house through breathlessness
- Signs and symptoms of right heart failure
- Combination of other factors, e.g. anorexia, previous ICU/non-invasive ventilation, resistant organism, depression

See also the other two possible triggers for supportive/palliative care and general indicators of end-stage illness on pages 251–252 (Gold Standards Framework 2006).

The main symptoms reported in the last year of life for patients with COPD and lung cancer in a study by Edmonds et al. (2001) are:

- Pain
- Breathlessness
- Cough
- Insomnia
- Low mood.

These symptoms apart from cough are dealt with in some detail in Chapter 13. However, it is important to look at specific treatments for breathlessness and physical and existential pain in breathlessness.

Smoking

Patients should be offered support to stop smoking.

Pulmonary rehabilitation

Pulmonary rehabilitation aims to maximise the patient's physical functioning. Studies have confirmed the value of these programmes in reducing dyspnoea, improving quality of life, increasing independence, extending exercise capacity and decreasing time in hospital (Lacasse et al. 1996). The programme should be tailored to the patient's individual needs and should include education about disease and management, physical training, and nutritional, psychological and behavioural intervention. It is not suitable for patients who are unable to walk, have unstable angina or have had a recent myocardial infarction (NICE 2004c). Successful pulmonary rehabilitation programmes require good multidisciplinary working. Programmes are usually headed up by a specialist nurse or a physiotherapist. An integrated approach to breathlessness is also discussed in Chapter 13.

Effective coughing

The role of the physiotherapist in helping the patient to develop an effective way of coughing is vital. Effective coughing is the best and obviously most constant way of helping to clear the airways of excessive mucus. The forced expiratory technique can be taught relatively easily and, done efficiently, can help clear the alveoli and small airways (Leach 2005). Patients with large volumes of secretion may need chest percussion, vibration and postural drainage performed by a physiotherapist. Towards the end of life, patients may decline active physiotherapy. It should be their choice.

Controlled breathing techniques

These techniques include pursed lip breathing and slow expiration, which is an important component of overcoming the feelings of panic that accompany breathlessness. In addition, there are very simple positive positions that can help reduce respiratory distress, which patients with COPD should be taught. All these techniques should be taught regardless of whether the patient is fit enough for a pulmonary rehabilitation programme. The physiotherapist will usually take responsibility for this.

Non-invasive ventilation

A Cochrane review looking at 14 good-quality, randomised controlled trials concluded that non-invasive ventilation (NIV) used in patients with acute exacerbations of COPD substantially improves recovery. It should be considered early in the course of respiratory failure before severe acidosis ensues, as a means of reducing the likelihood of endotracheal incubation, treatment failure and mortality (Ram et al. 2004). Therefore NIV, including negative and intermittent positive pressure ventilation (IPPV), should be used as a treatment of choice for persistent hypercapnic ventilatory failure during exacerbations of breathlessness not responding to medical therapy. It is important that it is delivered by staff who are well trained and experienced in its use and aware of its limitations. An advance care plan with ceilings of therapy should be agreed with the patient requiring NIV (NICE 2004c).

   A Cochrane review looking at the use of nocturnal NIV for at least 3 months in hypercapnic patients concluded that there was no consistent clinically or statistically significant effect on lung function, gas exchange, respiratory muscle strength, sleep efficiency or exercise tolerance. However, the authors also state that the small sample sizes of these studies preclude a definite conclusion about the effects of nocturnal NIV in COPD (Wijkstra et al. 2002).

Immunisation and antiviral therapy

Patients with COPD should be offered pneumococcal immunisation and an annual influenza immunisation. Zanamivir and oseltamivir, within their licensed indications, are recommended for at-risk patients who present with influenza-like illness within 48 hours of onset of symptoms. Patients with COPD should have a fast-acting bronchodilator available when taking zanamivir, because of the risk of bronchospasm (NICE 2004c).

Pharmacology

The criteria for evaluating the effectiveness of COPD treatments are to look for improvement in:

- Symptoms
- Activities of daily living
- Exercise capacity
- Lung function tests. This may not be appropriate in end stage disease.

Drugs used need to be expertly titrated by a chest physician, respiratory clinical nurse specialist or a team working with a clearly laid out protocol and access to specialist advice. Drugs used include:

- Inhaled bronchodilator therapy
- Theophylline
- Inhaled corticosteroids
- Combination therapies
- Delivery systems including inhalers, spacers and nebulisers.

During acute episodes bronchodilators may be given via a nebuliser and theophylline may be needed intravenously.

Oxygen therapy

Long term oxygen therapy is indicated in patients with PaO_2 (partial oxygen pressure in arterial blood) <7.3 kPa when stable or 7.3–8 kPa in patients with secondary polycythaemia, nocturnal hypoxaemia, peripheral oedema or pulmonary hypertension (NICE 2004c).

Ambulatory oxygen should be prescribed for patients using LTOT who want to continue with therapy outside the home. Short bursts of oxygen therapy should be considered only for episodes of severe breathlessness not relieved by other treatments.

Opioid use

The place of opioids in COPD is under-researched. In one study oral morphine reduced breathlessness and increased exercise tolerance but, with drowsiness, there was a fall in PaO_2 and increase in $PaCO_2$ as significant side effects (Light et al. 1989). A recent meta-analysis of a number of randomised controlled trials suggests that, again, opioids reduce the sensation of dyspnoea, although there are associated side effects (Jennings et al. 2002). That said, there is, however, a consensus (NICE 2004c; Leach 2005; Randall-Curtis and Rocker 2006) that the use of opioids is justified for the relief of breathlessness and restlessness in the terminal phase. Excessive concern about respiratory depression may well result in unnecessary patient suffering. Laxatives and stool softeners should be given with opioids and the subcutaneous route for opioids can be used when the oral route is not possible (Leach 2005). Randall-Curtis and Rocker (2006) state that opioid therapy should be considered not only at the end of life, but also in stable patients with COPD when breathlessness is severe and continues despite maximal bronchodilator therapy.

Cor pulmonale

Many patients with COPD will develop pulmonary hypertension that eventually leads to the right ventricle of the heart becoming hypertrophied and right side heart failure, i.e. congestive heart failure; secondary to COPD this is called cor pulmonale. In fact, this should always be considered, if not already diagnosed, during acute exacerbations.

Cor pulmonale should also be considered in patients with COPD who have peripheral oedema, a raised venous pressure, a systolic parasternal heart and/or a loud pulmonary second heart sound. Patients with cor pulmonale should be assessed for the need for LTOT and oedema should be treated with diuretics (NICE 2004c).

A new model of care?

About 72% of patients with COPD die in hospital after or during an acute exacerbation of their illness; 12% die at home and none in hospices (Edmonds et al. 2001). It is only in the latter years that specialist palliative care units are becoming involved in COPD management. There has been a recent move towards helping acute exacerbations at home. This hospital-at-home management has been demonstrated to be safe and cost-effective according to Cotton et al. (2000) and Ojoo et al. (2002). The patient's preference is difficult to assess. One study of 184 patients with acute exacerbation of COPD reported satisfaction with hospital-at-home care (Skwarska et al. 2000); another study demonstrated that patients expressed a preference for hospital care (Shepperd et al. 1998). A palliative approach for people who experience acute breathlessness is a challenge. These patients need to have faith in their carers.

Neurodegenerative diseases

There are a variety of neurodegenerative diseases that affect the adult and ageing population. In the main they cause a progressive deterioration of physical and sometimes cognitive functioning, leading to increasing disability and dependence on friends, relatives, carers and health professionals. The cause of many of these conditions is not as yet known and in general there are no known cures. O'Brien (2001) highlights that, as a result of this lack of knowledge and potential for cure, neurodegenerative diseases can evoke the most negative and despondent attitudes in the minds of health-care professionals. This attitude may readily transmit to patients and their families, which is regrettable. These patients need comprehensive physical and psychosocial care delivered by a cohesive multidisciplinary team. The aim is an optional level of palliation to help ensure the best possible quality of life, so there is a lot that can be done working in partnership with patients, relatives and friends.

This section highlights some of the more common neurodegenerative disorders occurring in adults. It does not provide a comprehensive text describing the characteristics of each disorder, but rather identifies common symptomatology and discusses these.

The more common neurodegenerative disorders in adults include:

- Strokes
- Multiple sclerosis (MS)
- Motor neurone disease (MND) – also know as Amyotrophic lateral sclerosis (ALS)
- Parkinson's disease
- Huntington's disease.

Prognosis

The time course for neurological disease varies from acute progressive with a prognosis of days or weeks to becoming a chronic disability (Table 14.3).

Neurological disorders are among the leading causes of death in the western world. Stroke alone counts for 60 deaths per 100 000 population in Europe. Other disorders that are also highly prevalent are MS and Parkinson's disease, and they ultimately lead to premature death, although death is usually recorded in terms of a terminal complication, e.g. pneumonia (Borasio et al. 2005).

Table 14.3 Time course for some neurodegenerative diseases

Subacute progressive (days–weeks)	Progressive stroke, meningitis/encephalitis, Creutzfeldt–Jakob disease
Chronic progressive (months–years)	MND/ALS, Huntington's disease, muscular dystrophies, MS (some), Alzheimer's disease
Chronic disability (± fluctuations)	Stroke, persistent vegetative state, MS (some), Parkinson's disease

ALS, amyotrophic lateral sclerosis; MND, motor neurone disease; MS, multiple sclerosis.
From Borasio et al. (2005). Reproduced with the permission of Oxford University Press.

Defining the palliative period

The clinical indicators for including patients on the supportive and palliative care register of the GSF are shown in Box 14.1.

Symptoms associated with chronic neurodegenerative disorders

Patients with chronic neurodegenerative disease will have the potential for multiple problems encompassing the 11 prevalent symptoms identified in Chapter 13.

The following symptoms have been highlighted by O'Brien (2001):

- Pain
- Dysphagia/nutritional problems
- Salivary dribbling
- Respiratory problems/breathlessness
- Dysarthria/anarthria/communication difficulties
- Bladder dysfunction
- Depression/anxiety.

Pain

Pain is reported in around 50% of patients with MS (Moulin 1989), 75% of people with MND/ALS (O'Brien et al. 1992) and 65% of stroke patients (Addington-Hall et al. 1995). Particular approaches for neuropathic pain are discussed in Chapter 13.

Pain may also be musculoskeletal in origin and associated with spasticity, gait disturbance and poor sitting posture. A lot can be done to prevent and alleviate this type of pain with early and continued physiotherapy and occupational therapy. Early passive exercises, advice on posture and positioning, and the introduction of appropriate aids can prove vital. All care settings would do well to have provisional plans for exercise, positioning and posture for patients admitted acutely with neurological problems or as a routine, as in respite care. Such a provisional plan provides a framework to prevent harm by negligence. The care can be tailored to the individual patient, when expert physiotherapy and occupational therapy are available. O'Brien (2001) highlights that pain associated with immobility and spasticity will usually respond well to anti-inflammatory agents in combination with low-dose opioids.

Dysphagia/nutritional problems

Many patients with a neurodegenerative illness develop difficulties in swallowing. This, of course, is very distressing for the patient, as well as their friends and relatives. As the illness progresses, the nutritional status of the patient will deteriorate, resulting in weight loss and fatigue. Attempts to carry on eating when swallowing is poor can result in choking episodes and aspiration pneumonia. A speech and language therapist should regularly assess swallowing and a dietitian the patient's nutritional status. This, with help from the physiotherapist and occupational therapist, should maintain independent eating and drinking for as long as possible.

Box 14.1   Clinical indicators in neurodegenerative disease

Stroke
- Persistent vegetative or minimal conscious state/dense paralysis/incontinence
- Medical complications
- Lack of improvement within 3 months of onset
- Cognitive impairment after stroke or dementia

MND
MND patients should be included from diagnosis, because it is a rapidly progressing condition. Indicators of rapid deterioration include:

- Evidence of disturbed sleep related to respiratory muscle weakness in addition to signs of dyspnoea at rest
- Barely intelligible speech
- Difficulty swallowing
- Poor nutritional status
- Needing assistance with ADLs
- Medical complications, e.g. pneumonia, sepsis
- A short interval between onset of symptoms and diagnosis
- A low vital capacity (<70% of predicted using standard spirometry)

Parkinson's disease
The presence of two or more of the criteria in Parkinson's disease should trigger inclusion on the register:

- Drug treatment is no longer as effective or there is an increasingly complex regimen of drug treatments
- Reduced independence, need for help with daily living
- Recognition that the condition has become less controlled and less predictable with 'off' periods
- Dyskinesias, mobility problems and falls
- Swallowing problems
- Psychiatric signs (depression, anxiety, hallucinations, psychosis)

MS
Indications of deterioration and inclusion on register are:

- Significant complex symptoms, e.g. pain
- Communication difficulties, e.g. dysarthria ± fatigue
- Cognitive difficulties
- Swallowing difficulties/poor nutritional status
- Breathlessness ± aspiration
- Medical complications, e.g. recurrent infection

See also the other two possible triggers for supportive/palliative care and general indicators of end-stage illness on pages 251–252 (Gold Standards Framework 2006)

ADLs, activities of daily living; MND, motor neurone disease; MS, multiple sclerosis

However, advance planning with the patient for when oral feeding is not viable is important.

If the patient cannot maintain an adequate nutritional status orally, consideration should be given to enteral feeding. It is important to discuss this relatively early with the patient and not wait until they are in a state of nutritional deficiency. This is because the usual preferred option is the insertion of a gastroscopy tube by endoscopic procedure, i.e. percutaneous endoscopic gastrostomy (PEG), and, if left too long, the patient may be too debilitated for the procedure. Sometimes a jejunal tube is used. The alternative, nasogastric feeding, is often unacceptable to patients. Specifically, assisted enteral feeding is indicated when (O'Brien 2001):

- patients are feeling hungry or thirsty
- there is weight loss of more than 10% of usual body weight
- meals are taking a long time to complete and become a burden for the patient
- patients are experiencing regular choking episodes.

Patients with gastroscopy feeding can continue to take oral fluids and foods, if they desire. In some centres patients opt to have an early gastroscopy, so that they can use it when they are ready. With the advice and support of the dietitian and speech and language therapist, patients can decide on the optimum regimen for them; it may be an overnight feed or by bolus every few hours. It will be individual to the patient. O'Brien (2001) recommends that patients requiring enteral feeding have access to support and advice on a 24-hour basis.

Salivary dribbling

On average, 2 l of saliva is produced each day. Therefore, when this cannot be swallowed, it presents a problem and can cause considerable embarrassment for the patient, impinging on quality of life. This problem is probably most common in patients with MND/ALS, who may have a specific bulbar palsy; however, it can be a feature in other neurodegenerative diseases as a result of general deterioration in swallowing. An empathic and creative approach from health professionals is needed in these circumstances.

Fortunately, this symptom can often be managed with medication; sublingual or transdermal hyoscine hydrobromide may be helpful. Other medications such as glycopyrronium bromide or amitriptyline may be useful. Radiotherapy has been tried in refractory cases. It is important, however, to achieve a balance between reducing secretions and leaving the patient with a dry uncomfortable mouth (O'Brien 2001).

Communication

Good communication is a vital part of health care in whatever setting. It can be argued that it is more important in palliative care because this is the 'last chance' to get things 'right'. In neurodegenerative disease, communication can be a challenge. It is imperative that early and continuing assessment and support from the speech and language therapist and occupational therapist are a routine part of care. The patient may be affected by dysphasia, which can disturb their comprehension of language, and/or dysarthria, a difficulty in speech articulation. Working together the patient, relatives, friends, speech and language therapist and occupational therapist can assess the difficulty and provide various aids to assist communication. The aids can range from picture charts to typewriters, some of which have a voice synthesiser.

As the patient weakens and speech becomes less intelligible it is still often possible for relatives, friends and carers to establish what the patient wants to communicate by facial expression. Often patients can 'point with their eyes' to a picture chart, for example. If it is not possible to ascertain what the patient is trying to communicate, it is best to be honest. The patient will know anyway as your response is likely to be inappropriate. This gives the patient a chance to rest and try again later.

Respiratory problems/breathlessness

As a result of immobility, poor cough reflex, malnutrition and weakened intercostal and diaphragmatic muscles, respiratory complications are relatively common in neurodegenerative disorders. Again teamwork with patient, relatives, friends and a physiotherapist can help to work out strategies to minimise and cope with this symptom. The strategies for an acute episode of breathlessness are outlined in Chapter 13.

Breathlessness at rest in the absence of heart failure or infection is a poor sign in neurodegenerative disorders. O'Brien (2001) states that, although symptoms may be minimised by attention to positioning and reassurance, pharmacological treatments may be added. O'Brien (2001) suggests a low-dose oral opioid, often in combination with a benzodiazepine, to help relieve subjective distress and anxiety.

Non-invasive ventilation

Patients with neurodegenerative disease may well suffer from the effect of hypoventilation. This is usually first apparent at night, because patients fail to eliminate CO_2 efficiently. Symptoms of disturbed sleep, nightmares, anxiety, morning headache, daytime fatigue and somnolence, and sometimes depression can impinge on quality of life. This is a particular feature of MND/ALS.

NIV is being used increasingly for patients with MND/ALS. Evidence from several retrospective studies and some prospective studies indicates that NIV may be associated with a gain in survival, improved quality of life and improved cognitive function (Leigh et al. 2003).

A Cochrane review of nocturnal mechanical ventilation for hypoventilation identified four randomised controlled trials, one of which included patients with MND/ALS. This review concluded that nocturnal ventilation may relieve chronic hypoventilation-related symptoms and prolong survival, but the quality of the studies was poor and the benefit of long-term ventilation needs more research (Annane 2003).

Tracheostomy with mechanical ventilation, i.e. invasive ventilation, can prolong survival for many years (Bach 1993; Cazzolli & Oppenheimer 1996); however, some people became 'locked in', i.e. unable to communicate on a day-to-day basis, and therefore not able to express wishes and preferences. Home ventilation is costly and exacts an emotional toll on carers (Moss et al. 1996). People affected by MND/ALS are becoming increasingly aware of this option (Leigh et al. 2003). Practice in offering ventilatory support varies worldwide and seems to be influenced more by culture and custom than by science (O'Brien 2001), e.g. in Japan, tracheostomy ventilation is undertaken more frequently than in Europe or North America.

O'Brien (2001) highlights that the role of ventilatory support raises complex practical, ethical and social issues for patients, families and health-care professionals. Advance care planning should fully explore and evaluate these issues before any mode of treatment is agreed or dismissed.

Bladder dysfunction

Continence may be jeopardised in patients with neurodegenerative diseases, by immobility. It is very poor care if this is allowed to become a chronic problem. Involving the occupational therapist to assess the patient in their usual environment is vital. Usually, plans and adaptations can be made to avoid unnecessary incontinence in this situation. Urinary tract infections are a potential for debilitated immobile patients. A good fluid intake will help to reduce the incidence.

Sphincter function is normally unaffected in MND/ALS. However, in MS, bladder dysfunction is more common. Detrusor hyperactivity is a common end-stage urodynamic pattern (O'Brien 2001). Symptoms may include urgency, hesitancy, retention and incontinence. It is wise to include the continence clinical nurse specialist in the management of this. Urinary frequency and urgency may be suppressed by the use of oxybutynin. Intermittent bladder catheterisation may be necessary if bladder emptying is a problem.

Palliation in neurodegenerative disease: the way forward?

Palliative care for patients with chronic neurodegenerative disease is under-researched and under-developed. The Regional Study for Care of the Dying is a study of 237 patients who died from a stroke (data collected from family, friends or officials about people who died of a stroke in 1990); it demonstrated that many patients did not receive optimal symptom control or 'sufficient' help to overcome psychological morbidity. In fact 65% were reported as experiencing pain and in 37% it was reported as being inadequately controlled. The report also demonstrated that 57% of patients had low mood, 56% urinary incontinence and 51% confusion. In addition 25% of respondents reported a feeling of insufficient choice about treatment (Addington-Hall and McCarthy 1995; Addington-Hall et al. 1995, 1998).

The *National Standards Framework for Long Term Conditions* (DH 2005) focuses on neurological conditions and its quality requirements are based on evidence from services for people with neurological conditions. However, it highlights that much of the guidance offered can apply to anyone living with a long-term condition. The framework sets out 11 quality requirements. Quality requirement number 11 states that people with long-term neurological conditions must have their specific neurological needs met when receiving treatment and care for other reasons in any health-care or social-care setting. People with neurological needs often have complex problems that need carefully integrated care plans, in order to maximise their full potential and avoid secondary complications, e.g. muscle contractures, pressure sores and incontinence. It is important in all care settings that the patient's care plan is understood and carried out. Often the patient and/or friends and relatives are key in helping this to happen. Anecdotally, many people with neurodegenerative disease fear admissions to other health-care settings. Often their care plans are not respected or understood and they experience deterioration in their ability to selfcare. This has been a problem for many years. Perhaps the health-care and social-care services of the twenty-first century can rise to this challenge.

The bottom line on the way forward for patients with neurodegenerative disease is that we have a long way to go. Quality standard number 9 of the *National Service Framework for Long Term Conditions* (DH 2005) is concerned with palliative care and recognises this. It spells out that there is a fundamental need for all health-care and social-care staff, be they generalists or specialists in palliative care, to integrate their services and learn from each other in both the formal and informal setting.

Dementia

Dementia is a cognitive impairment disorder characterised by difficulty in short- and long-term memory, impaired judgement and also potentially disturbance in higher cortical functions, e.g. aphasia and apraxia (Breitbart and Cohen 2000). There are over 50 different causes of dementia and it can occur in young people, e.g. Wilson's disease and myoclonic epilepsy. However, dementia is more commonly associated with older people. About 5% of the population aged over 65 in the UK have dementia (DH 2007a). The incidence of dementia increases with age and so, as the population ages, there will be an increase in dementia. By 2010, there will be an estimated 870 000 people in UK with dementia (Alzheimer's Society 2006). Currently, only a third of people with dementia receive a formal diagnosis at any time in their illness. Diagnosis is often made at a time of crisis and then it can be too late for those with the illness to make choices (DH 2007b). In a recent update of standard 7 from the NSF for Older People there is recognition from the government in the UK that the current system is failing too many dementia sufferers and their carers. Recently work has been started on producing the first ever national dementia strategy in response to 'one of the great challenges now facing society' (DH 2007b).

Defining the palliative period

The NICE *Guidelines for Dementia Care* (2006) recommend that a palliative care approach from diagnosis until death be adopted for people with dementia. That way there is a greater chance of the person being able to die with dignity in a place of their choosing. The clinical indicators for inclusion on the GSF supportive palliative care register are shown in Box 14.2.

Research

Potentially reversible dementias receive attention in the medical literature; this includes: development of new drugs; treating profound depression; correcting hypothyroidism and vitamin B_{12} deficiency; treating infection and anaemia; and

Box 14.2 Clinical indicators for end-stage dementia

Dementia
- Unable to walk without assistance and
- Urinary and faecal incontinence and
- No consistently meaningful verbal communication and
- Unable to dress without assistance
- Barthel's score <3
- Reduced ability to perform activities of daily living
- Plus any one of the following: 10% weight loss in previous 6 months without other causes, pyelonephritis or UTI, serum albumin 25 g/l, severe pressure sores, e.g. stage III/IV, recurrent fevers, reduced oral intake/weight loss, aspiration pneumonia

Patients with frailty and dementia
- Multiple comorbidities with signs of impairments in day-to-day functioning
- Deteriorating Karnofsky score
- Combination of at least three symptoms: weakness, slow walking speed, low physical activity, weight loss, self-reported exhaustion

See also the other two possible triggers for supportive/palliative care and general indicators of end-stage illness on pages 251–252 (Gold Standards Framework 2006)

diagnosing and treating subdural haematoma tumour (Ouslander et al. 1997). These approaches form a vital part of management, but will, however, often result in limiting further deterioration in mental status and not reverse cognitive impairment already present.

Symptoms

Patients with dementia often have concurrent physical symptoms that need attention to minimise impact on quality of life. The inherent difficulties with communication may make it more problematic for carers to pick up on these symptoms, so extra vigilance is needed. A study by McCarthy et al. (1997) looked retrospectively at symptoms of 170 patients in the last year of life with dementia:

- Mental confusion 83%
- Urinary incontinence 72%
- Pain 64%
- Low mood 61%
- Constipation and loss of appetite 57%.

These problems were similar to those reported by cancer patients; however, dementia patients experienced these for a longer duration. In a study of 47 patients by Luchins et al. (1997), 86% of patients had more than one physical complication:

- Swallowing problems 72%
- Decubitus ulcers 70%
- Aspiration pneumonia 55%
- Dehydration 57%
- Malnutrition 50%
- Urinary tract infections 37%.

These physical symptoms, in the main, have been dealt with in Chapter 13 and this includes the use of the Doloplus 2 pain assessment scale for elderly people who are unable to communicate.

Nutrition and hydration

Nutrition and hydration are clearly problematic areas and, to some extent, this is dealt with in the section on anorexia in Chapter 13. Patients with dementia probably need extra help and more care to be taken with their eating and drinking than patients without dementia. Early interventions from the speech and language therapist, dietitian and occupational therapist may help to support the patient in maintaining a balanced diet and good fluid intake. Clearly patients with swallowing problems need to have this assessed by their doctor and the speech and language therapist in the first instance. With good nutrition, urinary tract infections and decubitus ulcers would be less likely to occur.

Urinary incontinence

The incidence of urinary incontinence could quite simply be eliminated, or the incidence dramatically reduced, by a regular toileting regimen in which the patient is walked to the toilet and offered the opportunity to use it, at least 3 hourly during the day, last thing at night and immediately on waking in the morning, and if waking at night. These walks can be a time of sharing thoughts and promote camaraderie with the patient. In other words walking to the toilet can be a social event and not just a task. Seek advice from the promotion of continence team if a regular toileting regimen is not working

Decubitus ulcers

A 3-hourly toileting regimen would also help to prevent decubitus ulcers by regularly relieving sitting pressure and changing position. It would be good policy to use a pressure assessment risk tool, e.g. the Waterlow Scoring System, routinely in elderly demented patients. The Waterlow System also incorporates a pressure area care policy that should be followed. www.judy-waterlow.co.uk/waterlow_scale_references.htm.

Maintaining quality of life

A very large part of caring for patients with dementia is helping to maintain quality of life. Helping people with dementia to do this is not so very different from helping people with other illnesses; however because of an increased vulnerability that comes as mental abilities decline, people with dementia will almost certainly need more help with this than patients with a physical illness. The key is respect for the person and a genuinely person-centred approach. The Alzheimer's Society (2007) gives excellent guidance on achieving this.

Clearly a detailed assessment of the person, their history, social circumstances, preferences and abilities in performing ADLs is fundamental, as is working in partnership with the patient's family, friends and carers. People with dementia need reassurance and support from family, friends and professional carers (Alzheimer's Society 2007).

Helping someone with dementia to maintain their quality of life is set out under six headings by the Alzheimer's Society (2007). Each core component comes with a detailed carer's advice sheet, which gives very practical and achievable suggestions on how the core aims can be achieved (www.alzheimers.org.uk/caringforsomeonewithdementia/maintainingqualityoflife).

Core aims

1. Understanding and respecting the person with dementia: this aim emphasises the uniqueness of the person and reminds carers that dementia affects people in individual ways. It emphasises flexibility in approach and the importance of making time to listen, talk with and continue to show affection for and enjoy being with the person. It highlights the importance of cultural values, acting with courtesy, respecting privacy and offering simple choices. Guidance on helping patients to express feelings and tips for making the person feel good about him- or herself are included in the care advice sheet.
2. Maintaining skills: this advice sheet emphasises the importance of doing things with the person rather than for them and focused on what the person can do, rather than what they cannot.
3. Communicating: this section highlights the importance of listening carefully and reminds us that, when words are difficult, non-verbal communication becomes even more important. Being calm and having a relaxed body language can be helpful. If speech is difficult to understand, check back with the person to see if you have understood their meaning correctly. Use physical contact to reassure where appropriate.
4. Hobbies, pastimes and everyday activities: it is important to help the person for whom you are caring to find activities that they enjoy; this can be, for example, taking a walk, looking at photographs, taking part in group activities, either physical or sociable.
5. Memory loss: as dementia progresses the person may sometimes confuse facts with things that they have imagined. Usually it is best not to argue, but to focus on the feelings that are being expressed and relate to them.
6. Holidays: in this section, very practical advice and tips are given to friends and relatives who may be caring for a person with dementia, in an unfamiliar environment for that person, e.g. if on holiday.

The way forward?

The Alzheimer's Society has identified the following 12 points as key issues in end-of-life care for people with dementia:

1. It is well recognised that end-of-life care for people with dementia is an area that needs development (Sampson et al. 2006). This is well supported by anecdotal accounts from carers. The National Council for Palliative Care is working jointly with the Alzheimer's Society to develop an effective evidence-based service model for end-of-life care in dementia (Alzheimer's Society 2006).

2. Uncertainty in prognosis: the Alzheimer's Society suggests using the GSF checklist as included here and highlights this as an important initiative in care homes.

3. Communication: some aspects of communicating in dementia are dealt with in both Chapters 3 and 9; see also Chapter 13. Continuity of care and training of staff in some specifics of communicating in dementia are stressed (Alzheimer's Society 2006).

4. Pain: the under-recognition of pain in people with dementia has been discussed in this chapter and Chapter 13. The use of the Doloplus 2 Scale is highlighted.

5. Supporting relatives: Chapter 8 is concerned with supporting carers. Relatives of people with dementia report a 'huge amount of distress' when asked to consider decisions about treating infections and artificial nutrition or hydration towards the end of life (Alzheimer's Society 2006). Advance care planning is a key to quality provision at the end of life. Although these conversations are never easy to start, they can often result in a strengthening of relationships among professionals, patients, relatives and friends. Having these conversations early in the illness trajectory can empower the person with dementia to nominate a proxy to represent their wishes, when they lack the mental capacity to do so. This is discussed in more detail in Chapter 12.

6. Advocacy: in the absence of advance statements and decisions, and where the patient has not nominated another person with lasting power of attorney to make decisions on their behalf, the Alzheimer's Society (2006) would like to see an extension of the independent mental capacity advocate service to all decisions around end-of-life treatment. This is important because carers' views may differ from those of the patient.

7. Boredom and lack of activities: in many hospital wards and care homes patients are left under-stimulated. Guidelines for helping with this have already been highlighted in this chapter referring to: www.alzheimers.org.uk/caringforsomeonewithdementia/maintainingqualityoflife.

8. Spiritual care: Sampson et al. (2006) compared the notes of patients with and without dementia who died during an acute hospital admission. It was found that significantly fewer patients with dementia made any mention of their religious faith (40% vs 63%). This needs correcting.

9. Hospital care: the poor suitability of hospital care for patients with dementia is well documented. The research implicates that 60% of hospital beds are occupied by older people and that up to 40% of older people in hospital have dementia (Holmes et al. 2003). Dementia should become a core part of nurse training and continuing professional development. Strategies to avoid admission to hospital towards the end of life for patients with dementia should be developed (Alzheimer's Society 2006).

10. Caring at home: there is a long way to go before dying at home can be a realistic choice. Home-based emergency respite care has been reported as a positive by carers and supports them in carrying on caring. Carer education is valued.

11. Training of staff: it is vital that people with dementia are not excluded from specialist palliative care units, which are not equipped to care for such people. Education of specialist palliative care staff and care home staff is a priority. Care home staff is the biggest group of people caring for people with dementia at the end of their lives (Alzheimer's Society 2006). Working in care homes often equates with working with minimal staffing levels and attempting to achieve standards, which, on paper, are the ideals. The financial remuneration for unqualified staff, who represent most carers, is often little above the minimum wage. Society needs to place a higher value on caring in general.

12. Care coordination: the NICE (2004a) guidelines on support and palliative care recommend the idea of nominating a person to take the 'key role' to coordinate care. The NICE guidelines on dementia (2006) also suggest that specialist palliative care dementia nurses would be best placed to coordinate end-of-life care, in whichever location the individual was being cared for. The Alzheimer's Society (2006) supports these recommendations.

Examples of good practice

The self-fulfilling prophecy

The approach and outcome to caring for patients with dementia can speak volumes about the care staff and little about the people for whom they care. If there is an expectation that patients with dementia will not be able to communicate their needs effectively, this bias can decide the outcome; however, where the expectation is that patients with dementia can express their needs, they will.

A study exploring ways for staff to consult people with dementia about services included 40 practitioners (mainly qualified) and 31 people with dementia. The study highlighted the importance of providing opportunities for staff to reflect on and talk about their experiences. Against this background, the study demonstrated that it is possible for staff in busy service settings to undertake meaningful consultation work with people with dementia; even those who have significant difficulties in expressing their ideas, needs and preferences can express them in a caring respectful environment. The researcher suggests that ways forward include (Allan 2001):

- Reinforce service commitment to the centrality of communication throughout care practice.
- Help staff to develop self-esteem and confidence in the skills that they already have.
- Make a greater commitment to staff reflecting on their experience of working and communicating with people with dementia.
- Subject a range of organisational features of services to scrutiny in terms of how they affect communication and consultation practice.

Admiral nurses

A relative new development is the launch of a registered charity supporting 'Admiral nurses'. The model is based on the Macmillan nurse one. Admiral nurses are specialist dementia nurses, working in the community with families, carers and supporters of people with dementia. The Admiral nurse model was established as a direct result of the experiences of family carers. Admiral nurses are named after Joseph Levy, who had dementia. He was known to his family as 'Admiral Joe' because of his keen interest in sailing. The role of Admiral nurses is as follows:

- Promote best practice in person-centred dementia care
- Work with family carers as their prime focus
- Provide practical advice, emotional support, information and skills
- Deliver education and training in dementia care
- Provide consultancy to professionals working with people with dementia: www.fordementia.org.uk/admiral.htm.

HIV/AIDS in the UK

The human immunodeficiency virus (HIV) evolves over a period of years, into acquired immune deficiency syndrome (AIDS), which is uniformly fatal. However, in developed countries the progress made in researching antiretroviral therapy has had a big impact on the clinical course of HIV infection and AIDS. Antiretroviral drugs are used in combination. Collectively, these combinations are known as highly active antiretroviral therapy (HAART). Research into the optimal use of these drugs is ongoing as is the search for more effective drugs. According to Hirschtick and Von Roenn (2006), in affluent countries, although there is still associated morbidity and mortality associated with HIV infection, it has for many patients become a chronic manageable condition.

Brogan and George (2001) observed that some patients remain free of serious symptoms and complications until late in the illness. Others remain asymptomatic for years or even decades, and still others suffer debilitating malaise and frequent acute events.

AIDS in developing countries

In developing countries, the problem of AIDS is described by Brogan and George (2001) as assuming biblical proportions: 95% of the world's 40 million (UN AIDS 2001) people with AIDS live in developing countries where few people receive antibiotics for opportunistic infections, never mind antiretroviral therapy (Woodruff and Glare 2005). Overall, however, leadership and political action on AIDS have increased significantly since 2001. Internationally, in 2005 the UN's World Summit, the G8, industrialised countries and the African Union endorsed a policy of cooperation on HIV prevention, treatment, care and support (UN AIDS 2006). However, AIDS is still altering the demographics of countries in sub-Saharan Africa where 13 million children under the age of 15 have lost one or both parents to AIDS (Help the Hospices 2002).

Defining the palliative period

Clinical AIDS, sometimes called the last phase, is heralded when the CD4 lymphocyte count falls to <200 U/l or by the occurrence of AIDS-defining conditions, e.g. infections and cancers, some of which are included in the next section (Woodruff and Glare 2005). Before the use of antiretroviral therapy, when the CD4 lymphocyte count was <200 U/l survival time was 2–3 years but only 1 year after the first AIDS-defining condition (Woodruff and Glare 2005).

Associated infections

The progress of AIDS is characterised by a host of opportunistic infections. Some of these are: pneumocystis pneumonia, candida infection, tuberculosis and herpes simplex. There are many more. Much work has been done on developing treatment and prophylactic approaches to these infections. Updated expert recommendations are available on www.aidsinfo.nil.gov.

Associated cancers

There is an increased incidence of cancer in patients with HIV/AIDS. A quarter of patients with AIDS develop cancer and it is a major contributory cause of death in about 15% of patients (Woodruff and Glare 2005). The cancers that occur most frequently are Kaposi's sarcoma, non-Hodgkin's lymphoma, Hodgkin's disease, cervical cancer and anal cancer.

Neurological disease

Progressive neurological disease is listed as one of the most debilitating features of AIDS. At least 40% of patients have central nervous system (CNS) damage (Jellinger et al. 2000). Peripheral neuropathy and AIDS–dementia complex are among the neurological disorders.

Liver disease

Chronic liver disease is now among one of the most common causes of death for people infected with HIV. This is in large part the result of coinfection with hepatitis C virus (Hirschtick and Von Roenn 2006).

Late presenters

Some patients with HIV/AIDS come from marginalised groups in society, e.g. injecting drug users, refugees from countries where HIV/AIDS is endemic and those working in, and using, the sex industry. These minorities often take up services late, perhaps after the onset of an AIDS-defining illness.

Ten most common symptoms

Matthews et al. (2000) looked at data from 3000 American patients with AIDS and reported the following as the 10 most common symptoms:

1. Constitutional symptoms (fever, sweats, chills) 51%
2. Diarrhoea 51%
3. Nausea and anorexia 50%
4. Numbness, tingling/neuropathic pain in hands and feet 49%
5. Headaches 39%
6. Weight loss 37%
7. Vaginal symptoms 36%
8. Sinus symptoms 36%
9. Visual disturbances 32%
10. Cough or shortness of breath 30%.

Most of these symptoms are dealt with in some detail in Chapters 10 and 13. Brogan and George (2001) comment that these particular symptoms are not so very different from those found in other diseases. The ones that are not dealt with in this book, i.e. sinus symptoms, vaginal symptoms and visual disturbances, will need specialist input from professionals experienced in AIDS-related symptoms.

Challenges now and in the future

As for all patients receiving palliative care the challenge is to minimise symptom load and improve quality of living. Brogan and George (2001) also see that AIDS offers particular challenges in the following areas:

- Easily treatable symptoms can present atypically in this group of patients. Therefore new symptoms warrant investigation even towards the end of life.
- The only way of controlling some distressing symptoms, e.g. cancers and opportunistic infections, is by treating the underlying cause.
- To minimise symptoms many drugs used prophylactically may need to be continued to the end of life.
- The side effects of combination therapies can result in a heavy symptomatic load on the individual.

Expert symptom control and considerable expertise in psychosocial and spiritual care for AIDS patients often require the services of the specialist palliative care team, be they hands on or in a consultative role. The psychosocial and spiritual aspects of caring for dying people have been described in some detail in the earlier chapters. From their experience of caring for HIV/AIDS patients, Brogan and George (2001) note that existential issues are often very acute. Patients often demonstrate acute confusion and fear about dying; sometimes patients from Africa may express existential distress by using spiritual language, e.g. talk of spirits and devils. In these instances it is important to try to gain a mutual understanding of different cultural views (Brogan and George 2001).

Cancer

What is cancer?

Cancer can occur in any tissue of the body. It results from a change in certain cells that allow them to disrespect normal growth limits, i.e. they no longer obey the feedback controls that normally stop cellular growth and reproduction after a given number of cells have developed. Researchers have found that the genetic make-up of most, if not all, cancer cells is different from that of normal cells. This has led to the idea that cancer almost invariably results from mutation of the genetic system in the nucleus; cancerous cells will compete with normal tissues for nutrients and, because cancer cells continue to proliferate indefinitely, normal tissue gradually suffers nutritive death. Cancer can, of course, spread from the primary site to other parts of the body. A secondary cancer is called a metastasis. Cancer can spread by local invasion, lymphatic spread or to more distant sites via the bloodstream. In some instances metastases have formed before an initial diagnosis is made.

There are over 200 different cancers and their capacity to invade distant tissues varies. Likewise, a given tumour type has a different tendency to metastasise in different individuals (Souhami and Tobias 1998).

Staging of cancer and prognosis

A common method of staging tumours is the TNM system, developed by the American Joint Committee of Cancer Staging and End Result Reporting (Sobin and Wittekind 1997). It works as follows:

T = in some cancers the size of the tumour and in others the depth

N = the condition of the regional lymph nodes. Nodal involvement has important prognostic implications. In most types of cancers fixed (N3) lymph nodes that are surgically inaccessible carry a far worse prognosis than mobile ipsilateral (N1) nodes

M = the presence or absence of metastases. With very few exceptions (notably testicular tumours), the presence of metastases has considerable prognostic implications, usually proving fatal within months or a few years of diagnosis (Souhami and Tobias 1998)

The addition of numbers to TNM details the extent of the cancer, e.g. T1 N1 M0 denotes a localised small tumour, whereas T4 N3 MI represents a very large lesion that involves not only regional nodes but also distant sites.

In the UK one in three people will develop cancer at some stage in their lives. One in four will die of cancer (DH 2000b). Globally, for cancer, a third of cases are preventable and a third curable, if found early and standard therapies are available. For the remaining third, freedom from pain and other symptoms is possible. However, worldwide, most cancers when found are incurable and pain relief and symptom control, as we know it in this country, are often not available to many patients in developing countries with cancer (Stjernswärd and Clark 2005).

The western world

In the western world, the most common sites for cancers are:

* lung
* breast
* skin
* gut
* prostate
* blood
* ovary
* cervix
* pancreas.

The treatment consists of surgery, chemotherapy and radiotherapy, often in com-bination. *The NHS Cancer Plan* was published in 2000 (DH 2000b). It is a plan for reform. Despite the best efforts of NHS staff and cancer patients, the survival rates for many of the major cancers lagged behind those for the rest of Europe (DH 2000b). Cancer networks were identified as the organisational model for cancer services to implement the cancer plan. There are now 34 cancer networks in England. They have wide-reaching remits from education and screening to palliative care.

In terms of treatment of patients with cancer, the cancer plan aims to 'end the postcode lottery'. There is a programme of guidance setting national standards. In theory patients with a particular cancer should be offered the same treatment or combination of treatment, i.e. surgery, chemotherapy and radiotherapy, wherever they are in the country. To support local clinical governance arrangements there is a system of peer review for cancer services to monitor implementation of national guidance and help drive up quality (DH 2000b).

Defining the palliative period

The GSF PIG (2006) suggests the following criteria for predicting the palliative period in cancer:

> Any patient whose cancer is metastatic or not amendable to treatment, with some exceptions – this may include some cancer patients from diagnosis, e.g. lung cancer. 'The single most important predictive factor in cancer is performance status and functional ability' – if patients are spending more than 50% of their time in bed/lying down, prognosis is likely to be about 3 months or less. (See also pages 251–252.)

There are many different symptoms associated with the palliative care of cancer patients. Eleven of these symptoms were discussed in Chapter 13 and more are included in Chapter 15, i.e. palliative emergencies. This section is confined to a brief discussion on:

* palliative chemotherapy
* palliative radiotherapy
* symptoms resulting from local spread.

Palliative chemotherapy

The notion of palliative chemotherapy can cause some confusion for health-care professionals and patients alike. Chemotherapy is a term that is usually associated with cure. It is important that, when using palliative chemotherapy, the rationale is clearly understood by the patient, friends and relatives as well as associated health-care professionals. The possibility for palliative chemotherapy varies, of course, among different cancers. Some tumours have high sensitivity to chemotherapy, e.g. lymphoblastic leukaemia, testicular cancer, and others have a low sensitivity, e.g. oesophageal cancer, melanoma.

The aim of palliative chemotherapy is that, by the use of antineoplastic medications, the adverse signs and symptoms caused directly or indirectly by the malignant disease process can be reduced (Ellison 1998), and in many instances survival is prolonged. Tumour shrinkage induced by palliative chemotherapy can result, for example, in reduction in pain, breathlessness, coughing and bleeding in the bowel and genital tract (Wang and Kavanagh 2006).

The possible benefits of tumour response should be weighed up very carefully against the toxicity of the chemotherapy regimen. It is important that oncologists and palliative specialists work in harmony in terms of advising and supporting the patient in making choices about palliative chemotherapy. All too often disagreements between the two disciplines have the potential to maximise stress for the patient. The side effects of chemotherapy are well documented in other texts. The Cancerbacup factfile provides very helpful and practical information about these side effects and how to reduce their impact. Information is also available from their website.

Palliative radiotherapy

Radiotherapy is a relatively well-established palliative approach for relieving distressing symptoms, e.g. pain, breathlessness and bleeding caused by locally advanced and metastatic tumours. Its use in spinal cord compression to help reduce incidence of loss of sensation and function of spinal nerves is a clear example of its value (spinal cord compression is dealt with in Chapter 15).

Palliative radiotherapy is probably used most commonly for bone, lung and brain metastases. For palliation, a high total dose of radiotherapy is not required, so palliative fraction schedules can be shorter and use a higher dose per fraction. This serves to minimise patient visits to hospital for treatments and reduce treatment-related side effects (Barnes and Chow 2006).

Radiotherapy is used in the palliation of bone metastases for relief of pain, prevention of impending fractures and healing of pathological fractures. Palliation for bone metastases probably accounts for 40% of palliative radiotherapy courses (Barnes and Chow 2006).

Brain metastases are most commonly seen in patients with lung, breast and gastrointestinal primaries, and are seen in approximately 25% of cancer patients (Walker et al. 1985; Johnson and Young 1996). Here the goal of radiotherapy is to help with neurological symptom relief, allow corticosteroid tapering and perhaps prolong survival. Palliative radiotherapy also has a place in lung cancer, pelvic disease, and head and neck, oesophageal and skin cancer.

As radiotherapy is a local treatment, apart from fatigue side effects depend on the area treated. According to Barnes and Chow (2006) acute toxicity tends to resolve within 2 weeks of treatment completion. As with palliative chemotherapy, it is imperative that all health-care professionals, the patient, family and friends have a mutual understanding of the aims and limitations of the treatment plan.

Local spread

Patients can suffer very unpleasant symptoms as a result of local spread of cancer. An example of this is a fungating wound, seen sometimes in breast cancer, as a result of tumour infiltration of the epithelium and its surrounding blood and lymphatic vessels. These wounds can become necrotic and infected as a result of infarctions to the tumour. They can be malodorous and serve as a painful psychological reminder of the extent of metastatic disease. The primary aim is the promotion of comfort and quality of life. This can be a challenge and needs health-care professionals, complementary therapists and patients and their families to communicate well and work in harmony.

The expertise of a tissue viability nurse will be needed to advise as an ideal aim of healing through either local or systemic treatment. Radiotherapy may reduce bleeding and discharge. In some situations, surgery and skin grafting may be considered (Wessex Specialist Palliative Care Units 2007). Hormonal manipulation or chemotherapy is also an option. Whatever the option taken, wound management and the use of topical applications will be a constant, and it is vital that it is supervised by an experienced tissue viability nurse. A variety of dressings is available to deal with specific wound conditions and there will almost certainly be local policies that will dictate the approach. For localised pain at the site, morphine 10 mg can be mixed with intrasite gel. Short-acting opioid preparations may be helpful to reduce pain and discomfort as the wound is being attended (Wessex Specialist Palliative Care Units 2007).

The complementary therapist can play a key role. Regular massage can help the patient to feel cared for and nurtured. Teaching friends or relatives foot or hand massage can bring a new and caring dimension to relationships at this difficult time. Judicious use of aromatherapy may be able to help with malodour if present.

Head and neck cancer

Locally advanced head and neck cancer can present with a range of devastating symptoms. The cancer may be not only visible, but also interfere with fundamental functions such as swallowing, breathing and talking. These patients will need the expertise of the multidisciplinary specialist palliative care team to work with them and specialist head and neck surgical teams to devise a highly individual care plan to help minimise symptom distress.

Pelvic disease

Recurrent metastatic and locally advanced pelvic disease can also result in distressing symptoms. Symptoms include renal failure caused by ureteric obstruction, rectovaginal fistulae, lower extremity oedema and necrotic vaginal discharge. These symptoms again require the highly skilled and sensitive approach of an expert specialist palliative care team working with the patient, family and friends, doctors and surgeons.

CONCLUSION

This chapter has attempted to look at some of the main palliative care issues of patients dying from end stage heart disease, COPD, chronic neurodegenerative disease, dementia, AIDS and cancer. Of course it is in no way, shape or form all-inclusive. However, perhaps one of the most important aspects is to be able to recognise the palliative period; although we do have the prognostic indicators they do not necessarily take into account the spirit of the person – and in many instances that is the most striking element of a palliative period, i.e. it is determined as much by the personality and spirit of the person as by the prognostic indicators. This is what makes palliative care so interesting and challenging.

Examples of good practice have been highlighted. Replication of good practice initiatives takes commitment and enthusiasm. Many of our elderly people in need of supportive and palliative care are being cared for by family and friends who may be under enormous stress. They need help. Many are being cared for in care homes where written standards are high, staffing levels poor, training and support scant, and financial remuneration reflecting care not important. Achieving good supportive and palliative care for all is as much a political issue as a medical and caring one.

MAIN IMPLICATIONS FOR PRACTICE

- Palliative and supportive care should be based on need not disease.
- Prognostic indicators can help in defining the palliative period.
- Health professionals need good leadership to encourage the replication of good-practice initiatives.
- The Gold Standards Framework, Liverpool Care Pathway and Preferred Place of Care initiatives, i.e. the national End-of-Life Programme, provide a framework for a multidisciplinary approach to the care of dying people. Also the programme provides a forum for the sharing of evidence-based and good-practice initiatives. All health-care organisations would do well to sign up to this programme.
- Informal and formal education between specialists in health care and specialists in palliative care should be ongoing.
- All care staff in all settings need to be committed to integrating their services.
- Good standards of palliative care take commitment and enthusiasm. All carers need to feel valued. Financial remuneration should reflect that care is a valued commodity. Hence palliative care is also a political affair.

SUGGESTED FURTHER READING

Addington-Hall JM, Higginson IJ (2001) *Palliative Care for Non Cancer Patients*. Oxford: Oxford University Press.

NHS Confederation (2005) *Leading Edge*: *Improving end of life care*: Issue 12. London: NHS Confederation.

NICE (2000) *Cancer Services Guidance*. London: NICE. Available at: www.nice.org.

NICE (2003) *Chronic Heart Failure: Management of chronic heart failure in adults in primary and secondary care*. London: NICE. Available at: www.nice.org.

NICE (2004) *Chronic Obstructive Pulmonary Disease. Management of COPD in adults in primary and secondary care*. London: NICE. Available at: www.nice.org.

NICE (2004) *Improving Supportive and Palliative Care for Adults*. London: NICE. Available at: ww.nice.org.

NICE (2006) *Guideline on Dementia*. London: NICE. Available at: www.nice.org.

Websites

www.nice.org

Improving-chronic-disease–management@doh.gsi.gov.uk

www.cancerbackup.org.uk

Chapter 15
Palliative emergencies

KEY POINTS

- **Palliative emergencies**: to those not familiar with the palliative world the concept of a palliative emergency may seem surprising; however, there are situations which, handled promptly, can well lessen distress in all domains – physical, psychological, spiritual and social.

  The palliative emergencies dealt with briefly in this chapter are hypercalcaemia, spinal cord compression, superior vena cava obstruction, neutropenic crisis and haemorrhage.
- **Other symptoms**: within specialist palliative care many other treatments for a wide range of symptoms have evolved, e.g. excessive sweating and hiccups. These symptoms may seem obscure and it may not occur to some health professionals that there is anything that can help.
- **Make contact**: make contact with your local specialist palliative care team and ask for their handbook on symptom management. They will almost certainly have one.
- **Challenging symptom**: when faced with a difficult symptom in palliative care seek advice from your specialist team.

PALLIATIVE EMERGENCIES

Over the years in palliative care several medical conditions have become grouped as palliative emergencies. This applies to a situation where a calm but rapid response can minimise physical damage, e.g. as in spinal cord compression, and correction of distressing chemical imbalances, e.g. as in hypercalcaemia. Sometimes, the emergency response is strongly empathic and calm and, with the help of sedatives, aims to make a very distressing symptom less frightening for the patient and/or relatives and friends, e.g. as in acute haemorrhage. In a majority of patients experiencing repeated palliative emergencies such as hypercalcaemia, there may be a time when the likely benefits of treatment will be out weighed by the burden of it. This should be sensitively discussed with patients and carers to ascertain their wishes regarding treatment.

Here follows a 'very brief' inventory of palliative emergencies. They reflect the history of palliative care, i.e. in cancer care. No doubt, in a few years, other emergencies will be added to this list, which will reflect other terminal illnesses.

It is advisable to contact your local specialist palliative care unit for a copy of the local palliative handbook, which gives more details than here and includes dosage of drug therapies. The *Palliative Care Formulary* (Twycross and Wilcock 2007) is essential reading.

Hypercalcaemia

Hypercalcaemia is diagnosed when the correct serum calcium level is >2.7 mmol/l: symptoms are only troublesome usually at >2.9 mmol/l. Levels >4 mmol/l may be fatal. It is the most common metabolic emergency in cancer care.

Incidence

- Relatively common in patients with bone metastases
- Occurs in up to 50% of patients with myeloma and breast cancer
- Also relatively common in patients with squamous cell carcinoma of the lung and cancer of the head, neck, kidney, cervix or uterus.

Symptoms

- Have a high index of suspicion in patients, with the cancers mentioned previously, who become suddenly emotionally disturbed or confused
- Thirst and polyuria, resulting in dehydration
- Nausea, loss of appetite and excessive fatigue are also features, although, of course, these symptoms in advanced cancer may already feature.

Management

- Correct dehydration, usually an intravenous infusion is needed to give 2 litres of saline in 24 hours
- If serum calcium is >3 mmol/l use intravenous bisphosphonates.

This can be a very satisfying symptom to treat. Usually within 48 hours the patient can be restored to feeling much better and no longer confused.

However, despite treatments, hypercalcaemia is often heralding a terminal phase. Only 20% of patients will be alive after 12 months (Bower et al. 1997).

After the event education about the importance of keeping well hydrated may help avoid other occurrences.

Spinal cord compression

Spinal cord compression occurs in 3–5% of patients with advanced cancer. Cancer of the breast, bronchus and prostate accounts for 40% (Twycross and Wilcock 2001). Most occur in the thorax.

It is vital to have a high index of suspicion about this condition. Early signs, e.g. heaviness of the legs, can belie the dramatic consequences that this condition can have. Once paralysed, only 5% of the people will walk again, but some will survive for more than a year with sensory deficit and paralysis (Wessex Specialist Palliative Care Units 2007).

Symptoms

- Often back pain with or without radiation around the nerve root. Signs can be vague sensory changes, e.g. heaviness in legs, a lack of 'usual' sensation when opening bowels
- Urinary retention or hesitancy
- Loss of strength in legs.

Physical examination

This will reveal:

- decreased strength in extremities
- loss of sensation for touch and pain
- abnormal tendon reflexes
- decrease in muscle coordination
- unsteady gait
- tenderness over compressed site.

Treatment

Treatment needs to be prompt and will consist of the following:

- Dexamethasone ⎱
- Radiotherapy   ⎰ concurrently
- Urgent referral to clinical oncologist and discuss potential for surgery with neuro/spinal surgical team.

Superior vena cava obstruction

The cause of obstruction of the superior vena cava (SVC) is usually the extrinsic compression of upper mediastinal lymph nodes. In 80% of cases lung cancer is responsible and it occurs in around 15% of patients with lung cancer, particularly small cell (Twycross and Wilcock 2001).

Symptoms

- Breathlessness (caused by laryngeal oedema)
- Choking sensation
- Headache and/or feeling of fullness in the head
- Neck and facial swelling
- Trunk and arm swelling
- May be visual changes
- Dizziness.

Visual signs

These may include:

- dilated non-pulsatile neck veins
- dilated collateral veins of chest and arms
- engorged conjunctivae, periorbital oedema.

Seek specialist oncology or palliative help.

Management

- High-dose steroids e.g. dexamethasone
- Radiotherapy to the mediastinal lymph nodes
- Chemotherapy may be used for patients with lymphoma and small cell lung cancer
- In some cases a self-expanding metal stent can be introduced into the SVC via a brachiocephalic or femoral vein. Anticoagulation therapy with heparin will be needed before stent insertion.

Survival can be prolonged for several months; however, a recurrence will be more difficult to control.

Neutropenic crisis

Chemotherapy is a more common occurrence in palliative care than ever before. Depression in the activity of bone marrow leads to lowered white blood cell count, which in turn lowers the patient's resistance to infection. The second week after chemotherapy, i.e. days 7–14, is usually the most vulnerable time, sometimes referred to as the nadir. It is important that patients appreciate the risk of this and take sensible precautions to avoid unnecessary exposure to infection. Useful guidelines for this are provided in patient information sheets from Cancerbacup. www.cancerbackup.org.uk.

It is important for patients, relatives and professionals to appreciate that the usual signs of infection, i.e. raised temperature, raised pulse, sweating, fever, may be minimal or absent. Patients, relatives and friends should be educated to take seriously any change in condition, however minimal, e.g. the patient may simply feel more lethargic than the day before and reluctant to get out of bed.

Patients will be told to contact the clinical nurse oncology specialist or a member of the oncology medical team. It is usual for them to be admitted straight to an oncology unit as rapidly as possible to start antibiotic therapy. Thus they bypass their GP and accident and emergency department. These patients can rapidly became septicaemic and die. Vigilance and speed are of the essence.

Haemorrhage

Patients may have acute or non-acute bleeding problems, some potential causes/ aggravating factors can be:

- Infection that can cause or aggravate bleeding, e.g. per vaginum, haematuria, haemoptysis or from a fungating wound
- Tumour invasion, which can cause an arterial bleed
- Peptic ulceration
- Bleeding can be exacerbated by anticoagulation therapy, NSAIDs (non-steroidal anti-inflammatory drugs) or a generalised clotting deficiency.

Management of non-acute bleed

- Replacement of blood, clotting factors, plasma and vitamin B_{12} may help.
- Stop all drugs that may be exacerbating bleeding.
- Treat any aggravating infection.
- Radiotherapy may be useful where bleeding is caused by malignancy, in particular haemoptysis, haematuria or cutaneous (Wessex Specialist Palliative Care Units 2007).
- Tranexamic acid stabilises clots, but should be used with caution in haematuria because it may lead to clot retention (Wessex Specialist Palliative Care Units 2007).

Massive terminal bleeding

This occurs in approximately 6–10% of patients in a palliative care setting (Yennurajalingam and Bruera 2006); clearly, it has the potential to be an extremely distressing event. All health-care settings should have a policy on how to deal with this.

Patients will need a confident, kind professional to stay with them during the whole of this event. Physical touch and hand holding may be very comforting. Medications may include intramuscular or intravenous midazolam, perhaps with diamorphine, for the relief of psychological distress.

Relatives and friends will need support and reassurance from staff and debriefing after the event. Staff may also need the opportunity to debrief.

It is advisable to have dark-coloured towels around that can be used to help protect and clean in the event of a massive bleed. Blood looks far less dramatic on a dark than on a white towel.

OTHER SYMPTOMS

This book has looked at 11 prevalent symptoms in patients with a variety of diseases and 5 palliative emergency situations that have emerged from the history of palliative cancer care. Over the years a lot of work has been done to reduce the distress of a whole variety of troublesome symptoms, e.g.:

- Ascites
- Coughing

- Fistulae
- Fits
- Hiccups
- Intestinal obstruction (malignant)
- Itching
- Lymphoedema
- Mouth problems
- Raised intracranial pressure
- Restlessness
- Use of steroids
- Sweating.

There should be a specialist palliative care team in your locality. It is highly likely that they will have produced a pocket handbook that provides guidelines for helping with these symptoms, and much more besides. These books are usually free and a good specialist palliative care team will be very happy to supply copies. It is an important part of the end-of-life care strategy that generalists in palliative care liaise with and seek advice, when needed, from specialist palliative care teams. Thus, make sure that you have the local handbook and know how to contact the local team. This way provision of specialist palliative care in any care setting can be a reality. It is what we all want and deserve at the end of life.

MAIN IMPLICATIONS FOR PRACTICE

- Increase your knowledge about palliative emergencies.
- Have a good knowledge and a high index of suspicion with regard to palliative emergencies – it can do much to help maintain a good quality of life in end-of-life care.
- Do not hesitate to contact your local specialist team for advice when needed.
- Make sure that you have a copy of the local specialist team's handbook.

SUGGESTED FURTHER READING

Twycross R, Wilcock A (2001) *Symptom Management in Advanced Cancer*, 2nd edn. Oxford: Radcliffe Medical Press.
Twycross R, Wilcock A (2007) *Palliative Care Formulary*, 3rd edn. Nottingham. Available at: palliativedrugs.com.
Watson M, Lucas C, Hoy A, Back I (2006) *Oxford Handbook of Palliative Care*. Oxford: Oxford University Press.
Also your local specialist team's handbook.

References

Abbot NC (2000) Healing as a therapy for human disease: a systematic review. *J Altern Complement Med* **6**: 159–169.

Addington-Hall JM, McCarthy M (1995) The regional study of care for the dying: methods and sample characteristics. *Palliative Med* **9**: 27–35.

Addington-Hall J, Lay M, Altmann D, McCarthy M (1995) Symptom control, communication with health professionals, and hospital care of stroke patients in the last year of life as reported by surviving family, friends and officials. *Stroke* **26**: 2242–8.

Addington-Hall JM, Lay M, Altmann D, McCarthy M (1998) Community care for stroke patients in the last year of life: results of a national retrospective survey of surviving family, friends and officials. *Health Social Care Commun* **6**: 112–19.

Ahlberg K, Ekman T, Garston-Johansson F, Mock V (2003) Assessment and management of cancer related fatigue in adults. *Lancet* **362**: 640–9.

Aldridge D (1999) *Music Therapy in Palliative Care. New Voices.* London: Jessica Kingsley Publications.

Allan K (2001) *Communication and Consultation: Exploring ways for staff to involve people with dementia in developing services.* Bristol: The Policy Press.

Allan K, Killick J (2001) *Communication and the Care of People with Dementia.* Milton Keynes, Bucks: Open University Press.

Allan SG (1993) Nausea and vomiting. In: Doyle D, Hanks GW, MacDonald N (eds), *Oxford Textbook of Palliative Medicine.* Oxford: Oxford University Press, 282–90.

Allum WH, Brearley S, Wheatley KE (1990) Acute haemorrhage from gastric malignancy. *Br J Surg* **77**: 19–20.

Alzheimer's Society (2006) Memorandum to Professor Mike Richards, 31 August 2006. Available at: www.alzheimers.org.uk (accessed August 2007).

Alzheimer's Society (2007) Maintaining Quality of Life. London: Alzheimer's Society. Available at: www.alzheimers.org.uk/caringforsomeonedementia/maintingqualityoflife (accessed 25 August 2007).

American Psychiatric Association (1994) *Diagnostic and Statistical Manual of Mental Disorders,* 4th edn. Washington DC: American Psychiatric Association.

American Thoracic Society (1999a) Dyspnea. Mechanisms, assessment, and management: a consensus statement. *Am J Respir Crit Med* **159**: 321–40.

American Thoracic Society (1999b) Pulmonary rehabilitation. *Am J Respir Crit Care* **159**: 1666–82.

Andershed B, Ternestedt B (2001) Development of a theoretical framework describing relatives' involvement in palliative care. *J Adv Nursing* **34**: 554–62.

Anderson DM (2002) *Mosby's Medical, Nursing and Allied Health Dictionary,* 6th edn. London: Harcourt Health Sciences Co.

Anker S, Ponikowski P, Varney S et al. (1997) Wasting as an independent risk factor for mortality in chronic heart failure. *Lancet* **349**: 1050–3.

Annane D (2003) Mechanical ventilation for amyotrophic lateral sclerosis/motor neurone disease. *Cochrane Database of Systemic Reviews* Issue 4.

Archibald CJ, McGrath PG, Ritvo PG et al. (1994) Pain prevalence, severity and impact in a clinic sample of MS patients. *Pain* **58**: 89–93.

Argyle M (1978) *The Psychology of Interpersonal Behaviour*. London: Methuen & Colt.

Aries P (1983) *The Hour of Death*. London: Peregrine Books.

Arora R, Chou T, Jain D (1999) The multicenter study of enhanced external counterpulsation (MUST-EECP): effect of EECP on exercise induced myocardial ischemia and anginal episodes. *J Am Coll Cardiol* **33**: 1833–40.

Audit Commission (1993) *Making Time for Patients: A handbook for ward sisters*. London: HMSO.

Bach JR (1993) Amyotrophic lateral sclerosis. Communication status and survival with ventilatory support. *American Journal of Physical Medicine and Rehabilitation* **72**(6): 343–9 (MEDLINE 94082-77).

Bailey K, Wilkinson S (1998) Patients' views on nurses' communication skills: a pilot study. *Int J Palliative Nurs* **4**: 300–5.

Banks P, Cheeseman C (2000) *Taking Action To Support Carers: A carers' impact guide for commissioners and managers*. London: King's Fund.

Barakzoy AS, Moss AH (2006) Efficacy of the World Health Organization ladder to treat pain in end stage renal disease. *J Am Soc Nephrol* **17**: 3198–203.

Barnes EA, Chow E (2006) Cancer: radiotherapy. In: Bruera E, Higginson I, Ripamonti C, Von Gunten C (eds), *Textbook of Palliative Medicine*. London: Hodder Arnold, 871–9.

Barraclough J (1994) *Cancer and Emotion*. London: Radcliffe Medical Press.

Beaver K, Luker K, Woods S (1999) The views of terminally ill people and lay carers on primary care services. *Int J Palliative Nurs* **5**: 266–74.

Beebe A, McCaffery M (1994) *Pain Clinical Management for Nursing Practice*. London: Mosby.

Beecher HK (1959) *Measurement of Subjective Responses*. New York: Oxford University Press.

Benor DJ (2001) *Spiritual Healing: Scientific validation of a healing revolution*. Michigan, MI: Vision Publications.

Bercovitch M, Waller A (2005) Transcutaneous electrical nerve stimulation (TENS). In: Doyle D, Hanks G, Cherny N, Calman K (eds), *Oxford Textbook of Palliative Medicine*, 3rd edn. Oxford: Oxford University Press, 405–10.

Berglund G, Bolund C, Gustafasson UK et al. (1994) A randomised study of a rehabilitation programme for cancer patients: the 'starting again group'. *Psycho-Oncology* **3**: 109–20.

Bezein E, Norberg A, Saveman BI (2001) The meaning of the lived experience of hope in patients with cancer in palliative home care. *Palliative Med* **15**: 117–26.

Birch SJ, Felt RL (1999) *Understanding Acupuncture*. London: Churchill Livingstone.

Blackman N (2003) *Loss and Learning Disability*. London: Worth Publishing Ltd.

Blinderman CD, Cherny NI (2005) Existential issues do not necessarily result in existential suffering: lessons from cancer patients in Israel. *Palliative Med* **19**: 371–80.

Bluglass K (2003) *Hidden from the Holocaust*. Westport, CT: Praeger.

Bond C (2004) *Concordance – A partnership in medicine taking*. London: Pharmaceutical Press.

Bondly C, Jatoi A (2006) Overview of the management the anorexia/weight loss syndrome. In: Bruera E, Higginson IJ, Ripamonti C, Von Gunten C (eds), *Textbook of Palliative Medicine*. London: Hodder Arnold, 538–45.

Bonica JJ (1953) *The Management of Pain*. Philadelphia: Lea & Febiger.

Bonica JJ (1979) Importance of the problem. In: Bonica JJ, Ventafridda V (eds), *Proceedings of the First International Congress on Cancer Pain. Advances in pain research and therapy*, Vol 2. New York: Raven Press, 1–12.

Boore J (1978) *Prescription for Recovery: the effect of preoperative preparation of surgical patients an postoperative stress*. London: Royal College of Nursing.

Borasio DM, Rogers A, Voltz R (2005) Palliative medicine in non-malignant neurological disorders. In: Doyle D, Hanks G, Cherny N, Calman K (eds), *Oxford Textbook of Palliative Medicine*, 3rd edn. Oxford: Oxford University Press, 925–35.

Borg G (1970) Perceived exertion as an indicator of somatic stress. *Scand J Rehabil Med* **2**: 92–8.

Borg G (1978) Subjective effort and physical activities. *Scandinavian Journal of Rehabilitation Medicine* **6**: 108–13.

Botting D (1997) Review of literature on the effectiveness of reflexology. *Complementary Therapies in Nursing and Midwifery* **5**: 123–30.

Boud D, Keogh R, Walker D (1985) *Reflection: Turning experience into learning*. London: Kogan Page.

Bower M et al. (1997) Endocrine and metabolic complications of advanced cancer. In: Doyle D, Hanks G, MacDonald N (eds) *Oxford Textbook of Palliative Medicine*. Oxford: Oxford University Press, 447–60.

Bowlby J (1980) *Attachment and Loss: Loss, sadness, and depression*, vol III. New York: Basic Books.

Bowman GS, Thompson DR (1995) Strategies for organising care. In: Schober JE, Hinchliff SM (eds), *Towards Advanced Nursing Practice*. London: Arnold, 222–52.

Bowsher D (1995) Pain management in nursing. In: Carroll D, Bowsher D (eds), *Pain Management and Nursing Care*. Oxford: Butterworth Heinemann: 5–16.

Boyle M, Carter D (1998) Death anxiety amongst nurses. *Int J Palliative Nurs* **4**: 37–43.

Bredin M, Corner J, Krishasamy M, Plant H, Bailey C, A'Hern R (1999) Multi-centred randomised controlled trial of nursing intervention for breathlessness in patients with lung cancer *BMJ* **318**: 901–4.

Breitbart W, Cohen K (2000) Delirium in the terminally ill. In: Chochinov HM, Breitbart W (eds), *Handbook of Psychiatry in Palliative Medicine*. Oxford: Oxford University Press, 75–90.

Breitbart W, Patt R (1994) Pain management in the patient with AIDS. *Haematol/Oncol Ann* **2**: 391–9.

Breitbart W, Levenson JA, Passik SD (1993) Terminally ill cancer patients. In: Breitbart W, Holland JC (eds), *Psychiatric Aspects of Symptom Management in Cancer Patients*. Washington DC: American Psychiatric Press, 192–4.

Breitbart W, Rosenfield B, Pessin H et al. (2000) Depression, hopeless, and desire for hastened death in terminally ill people with cancer. *JAMA* **284**: 2907–11.

Breitbart W, Chochinov HM, Passik SD (2005a) Psychiatric symptoms in palliative medicine. In: Doyle D, Hanks G, Cherny N, Calman K (eds), *Oxford Textbook of Palliative Medicine*, 3rd edn. Oxford: Oxford University Press, 746–71.

Breitbart W, Payne D, Passik SD (2005b) Psychological and psychiatric interventions in pain control. In: Doyle D, Hanks G, Cherny N, Calman K (eds), *Oxford Textbook of Palliative Medicine*, 3rd edn. Oxford: Oxford University Press, 424–38.

Brewin T (1996) *The Friendly Professional*. Bognor Regis: Eurocommunia.

Bridge LR, Benson P, Pietroni P, Priest RG (1988) Relaxation and imagery in the treatment of breast cancer. *BMJ* **297**: 1169–72.

Britten N, Weiss M (2004) What is concordance? In: Bond C (ed.), *Concordance*. London: Pharmaceutical Press, 9–25.

Brogan G, George R (2001) HIV / AIDS In: Addington–Hall J, Higginson IJ (eds), *Palliative Care for Non Cancer Patients*. Oxford: Oxford University Press, 137–45.

Broqvist M, Arnqvist H, Dahlstrom U et al. (1994) Nutritional assessment and muscle energy metabolism in severe chronic congestive heart failure. *Eur Heart J* **15**: 1641–50.

Brown CK (1998) The integration of healing and spirituality into health care. *J Interprof Care* **12**: 373–81.

Brown GW, Harris T (1978) Social origins of depression. In: *A Study of Psychiatric Disorder in Women.* London: Tavistock.

Bruera E, Fadul N (2006) Constipation and diarrhea. In: Bruera E, Higginson IJ, Ripamonti C, Von Gunten C (eds), *Textbook of Palliative Medicine.* London: Hodder Arnold, 554–70.

Bruera E, Pituskin E, Calder K, Neumann CM, Hanson J (1999) The addition of an audiocassette recording of a consultation to written recommendations for patients with advanced cancer: a randomised controlled trial. *Cancer* **86**: 2420–5.

Bryan K (2007) Communicating with people in the later stages of dementia. Journal of Dementia Care Conference: Care matters for people with advanced dementia: best practice at the end of life. University of Surrey, Guildford.

Buckle J (2003) *Clinical Aromatherapy: Essential oils in practice*, 2nd edn. Edinburgh: Churchill Livingstone.

Buckley J (1998) An investigation to promote an understanding of hope and how to foster hope for people receiving palliative care. Unpublished MA thesis. Available from St Wilfrid's Hospice Library, Grosvenor Road, Chichester, West Sussex PO19 8FP.

Buckley J (2002a) Holism and a health-promoting approach to palliative care. *Int J Palliative Nurs* **8**: 505–8.

Buckley J (2002b) Massage and aromatherapy massage: nursing art and science. *Int J Palliative Nurs* **8**: 276–80.

Buckley J, Herth K (2004) Fostering hope in terminally ill patients. *Nursing Stand* **19**(10): 33–41.

Buckman R (1993a) *How To Break Bad News – A guide for healthcare professionals.* London: Macmillan Medical.

Buckman R (1993b) Communication in palliative care: a practical guide. In: Doyle D, Hanks G, Macdonald N (eds), *Oxford Textbook of Palliative Medicine.* Oxford: Oxford University Press, 47–61.

Buckman R (2005) Communication in palliative care. In: Dickenson D, Johnson M, Katz JS (eds), *Death, Dying and Bereavement.* London: Open University Press, in association with Sage Publications, 146–73.

Burden B, Herron-Marx S, Clifford C (2005) The increasing use of reiki as a complementary therapy in palliative care. *Int J Palliative Nurs* **11**: 248–53.

Burge F (1993) Dehydration symptoms of palliative care. *J Palliative Care* **8**(3): 68–79.

Burgess KR, Whitelaw WA (1988) Effects of nasal cold receptors on pattern of breathing. *J Appl Physiol* **64**: 371–6.

Burish TG, Carey MP, Redd WH, Krozely MC (1983) Behavioural relaxation techniques in reducing the distress of cancer chemotherapy patients. *Oncol Nurs Forum* **10**(3): 32–5.

Burman R (2006) Neurological diseases. In: Bruera E, Higginson IJ, Ripamonti C, Von Gunten C (eds), *Textbook of Palliative Medicine.* London: Hodder Arnold, 911–17.

Burnard P (1992) *Know Yourself! Self awareness activities for nurses.* Harrow: Scutari Press.

Byrd R (1988) The integration of healing and spirituality in health care. *J Interprof Care* **12**: 373–81.

Calde K, Classen C, Spiegel D (2002) Can psychosocial interventions extend survival? A critical evaluation of clinical trials of group and individual therapies. In: Lewis CE, O'Brien RM, Barraclough J (eds), *The Psychoimmunology of Cancer*, 2nd edn. Oxford: Oxford University Press, 182–209.

Calman K, Hine D (1995) *A Policy Framework for Commissioning Cancer Services.* London: Department of Health and Welsh Office.

Cancer Action Team NHS (2007) *Advanced Communications in Cancer Care. Better communication improves patient care.* Available from National Cancer Action Team, St Thomas' Hospital, Lambeth Palace Road, London SE1 7EH.

Cantwell BM, Ramirez AJ (1997) Doctor–patient communication: A study of junior house officers. *Med Educ* **31**: 17–21.

Capeda MS, Carr DB, Lau J, Alvarez H (2006) Music for pain relief. *Cochrane Database Syst Rev* **3**: CD004843.

Caplan G (1961) *An Approach to Community Mental Health.* London: Tavistock.

Capra S, Ferguson M, Reid K (2001) Cancer: impact of nutrition intervention outcome – nutrition issues for patients. *Nutrition* **17**: 769–72.

Carroll D, Bowsher D, eds (1995) *Pain Management and Nursing Care.* Oxford: Butterworth Heinemann.

Cartwright A, Hockey L, Anderson JL (1973) *Life Before Death.* London: Routledge & Kegan Paul.

Casey P (1994) Depression in the dying – disorder or distress. *Prog Palliative Care* **2**: 1–3.

Cassell EJ (1991) *The Nature of Suffering and the Goals of Medicine.* Oxford: Oxford University Press.

Cassileth BR, Schulman G (2005) Complementary therapies in palliative medicine, In: Doyle D, Hanks G, Cherny N, Calman K (eds), *Oxford Textbook of Palliative Medicine*, 3rd edn. Oxford: Oxford University Press, 1087–93.

Cassileth BR, Vickers J (2004) Massage therapy for symptom control: outcome study at a major cancer centre. *J Pain Symptom Manage* **28**: 244–9.

Caven L (1959) *Twice a Victim.* London: Faber & Faber.

Cazzolli PA, Oppenheimer EA (1996) Home mechanical ventilation for amyotrophic lateral sclerosis: nasal compared to tracheostomy – intermittent positive pressure ventilation. *J Neuro Sciences* **139** (suppl): 123-8.

Chambers P (1997) Why are Most Churchgoers Women? A Welsh perspective. Conference paper, Network for the Study of Implicit Religion, Winterbourne, May 1997.

Chapario SL, the DOLOPLUS group (2001) The Doloplus 2 Scale – evaluating pain in the elderly. *Eur J Palliative Care* **8**: 191–4.

Charman RA (1995) Physiotherapy for the relief of pain. In: Carroll D, Bowsher D (eds), *Pain Management and Nursing Care.* Oxford: Butterworth Heinemann, 146–66.

Charmaz K (1983) Loss of self: a fundamental form of suffering in the chronically ill. *Sociol Health Illness* **5**: 168–95.

Charnock D, Shepperd S (2004) Learning to DISCERN on line: applying an appraisal tool to health websites in a workshop setting. *Health Educ Res* **19**: 440–6 (epup 20 May).

Cheshire and Merseyside Specialist Palliative Care and Cardiac Clinical Networks (2005) Symptom control guidelines for patients with end stage heart failure and criteria for referral to specialist palliative care. Available at: www.cmcn.nhs.uk (accessed July 2007).

Cheston R, Bender M (1999) *Understanding Dementia.* London: Jessica Kingsley Publishers.

Child Bereavement Trust (2003) Handout available from The Child Bereavement Trust, Aston House, High Street, West Wycombe, Bucks HP14 3AG.

Chochinov HM, Breitbart W (2000) *Handbook of Psychiatry in Palliative Medicine.* Oxford: Oxford University Press.

Chochinov HM, Wilson KG, Enns M et al. (1995) Desire for death in the terminally ill. *Am J Psychiatry* **152**: 1185–91.

Claessens MT, Lynn J, Zhong Z et al. (2000) Dying with lung cancer or chronic obstructive pulmonary disease: Insights from SUPPORT. Study to understand prognoses and preferences for outcomes and risks of treatment. *Am J Geriatr Soc* **48**(5): 146–53.

Clark D (2004) History, gender and culture in the rise of palliative care. In: Payne S, Seymour J, Ingleton C (eds), *Palliative Care Nursing – Principles and evidence for practice.* Milton Keynes, Bucks: Open University Press, 39–55.

Clark D (2005a) *Cicely Saunders Founder of the Hospice Movement: Selected letters 1959–1999.* Oxford: Oxford University Press.

Clark D (2005b) Death in Staithes. In: Dickenson D, Johnson M, Katz JS (eds), *Death, Dying and Bereavement*. London: Open University Press, 4–9.

Clark D, ed. (2006) *Cicely Saunders Selected Writings 1958–2004*. Oxford: Oxford University Press.

Clinical Standards Advisory Group (CSAG) (2003) *Services for Patients in Pain*. Cited in Prince of Wales' Foundation for Integrated Health (2003).

Cobb M (2001) *The Dying Soul: Spiritual care at the end of* life. Milton Keynes, Bucks: Open University Press.

Cole K, Vaughan FL (2005) The feasibility of cognitive behavioural therapy for depression associated with Parkinson disease: a literature review. *Parkinsonism Related Disord* **11**: 269–76.

Cole W (1956) Foreword. In: Schiffin MJ (ed.), *The Management of Pain in Cancer*. Chicago: Year Book.

Connor SR (1992) Denial in terminal illness: to intervene or not to intervene. *Hospice J* **8**: 1–15.

CONSENSUS Trial Study Investigators (1987) Effects of enalapril on mortality in severe congestive heart failure. Results of the cooperative north Scandinavian enalaupril study. *N Engl J Med* **316**: 1429–35.

Cooper P, Osborn M, Gath D, Feggetter G (1982) Evaluation of a modified self report measure of social adjustment. *Br J Psychiatry* **141**: 69–75.

Copp G, Field D (2002) Open awareness and dying: the use of denial and acceptance as coping strategies by hospice patients. *NT Res* **7**: 188–227.

Corcoran C, Grinspoon S (1999) Treatments for wasting in patients with acquired immuno-deficiency syndrome. *N Engl J Med* **340**: 1740–50.

Corner J (2004) Working with difficult symptoms. In: Payne S, Seymour J, Ingleton C (eds), *Palliative Care Nursing*. Milton Keynes, Bucks: Open University Press, 241–60.

Corner J, Crawley N, Hilderbrand S (1995) An evaluation of the use of massage and essential oils on the wellbeing of cancer patients. *Int J Palliative Nurs* **1**(2): 67–73.

Coronary Heart Disease (2005) Collaborative supportive and palliative care for advanced heart failure. Available at: www.modern.nhs.uk/chd (accessed July 2007).

Coser RL (1965) Some functions of laughter. In: Skipper JK, Leonard RC (eds), *Social Interaction and Patient Care*. Philadelphia: Lippincott.

Costello J (1999) Anticipatory grief: coping with the impending death of a partner. *Int J Palliative Nurs* **5**: 223–31.

Cotton MM et al. (2000) Early discharge for patients with exacerbations of chronic obstructive pulmonary disease: a randomised controlled trial. *Thorax* **55**: 902–6.

Coulter A (1999) Paternalism or partnership? Patients have grown up – and there's no going back. *BMJ* **319**: 719–20.

Courneya KS, Vallance JKH, McNeely ML, Peddle CJ (2006) Exercise, physical function and fatigue in palliative care. In: Bruera E, Higginson IJ, Ripamonti C, Von Gunten C (eds), *Textbook of Palliative Medicine*. London: Hodder Arnold, 629–39.

Cox J, Holden J, Sagovsky R (1987) Detection of postnatal depression: development of 10 item Edinburgh Postnatal Depression Scale. *Br J Psychiatry* **150**: 782–6.

Cruess DG, Antoni MH, Kumar M, Schneiderman (2000) Reductions in salivary cortisol are associated with mood improvement during relaxation training among HIV seropositive men. *J Behav Med* **23**: 107–22.

Curran SL, Andrykowski MA, Studts JL (1995) Short form of the profile of moods state (POMS-SF): psychometric information. *Psychol Assess* **7**: 80–3.

Cutcliffe J (1995) How do nurses inspire and instil hope in terminally ill HIV patients? *J Adv Nurs* **22**: 888–95.

Daley A, Matthews C, Williams A (2006) Heart failure and palliative care services working in partnership: report of a new model of care. *Palliative Med* **20**: 593–601.

Daniel R (2001a) *The Cancer Prevention Book*. London: Simon & Schuster.

Daniel R (2001b) Holistic approaches to cancer: general principles and assessment of the patient. In: Barraclough J (ed.), *Integrated Cancer Care*. Oxford: Oxford University Press, 18–30.

Daniel R, Fawzy NW (1994) A structured psychoeducational intervention for cancer patients. *General Hosp Psychiatry* **16**: 149–92.

Dargie HJ, McMurray JJV (1992) Chronic heart failure: epidemiology, aetiology, pathophysiology and treatment. In: Rowlands D (ed.), *Recent Advances in Cardiology II*, 2nd edn. Edinburgh: Churchill Livingstone, 73–114.

Daut RL, Cleeland CS, Flanery RC (1983) Development of the Wisconsin Brief Pain Questionnaire to Assess Pain in Cancer and Other Diseases. *Pain* **17**: 197–210.

de Beauvoir S (1965) *A Very Easy Death*. New York: Pantheon Books.

de Haes JCJM, van Knippenberg FCE, Neijt JP (1990) Measuring psychological and physical distress in cancer patients: structure and application of the Rotterdam Symptom Checklist. *Br J Cancer* **62**: 1034–8.

De Lima L (2006) Palliative care: global situations and initiatives. In: Bruera E, Higginson IJ, Ripamonti C, Von Gunten C (eds), *Textbook of Palliative Medicine*. London: Hodder Arnold, 117–26.

de Vries K (2007) Matters of the heart: the CHMN and palliative care. In: Keady J, Clarke CL, Page S (eds), *Partnerships in Community Mental Health Nursing and Dementia Care*. Milton Keynes, Bucks: Open University Press, 260–71.

Dein S (2005) Working with the patient who is in denial. *Eur J Palliative Care* **12**: 251–3.

Department of Health (1987) *Promoting Better Health*. London: The Stationery Office.

Department of Health (1991a) *The Health of the Nation*. London: The Stationery Office.

Department of Health (1991b) *The Patients' Charter*. London: Department of Health.

Department of Health (1997) *The New NHS: Modern, Dependable*. London: The Stationery Office.

Department of Health (1998) *A First Class Service – Quality in the NHS*. London: HMSO.

Department of Health (1999a) *Saving Lives: Our healthier nation*. London: The Stationery Office.

Department of Health (1999b) *Caring about Carers. A National Strategy for Carers*. London: The Stationery Office.

Department of Health (2000a) *Manual of Cancer Service Standards*. London: Department of Health.

Department of Health (2000b) *The NHS Cancer Plan: A plan for investment, a plan for reform*. London: HMSO.

Department of Health (2000c) *Cancer Plan – Sharing our Practice*. London: DH.

Department of Health (2001) *The Expert Patient: A new approach to chronic disease management for the 21st century*. London: DH.

Department of Health (2003a) *Building on the Best: Choice, responsiveness and equity in the NHS*. London: DH.

Department of Health (2003b) Commission for Patient and Public Involvement in Health. Available at: www.cppih.org (accessed 24 March 2008).

Department of Health (2004a) *The Priorities of Care Explained*. London: HMSO. Available at: www.cancerlancashire.org.uk (accessed 24 March 2008).

Department of Health (2004b) *The Preferred Place of Care Explained: Patient information leaflet*. London: DH.

Department of Health (2004c) *Choosing Health: Making healthy choices easier*. London: The Stationery Office.

Department of Health (2005) *National Service Framework for Long Term Conditions*. London: DH. Available at: www.dh.gov.uk.

Department of Health (2006) *Our Health, Our Care, Our Say: A new direction for community services*. London: DH.

Department of Health (2007a) *Standard Seven – Mental health in older people*. Available at: www. dh.gov.uk/en/policyandsocialcaretopics/olderpeoples Gateway reference 2111 (accessed 24 March 2008).

Department of Health (2007b) Government project to produce the first ever dementia strategy: work programme. Available at: www.dh.gov.uk/en/policyandsocialcaretopics/older-peoples Gateway reference 8634 (accessed August 2007).

Derby S, Portenoy RK (1997) Assessment and management of opioid induced constipation. In: Portenoy RK, Bruera E eds (eds), *Topics in Palliative Care*. Oxford: Oxford University Press, 95–112.

Derogatis LR, Spencer PM (1982) *Administration and procedures BSI manual*. Baltimore, MD: Clinical Psychometric Research.

Devito A (1990) Dyspnoea during hospitalisation for acute phase of illness as recalled by patients with chronic obstructive pulmonary disease. *Heart Lung* 19: 186–91.

Dewys WD, Begg C, Lavin PT et al. (1980) Prognostic effect of weight loss prior to chemotherapy in cancer patients. Eastern Cooperative Oncology group. *Am J Med* 69: 491–7.

Dibble SL, Chapman J, Mack KA, Shih AS (2000) Acupressure for nausea: results of a pilot study. *Oncol Nurs Forum* 27: 41–7.

Dorman S, Byrne A, Edwards A (2007) Which measurement scales should we use to assess breathlessness in palliative care? A systematic review. *Palliative Med* 21: 177–91.

Douglas DB (1999) Hypnosis: useful, neglected, available. *Am J Hospice Palliative Care* 16: 665–70.

Downie RS, Randall F (2006) *The Philosophy of Palliative Care*. Oxford: Oxford University Press.

Doyle D, Hanks G, Cherny N, Calman K, eds (2005) *Oxford Textbook of Palliative Medicine*, 3rd edn. Oxford: Oxford University Press.

Duggleby W, Wright K (2005) Transforming hope: how elderly people live with hope. *Can J Nurs Res* 37(2): 70–84.

Duncan ER, Shah AM, Kearney MT (2006) End stage congestive cardiac failure. In: Bruera E, Higginson IJ, Ripamonti C, Von Gunten C (eds), *Textbook of Palliative Medicine*. London: Hodder Arnold, 918–23.

Dundee JW, Ghaly RG, Fitzpatrick KTJ, Lynch GA, Abram WP (1987) Acupuncture to prevent cisplatin associated vomiting. *Lancet* i: 1083.

Dunlop GM (1989) A study of the relative frequency of importance of gastrointestinal symptoms and weakness in patients with far advanced cancer. *Palliative Med* 4: 37–43.

Dunman M, Farell C (2000) *The Practicalities of Producing Patient Information. The POPPI guide*. London: King's Fund.

Dunn SM, Butow PN, Tattershall MHN et al. (1993) General information tapes inhibit recall of the cancer consultation. *J Clin Oncol* 11: 2279–85.

Dunniece U, Slevin E (2000) Nurses' experience of being present with a patient receiving a diagnosis of cancer. *J Adv Nurs* 32: 611–18.

Dunniece U, Slevin E (2002) Giving voice to the less articulate knowledge of palliative nursing: an interpretive study. *Int J Palliative Nurs* 8: 13–20.

Dunphy K (2000) Futilitarianism: knowing how much is enough in end of life care. *Palliative Med* 14: 313–22.

Dunwoody L, Smyth A, Davidson R (2002) Cancer patients' experiences and evaluations of aromatherapy massage in palliative care. *Int J Palliative Nurs* 8: 497–504.

Dutton YC, Zisook S (2005) Adaptation to bereavement. *Death Studies* 19: 877–903.

Dyer WG (1984) *Strategies for Managing Change*. New York: Addison Wesley.

Dyregov A (1991) *Grief in Children*. London: Jessica Kingsley.

Eakes G (1985) The relationship between death anxiety and attitudes towards the elderly amongst nursing staff. *Death Studies* **9**: 163–72.

Eccles M, Mason J (2001) How to develop cost-conscious guidelines. *Health Technol Assess* **5**(16): 1–69.

Edmonds P, Karlson S, Khan S et al. (2001) A comparison of the palliative care needs of patients dying from respiratory disease and lung cancer. *Palliative Med* **15**: 287–95.

Ehman JW, Ott BB, Short TH, Ciarupa RC, Hansen-Flaschen J (1999) Do patients want physicians to inquire about their spiritual or religious beliefs if they became gravely ill? *Arch Int Med* **23**: 1803–6.

Ekwall AK, Sivberg B, Hallberg IR (2007) Older caregivers' coping strategies and sense of coherence in relation to quality of life. *J Adv Nurs* **57**: 584–96.

Ellershaw JE, Murphy D (2005) The Liverpool Care Pathway (LCP): Influencing the UK national agenda on care of the dying. *Int J Palliative Nurs* **11**: 132–4.

Ellershaw JE, Sutcliffe JM (1995) The dying patient and dehydration. *J Pain Symptom Man* **10**: 192–7.

Ellershaw J, Wilkinson S (2003) *Care of the Dying: A pathway to excellence*. Oxford: Oxford University Press.

Ellison NM (1998) Palliative chemotherapy. In: Berger AM, Portenoy D, Weissman D (eds), *Principles and Practice of Supportive Oncology*. Philadelphia: Lippincott-Raven, 667–9.

Enzer SV (2000) *Reflexology: A tool for midwives in Australia*. Self-published.

Epstein NB, Baldwin LM, Bishop DS (1983) The McMaster Family Assessment Device. *J Mar Fam Ther* **9**: 171–80.

Ernst E (1999) Abdominal massage therapy for chronic constipation: A systematic review of controlled trials. *Forsch Komplementarmed* **6**: 149–51.

Ernst E (2001) *The Desktop Guide to Complementary and Alternative Therapies*. London: Harcourt Publishers Ltd.

Ezzone S, Baker C, Rosselet R, Terepka E (1998) Music as an adjunct to antiemetic therapy. *Oncol Nurs Forum* **25**: 1551–6.

Fainsinger R (2006) Non oral hydration in palliative care. *J Palliative Med* **9**: 206–8.

Faller H, Lang H, Schilling S (1995) Emotional distress and hope in lung cancer patients, as perceived by patients, relatives, physicians, nurses and interviewers. *Psycho-Oncology* **4**: 21–31.

Fallon M, Hanks G (2006) *ABC of Palliative Care*, 2nd edn. Oxford: Blackwell Publishing.

Fallowfield L (1993) Giving sad and bad news. *Lancet* **341**: 476–8.

Fallowfield L (1995) Communication skills for oncologists. *Clin Med* **5**(1): 99–103.

Fallowfield L, Jenkins V (1999) Effective communication skills are the key to good cancer care. *Eur J Cancer* **35**: 1592–7.

Fallowfield LJ, Hall A, Maguire GP, Baum M (1990) Psychological outcomes of different treatment policies in women with early breast cancer outside clinical trials. *BMJ* **301**: 575–80.

Fallowfield L, Saul J, Gilligan B (2001) Teaching senior nurses how to teach communication skills in oncology. *Cancer Nurs* **24**: 185–91.

Fallowfield L, Jenkins V, Farewell V et al. (2002) Efficacy of a Cancer Research UK communication skills training model for oncologists: a randomised controlled trial. *Lancet* **359**: 650–6.

Farran CJ, Herth KA, Popovich JM (1995) Hope and Hopelessness. Critical Clinical constructs. London: Sage Publication.

Farrell T (1992) A process of mutual support. *Professional Nurse* **8**(1): 10–14.

Faulkner A (1979) Monitoring nurse patient conversations in a ward. *Nursing Times* **5**: 95–6.

Faulkner A (1992) The evaluation of training programs for communication skills in palliative care. *J Cancer Care* **1**: 75–8.

Faulkner A, Maguire P (1994) *Talking to Cancer Patients*. Oxford: Oxford University Press.

Fawzy I, Fawzy NW (1994) A structured psychoeducational intervention for cancer patients. *Gen Hosp Psychiatry* **16**: 149–92.

Fawzy FI, Cousins N, Fawzy NW et al. (1990) A structured psychiatric intervention for cancer patients: changes over time in methods of coping and affective disturbance. *Arch Gen Psychiatry* **47**: 720–5.

Fawzy FI, Cousins N, Fawzy NW et al. (2003) Assessment and management of cancer related fatigue in adults. *Lancet* **362**: 640–50.

Fellowes D, Gambles MA, Lockhart-Wood K, Wilkinson SM (2001) Reflexology for symptom relief in patients with cancer. (Protocol for a Cochrane Review.) *The Cochrane Library*, Issue 2. Oxford: Update Software.

Fellowes D, Barnes K, Wilkinson S (2004) Aromatherapy and massage for symptom relief in patients with cancer. *Cochrane Database Syst Rev* **3**: CD02287.

Fielding R, Hunt J (1996) Preferences for information and involvement in decisions during cancer care among Hong Kong Chinese population. *Psycho-Oncology* **5**: 321–9.

Filshie J (1990) Acupuncture for malignant pain. *Acupuncture Med* **8**(20): 38–9.

Filshie J, Redman D (1985) Acupuncture and malignant pain problems. *Eur J Surg Oncol* **11**: 389–94.

Filshie J, Thompson J (2005) Acupuncture. In: Doyle D, Hanks G, Cherny N, Calman K (eds), *Oxford Textbook of Palliative Medicine*. Oxford: Oxford University Press, 410–24.

Filshie J, Penn K, Ashley S, Davis CL (1996) Acupuncture for the relief of cancer related breathlessness. *Palliative Med* **10**: 145–50.

Firth S (2001) *Wider Horizons: Care of the dying in a multicultural society*. London: National Council for Hospice and Specialist Palliative Care Services.

Flemming K (1997) The meaning of hope to palliative care cancer patients. *Int J Palliative Nurs* **3**(1): 14–18.

Fletcher CM, Elmes PC, Fairbairn MB et al. (1959) The significance of respiratory symptoms and the diagnosis of chronic bronchitis in a working population. *British Medical Journal* **2**: 257–66.

Foley KM (2006) Appraising the WHO Analgesic Ladder on its 20th Anniversary. Online interview with Katherine Foley. Available at: www.whocancerpain.wise.edu/eng/19–1 (accessed 22 April 2007).

Forbes S, Bern-Klug M, Gessert C (2000) End-of-life decision making for nursing home residents with dementia. *J Nurs Scholarship* **32**: 251–8.

Foundation for Integrated Medicine (1997) *Integrated Health Care – A way forward for the next five years?* London: Foundation for Integrated Medicine (now the Prince of Wales's Foundation for Integrated Health).

Frank BA (1995) People with dementia can communicate – if we are able to hear. In: Kitwood T, Benson S (eds), *The New Culture of Dementia Care*. London: Hawker.

Frankl V (1946) *Man's Search for Meaning*. London: Hodder & Stoughton.

Freud S (1915) *Instincts and Their Vicissitudes. Collected Papers*. New York: Basic Books.

Freud S (1917) Mourning and melancholia. In: Strachey J (ed.), *Standard Edition of the Complete Psychological Works of Sigmund Freud*, Vol 14. New York: Norton.

Friedman T, Lloyd-Williams M, Rudd N (1999) A survey of psychosocial service provision within hospices. *Palliative Med* **13**: 431–2.

Fulton C (1998) The prevalence and detection of psychiatric morbidity in patients with metastatic breast cancer. *Eur J Cancer Care* **7**: 232–9.

Gambles M, Cooke M, Wilkinson S (2002) Evaluation of a hospice based reflexology service: a qualitative audit of patients' perceptions. *Eur J Oncol Nurs* **6**(1): 37–44.

Garmatis CJ, Chu F (1978) The effectiveness of radiotherapy in the treatment of bone metastases from breast cancer. *Radiology* **16**: 235–7.

Gessert CE, Forbes S, Bern-Klug M (2001) Planning end-of-life care for families with dementia: roles of families and health professionals. *Omega: J Death Dying* **42**: 273–91.

Gibbs G (1988) *Learning by Doing: A guide to teaching and learning methods*. Oxford: Further Education Unit, Oxford Polytechnic (now Oxford Brookes University).

Gibbs LME, Addington-Hall J, Gibbs JS (1998) Dying from heart failure: lessons from palliative care. *BMJ* **317**: 961–2.

Gift AG, Narsavage G (1998) Validity of the numeric rating scale as a measure of dyspnea. *Am J Crit Care* **7**: 200–4.

Gift A, Moore T, Soeken K (1992) Relaxation to reduce dyspnoea and anxiety in COPD patients. *Nurs Res* **41**: 242–6.

Gilbert HA, Kagan AR, Nussbaum H et al. (1977) Evaluation of radiation for bone metastases: pain relief and quality of life. *Am J Roentgenol* **129**: 1095–8.

Gillard Y (1988) Reflexology and radiotherapy. *Footprints* July: 6–17.

Gilley J (1988) Intimacy and terminal care. *J R Coll GP* **38**: 121–2.

Gilron I, Bailey JM, Dongsheng T et al. (2005) Morphine, gabapentin or their combination for neuropathic pain. *N Engl J Med* **352**: 1324–34.

Glare P, Christakis N (2005) Predicting survival in patients with advanced disease. In: Doyle D, Hanks G, Cherny N, Calman K (eds), *Oxford Textbook of Palliative Medicine*. Oxford: Oxford University Press, 29–42.

Glover J, Dibble S, Dodd M et al. (1995) Mood states of oncology outpatients: does pain make a difference? *J Pain Symptom Man* **10**: 120–8.

Gold Standards Framework (2006) Prognostic Indicator Guidance Version 2.25. Available at: www.goldstandardsframework.nhs.uk (accessed August 2007).

Gold Standards Framework (2007) Advance Care Planning. Available at: www.goldstandardsframework.nhs.uk/_advanced_care.php (accessed July 2007).

Goldberg B (1998) Connection: an exploration of spirituality in nursing care. *J Adv Nurs* **17**: 836–42.

Gorer CT (1955) *The Pornography of Death, Grief and Mourning in Contemporary Britain*. London: Cresset.

Gould D, Thomas V (1997) Pain mechanisms: The reurophysiology and neuropsychology of pain perceptions. In: Thomas V (ed.), *Pain: Its nature and management*. London: Baillière Tindall, 20–35.

Graham F, Clark D (2005) The syringe driver and the subcutaneous route in palliative care: the inventor, the history and the implications. *J Pain Symptom Man* **29**: 32–40.

Grealish L, Lomasney A, Whiteman B (2000) Foot massage. *Cancer Nurs* **23**: 237–43.

Grollman EA (1993) *Straight Talk About Death for Teenagers*. Boston, MA: Beacon Press.

Guyatt GH, Berman LB, Townsend M, Pugsley SO, Chambers LW (1987) A measure of the quality of life for clinical trials in chronic lung disease. *Thorax* **42**: 773–8.

Haas F (1994) In the patient's best interests? Dehydration in dying patients. *Professional Nurse* **10**(2): 82–7.

Hallett A (2003) Unpublished Interim Audit Ipswich Hospital NHS Trust. Cited in Prince of Wales's Foundation for Integrated Health (2003).

Hanks G, Cherny NI, Fallon M (2005) Opioid analgesic therapy. In: Doyle D, Hanks G, Cherny NI, Calman K (eds), *Oxford Textbook of Palliative Medicine*, 3rd edn. Oxford: Oxford University Press, 316–41.

Harding R, Higginson I (2001) Working with ambivalence: informal care givers of patients at the end of life. *Supportive Care Cancer* **9**: 642–5.

Hardwick C, Lawson N (1995) The information and learning needs of the caregiving family of the adult patient with cancer. *Eur J Cancer Care* **4**: 118–21.

Harris KA (1998) The informational needs of patients with cancer and their families. *Cancer Practice* **6**(10): 39–46.

Harris R (2004) Clinical aromatherapy – essential oils in practice. *Int J Clin Aromatherapy* **14**: 95–6.

Hauri PJ, Sateia MJ (1985) Non pharmacological treatment of sleep disorders. In: Hales RE, Frances AJ (eds), *American Psychiatric Association Annual Review*, 4. Washington DC: American Psychiatric Press, 361–78.

Hayward J (1975) *Information: A prescription against pain*. London: RCN. Reprinted in 1995 by Scutari Press.

Heaven C, Maguire P (2003) Communication issues. In: Lloyd-Williams M (ed.), *Psychosocial Issues in Palliative Care*. Oxford: Oxford University Press, 13–34.

Heinzer MMV, Bish C, Detwiler R (2003) Acute dyspnoea as perceived by patients with chronic obstructive pulmonary disease. *Clin Nurs Res* **12**(1): 85–101.

Helig S (1988) The San Francisco Medical Society euthanasia survey. *San Francisco Medicine* **61**: 24–34.

Help the Hospices (2002) *Children on the Brink: A joint report on orphan estimates and program strategies USAID, UNAIDS, UNICEF in suffering at the end of life: the state of the world*. London: Help the Hospices.

Help the Hospices (2005) *Suffering at the End of Life: The state of the world*. London: Help the Hospices.

Help the Hospices (2006) International Palliative Care Reference Group. Available at: www.helpthehospices.org.uk/international/index.asp (accessed 24 March 2008).

Helsing K, Comstock G, Szklo M (1982) Causes of death in a widowed population. *Am J Epidemiol* **116**: 524–32.

Herr K, Bjoro K, Decker S (2004) Tools for assessment of pain in nonverbal adults with dementia: a state-of-the science review. *J Pain Symptom Man* **31**: 170–92.

Herth K (1990a) Fostering hope in terminally ill people. *J Adv Nurs* **15**: 1250–9.

Herth K (1990b) Contributions of humour as perceived by the terminally ill. *Am J Hospice Care* **7**(1): 36–40.

Herth K, Cutcliffe J (2002) The concept of hope in nursing: hope and palliative care nursing. *Br J Nurs* **11**: 977–83.

Hesketh PJ, Gralla RJ, duBois A et al. (1998) Methodology of antiemetic trials: response assessment, evaluation of new agents and definition of chemotherapy emetogenicity. *Support Cancer Care* **6**: 221–7.

Hicks F, Corcoran G (1993) Should hospices offer admissions to patients with motor neurone disease? *Palliative Med* **7**: 145–50.

Higginson IJ (2002) Palliative care and progressive illness. The Development Forum. www.devforum.org.uk/uploads/palliative_care_irenehigginson.doc. (accessed 11 July 2003).

Highfield M, Cason C (1983) Spiritual needs of patients: are they recognised? *Cancer Nurs* **6**: 187–92.

Hill D, Penso D (1995) *Opening Doors: Improving access to hospice and specialist palliative care services by members of the black and ethnic minority communities*. London: National Council for Hospice and Specialist Palliative Care Services.

Hills HM, Taylor EE (2001) *Complementary Therapies in Palliative Care: Audit Report 2001–2002*. East Lancashire Integrated Health Care Centre. Available via The Prince of Wales's Foundation for Integrated Health.

Hinds P, Martin J (1988) Hopefulness and the self–sustaining process in adolescents with cancer. *Nurs Res* **37**: 336–9.

Hirschtick RE, Von Roenn JH (2006) Human immunodeficiency virus in palliative care. In: Bruera E, Higginson IJ, Rapamonti C, Von Gunten C (eds), *Textbook of Palliative Medicine*. London: Hodder Arnold, 903–10.

Hockey J (1990) *Experiences of Death: An anthropological account*. Edinburgh: Edinburgh University Press.

Hodgson H (2000) Does reflexology impact on cancer patients' quality of life? *Nursing Standard* **14**(31): 33–8.

Hollins S, Esterhuyzen A (1997) Bereavement and grief in adults with learning disabilities. *Br J Psychiatry* **170**: 497–501.

Holmberg L (2006) Communication in palliative home care. *J Hospice Palliative Nurs* **8**: 15–24.

Holmes S, Dickerson J (1987) The quality of life design and evaluation of a self assessment instrument for use with cancer patients. *Int J Nurs Studies* **24**(10): 15–24.

Holmes J, Bently K, Cameron I (2003) A UK survey of psychiatric services for older people in general hospitals. International Journal of Geriatric Psychiatry **18**: 716–21.

Hoskins PJ (2005) Radiotherapy in symptom management. In: Doyle D, Hanks G, Cherny N, Calman K (eds), Ox*ford Textbook of Palliative Medicine*. Oxford: Oxford University Press, 239–55.

Hunt M (1991) Being friendly and informal: reflected in nurses', terminally ill patients' and relatives' conversations at home. *J Adv Nurs* **16**: 929–38.

Hutchinson T, Scherman A (1992) Didactic and experiential death and dying training: impact upon death anxiety. *Death Studies* **16**: 317–30.

Ibbotson T, Maguire P, Shelby P, Priestman T, Wallace L (1994) Screening for anxiety and depression in cancer patients: the effects of disease and treatment. *Eur J Cancer* **30**A: 37–40.

Ihilevich D, Gleser GC (1986) *Defence Mechanisms: Their classification, correlates, and measurements with the defence mechanism inventory*. Odessa, FL: Psychological Assessment Resource.

Illich I (1975) *Medical Nemesis*. London: Penguin.

International Association for the Study of Pain (1986) Classification of chronic pain. Description of chronic pain syndromes and definitions of pain terms. *Pain* (suppl 3).

International Association for the Study of Pain (1995) Cited in Carroll and Bowsher (1995).

Jacobs S (1993) An analysis of the concept of grief. *J Adv Nurs* **18**: 1787–94.

Jellinger KA et al. (2000) Neuropathology and general autopsy findings in AIDS during the last 15 years. *Acta Neuropathol (Berlin)* **100**: 213–20.

Jenkins V, Fallowfield L, Saul J (2001) Information needs of patients with cancer: results from a large study of UK cancer centres. *Br J Cancer* **84**: 48–51.

Jennings AL, Davies AN, Higgins JP et al. (2002) A systematic review of the use of opioids in the management of dyspnoea. *Thorax:* **57**: 939–44.

Johns C (2002) *Guided Reflection: Advancing practice*. Oxford: Blackwell Publishing.

Johns C (2004) *Becoming a Reflective Practitioner*, 2nd edn. Oxford: Blackwell Publishing.

Johns C (2006a) *Being Mindful, Easing Suffering*. London: Jessica Kingsley Publishers.

Johns C (2006b) *Engaging Reflection in Practice – A narrative approach*. Oxford: Blackwell Publishing.

Johnson JD, Young B (1996) Demographics of brain metastasis. *Neurosurg Clin North Am* **7**: 337–44.

Johnston G (2004) Social death. The impact of protracted dying. In: Payne S, Seymour J, Ingelton C (eds), *Palliative Care Nursing*. Milton Keynes, Bucks: Open University Press, 351–63.

Jones AC (2005) The role of hope in serious illness and dying. *Eur J Palliative Care* **12**(1): 28–31.

Jones R, Pearson J, MacGregor S et al. (1999) Randomised trial of personalised computer information based information for cancer patients. *BMJ* **319**: 1241–7.

Jones R, Tweddle S, Hampshire M et al. (2000) Effective health care. Informing, communicating and sharing decisions with people who have cancer. *NHS Centre for Reviews and Dissemination* **6**(6): 1–8.

Jordan J, Neimeyer R (2003) Does grief counselling work? *Death Studies* **27**: 765–86.

Jordan JR, Baker J, Matteis M, Rosenthal S, Ware E (2005) The grief evaluation measure (GEM): an initial validation study. *Death Studies* **29**: 301–32.

Joyce M, Richardson R (1997) Reflexology can help MS. *Int J Alternative Complementary Med* **15**(7): 10–12.

Kafetz K (2002) What happens when elderly people die? *JRSoc Med* **95**: 536–8.

Kastenbaum R (2000) *The Psychology of Death*. New York: Springer.

Katz JS, Pearce S (2003) *End of Life in Care Homes – A palliative approach*. Oxford: Oxford University Press.

Kaye P (2003) *A–Z Pocketbook of Symptom Control*, 2nd edn. Northampton: EPL Publications.

Kearney M (2000) *A Place of Healing: Working with suffering in living and dying*. Oxford: Oxford University Press.

Kellehear A (2000) Spirituality and palliative care: A model of needs. *Palliative Med* **14**(20): 149–55.

Kettering T (1993) In: Grollman EA (ed.), *Straight Talk About Death For Teenagers*. Boston, MA: Beacon Press.

Kindell J, Griffiths H (2006) Speech and language therapy intervention for people with Alzheimer's disease. In: Bryan K, Maxim J (eds), *Communication Disability in the Dementias*. Chichester: Wiley, 201–37.

Kirk K (1992) Confidence as a factor in chronic illness care. *J Advanced Nurs* **17**: 1238–42.

Kirkpatrick EM, ed. (1983) *Chambers Twentieth Century Dictionary*, new edn. Edinburgh: Chambers.

Kirsch I, Montgomery G, Sapirstein G (1995) Hypnosis as an adjunct to cognitive behavioural psychotherapy, a meta analysis. *J Consult Clin Psychol* **63**: 214–20.

Kissane DW (2005) Bereavement. In: Doyle D, Hanks G, Cherny N, Calman K (eds), *Oxford Textbook of Palliative Medicine*, 3rd edn. Oxford: Oxford University Press, 1137–51.

Kissane D, Clarke D, Street A (2001) Demoralisation syndrome: a relevant psychiatric diagnosis in palliative care. *J Palliative Care* **17**: 12–21.

Kissane DW, McKenzie M, McKenzie DP et al. (2003) Psycho social morbidity associated with patterns of family functioning in palliative care: baseline data from the family focused grief therapy controlled trial. *Palliative Med* **17**: 527–37.

Knaus WA et al. (1995) The SUPPORT prognostic model: objective estimates of survival of seriously ill hospitalised adults. *Ann Intern Med* **122**: 191–203.

Knaus WA, Wagner DP, Draper EA et al. (1991) The APACHE III prognostic system. Risk prediction of hospital mortality for critically ill hospitalized adults. *Chest* **100**: 1619–35.

Knox TA et al. (2000) Diarrhea and abnormalities of gastrointestinal function in a cohort of men and women with HIV infection. *Am J Gastroenterol* **95**: 3482–9.

Kohn M (1999) Complementary therapies in palliative care: abridged report of a study produced for Macmillan Cancer Relief. Available from Complementary Therapies Medical Advisor, Macmillan Cancer Relief, 89 Albert Embankment, London SE1 7UO.

Korner I (1970) Hope as a method of coping. *J Consulting Clin Psychol* **34**: 134–9.

Kotler D, Tierney AR, Culpepper-Morgan JA et al. (1990) Effect of home total parenteral nutrition on body composition in patients with acquired immunodeficiency syndrome. *J Parent Ent Nutr* **14**: 454–8.

Kovach CR, Weissman DE, Griffie K, Matson S, Muchkas (1999) Assessment and treatment of discomfort for people with late stage dementia. *Pain Symptom Man* **18**: 412–19.

Kristjanson LJ, Cousins K, Smith J, Lewin G (2005) Evaluation of the Bereavement Risk Index (BRI): a community hospice care protocol. *Int J Palliative Nurs* **11**: 610–18.

Kübler-Ross E (1969) *On Death and Dying*. London: Tavistock Press.

Kübler-Ross E (1970) *On Death and Dying*, 2nd edn. London: Tavistock Publications. Reprinted 1989, 1991, 1992, 1995 – London: Routledge.

Kübler-Ross E (1993) *Questions and Answers on Death and Dying*. New York: Macmillan.

Kübler-Ross E, Kessler D (2005) *On Grief and Grieving: Finding the meaning of grief through the fine stages of loss*. London: Simon & Schuster.

Lacasse Y, Wong E, Guyatt GH et al. (1996) Meta-analysis of respiratory rehabilitation in chronic obstructive pulmonary disease. *Lancet* **348**: 1115–19.

Lake T (1984) *Living with Grief*. London: Sheldon Press.

Lanceley A (1995) Emotional disclosure between cancer patients and nurses. In: Richardson A, Wilson-Barnett J (eds), *Nursing Research in Cancer Care*. Glasgow: Scutari Press, 167–89.

Langewitz WA, Eich P, Kiss A, Wossmer B (1998) Improving communication skills – A randomised controlled behaviourally oriented intervention study for residents in internal medicine. *Psychosom Med* **60**: 268–76.

Leach RM (2005) Palliative medicine and non malignant, end stage respiratory disease. In: Doyle D, Hanks G, Cherny N, Calman K (eds), *Oxford Textbook of Palliative Medicine,* 3rd edn. Oxford: Oxford University Press, 895–916.

Lefebvre-Chapiro S, Sebag-Lanoë R (1996) Le traitement des douleurs chez le vieillard. *Le Concours Medical* **118**: 81–4.

Leigh PN, Annane D, Jewitt K, Mustfa N (2003) Mechanical ventilation for amyotrophic lateral sclerosis/motor neurone disease. *Cochrane Database Syst Rev* **4**: CD004427.

Lesher EL, Berger KJ (1988) Bereaved elderly mourners: Changes in health, functional activity, family cohesion and psychological well being. *Int J Aging Human Dev* **26**(2): 81-90.

Leszcz M, Goodwin PJ (1998) The rationale and foundations of group psychotherapy for women with metastatic breast cancer. *Int J Group Psychotherapy* **48**: 245–73.

Lett A (2000) *Reflex Zone Therapy for Health Professionals*. London: Churchill Livingstone.

Ley P (1988) *Communicating with Patients: Improving communication satisfaction and compliance*. London: Croom Helm.

Ley P, Florino T (1996) The use of reading formulas in health care. *Psychology, Health Med* **1**(1): 7–28.

Ley P, Spelman M (1967) *Communicating with the Patient*. St Albans: Staples Press.

Light RW, Muro JR, Stansbury DW et al. (1989) Effects of oral morphine on breathlessness and exercise tolerance in patients with chronic obstructive pulmonary disease. *Am Rev Respir Dis* **139**: 126–33.

Lindemann E (1944) Symptomatology and management of acute grief. *Am J Psychiatry* **101**: 141–8.

Liossi C, White P (2001) Efficacy of clinical hypnosis in the enhancement of quality of life of terminally ill cancer patients. *Contemp Hypnosis* **18**: 145–60.

Lipton SA (1994) HIV-related neuronal injury. Potential therapeutic intervention with calcium channel antagonists and NMDA antagonists. *Mol Neurobiol* **8**: 181–96.

Liss HP, Grant BJ (1988) The effect of nasal flow on breathlessness in patients with chronic obstructive pulmonary disease. *Am Rev Respir Dis* **137**: 1285–8.

Lloyd-Williams M, ed. (2006) *Psychosocial Issues in Palliative Care*. Oxford: Oxford University Press.

Lloyd-Williams M, Friedman T, Rudd N (1999a) A survey of psychosocial services provision within hospices. *Palliative Med* **13**: 43–2.

Lloyd-Williams M, Friedman T, Rudd N (1999b) A survey of antidepressant prescribing in the terminally ill. *Palliative Med:* **13**: 243–8.

Lloyd-Williams M, Friedman T, Rudd N (2000) Criterion validation of the Edinburgh Postnatal Depression Scale as a screening tool for depression in patients with advanced metastatic cancer. *J Pain Symptom Man* **20**: 990–6.

Lloyd-Williams M, Spiller J, Ward J (2003) Which depression screening tools should be used in palliative care? *Pall Med* **17**(1): 40–3.

Loge JH (2006) Assessment of fatigue in palliative care. In: Bruera E, Higginson IJ, Ripamonti C, Von Gunten C (eds), *Textbook of Palliative Medicine*. London: Hodder Arnold, 621–9.

Luchins DJ, Hanrahan P, Murphy K (1997) Criteria for enrolling dementia patients in hospice. *J Am Geriatr Soc* **45**: 1054–9.

Lynch ME (1995) The assessment and prevalence of affective disorders in advanced cancer. *J Palliative Care* **11**: 10–18.

Ma KW (1992) The roots and development of Chinese acupuncture: from pre history to 20th century. *Acupuncture Med* **10**(suppl): 92–9.

McCaffery M, Beebe A (1994) *Pain. Clinical manual for nursing practice*. London: Mosby.

McCain, Nancy L, Zeller et al. (1996) The influence of stress management training on HIV disease. *Nursing Res* **45**: 246–53.

McCarthy M, Addington-Hall J, Altmann D (1997) The experience of dying with dementia: a retrospective study. *Int J Geriatr Psychiatry* **12**: 404–9.

Macdonald E (2004) *Difficult Conversations in Medicine*. Oxford: Oxford University Press.

McGavigan A, Dunn FG (2005) Palliative medicine for patients with end-stage heart disease. In: Doyle D, Hanks G, Cherney N, Calman K (eds), *Oxford Textbook of Palliative Medicine*, 3rd edn. Oxford: Oxford University Press, 917–24.

McGee R (1984) Hope: a factor in influencing crisis resolution *Adv Nurs Sci* **6**(4): 34–44.

McGuire DB (1989) Cancer pain. Pathophysiology of pain in cancer. *Cancer Nursing* **12**: 310–15.

McHale J, Tingle J (2002) *The Law and Nursing*. Oxford: Butterworth-Heinemann.

McHugh P, Lewis S, Ford S et al. (1995) The efficacy of audiotapes in promoting psychological well–being in cancer patients: a randomised controlled trial. *Br J Cancer* **71**: 388–92.

McIlfatrick S (2007) Assessing palliative care needs: views of patients, informal carers and health care professionals. *J Adv Nurs* **57**: 77–86.

McKee P et al. (1971) The natural history of congestive heart failure: the Framingham study. *N Engl J Med* **285**: 1141–6.

Macleod-Clark J (1981) Communication in nursing. *Nursing Times* **77**: 12–18.

Macmillan Cancer Relief (2002) *Directory of Complementary Therapy Services in UK Cancer Care*. London: Macmillan Cancer Relief.

Maguire P (1985) For debate. Barriers to the psychological care of the dying. *BMJ* **291**: 1711–13.

Maguire P (1990) Can communication skills be taught? *Br J Hosp Med* **43**: 215–16.

Maguire P (2000) Communication with terminally ill patients and their relatives. In: Chochinov H, Breitbart W (eds), *Handbook of Psychiatry in Palliative Medicine*. Oxford: Oxford University Press, 291–301.

Maguire P, Faulkner A (1988) Communicate with cancer patients: 1 Handling bad news and difficult questions. *BMJ* **279**: 907–9.

Maguire P, Howell A (1992) Priorities in the psychological care cancer patients. In: Lloyd-Williams M (ed.), *Int Rev of Psychiatry* **4**(1): 35–44.

Maguire P, Hopwood P, Tarrier N, Howell T (1985) Treatment of depression in cancer patients. *Acta Psychiatr Scand Suppl* **320**: 81–4.

Maguire P, Booth K, Elliot C, Jones B (1996) Helping health professionals involved in cancer care acquire key interviewing skills – the impact of workshops. *Eur J Cancer Care* **32A**: 1486–9.

Mannix KA (2005) Palliation of nausea and vomiting. In: Doyle D, Hanks G, Cherney N, Calman K (eds), *Oxford Textbook of Palliative Medicine*, 3rd edn. Oxford: Oxford University Press, 459–68.

Mannix K, Blackborn IM, Garland A et al. (2006) Effectiveness of brief training in cognitive behaviour therapy technique for palliative care practitioners. *Palliative Med* **20**: 579–84.

Mansour AA, Beuche M, Laing G, Leis A, Nurse J (1999) A study to test the effectiveness of placebo Reiki standardised procedures developed for planned Reiki efficacy study. *J Alternative Med* **5**: 153–63.

Marie Curie Cancer Care (2003) *Spiritual and Religious Care Competencies for Specialist Palliative Care*. London: Marie Curie Cancer Care.

Marwitt SJ, Klass D (1995) Grief and the role of the inner representation of the deceased. *Omega* **30**: 283–98.

Masand PS, Tesar GE (1996) Use of stimulants in the medically ill. *Psychiatric Clin North Am* **19**: 515–47.

Massie MJ (1989) Depression. In: Holland JC, Rowland JH (eds) *Handbook of Psycho-Oncology: Psychological care of the patient with cancer*. New York: Oxford University Press, 283–90.

Matthews W, McCutcheon JA, Asch S et al. (2000) National estimates of HIV-related symptom prevalence from HIV Cost and Services Utilization Study. *Med Care* **38**: 750–62.

Meldrum M (2005) The ladder and the clock: cancer pain and public policy at the end of the twentieth century. *J Pain Symptom Man* **29**: 41–54.

Mellström D, Nilsson A, Oden A, Svanborg A (1982) Mortality among the widowed in Sweden. *Scand J Social Med* **10**: 33–41.

Melzack R (1987) The McGill Short Form Pain Questionnaire. *Pain* **30**: 191–7.

Melzack R, Wall P (1996) *The Challenge of Pain*, 2nd edn. London: Penguin Books.

Mendoza TR, Wang XS, Cleeland CS et al. (1999) The rapid assessment of fatigue severity in cancer patients: use of the Brief Fatigue Inventory. *Cancer* **85**: 1186–96.

Mental Capacity Act (2005) Department of Constitutional Affairs. London: The Stationery Office.

Menzies-Lyth (1988) A case study in the functioning of social systems as a defence against anxiety. In: *Containing Anxiety in Institutions: selected essays*. London: Free Association Books, 44–85.

Miesen BML (1997) Awareness in dementia patients and family grieving: a practical perspective. In: Miesen BML, Jones GMM (eds), *Care-giving in Dementia: Research and applications*, Vol 2. London: Routledge, 67–79.

Miesen BML (1999) *Dementia in Close-up: Understanding and caring for people with dementia* (transl GMM Jones). London: Routledge.

Milligan M, Fanning M, Harter S, Tadjali M, Stevens E (2002) Reflexology audit: patient satisfaction, impact on quality of life available in Scottish hospice. *Int J Palliative Nurs* **8**: 489–96.

Mills ME, Sullivan K (1999) The importance of information giving for patients newly diagnosed with cancer: a review of the literature. *J Clin Nurs* **8**: 631–42.

Mirando S (2005) Introducing an integrated care pathway for the last days of life. *Palliative Med* **19**: 33–9.

Mock V, Atkinson A, Barsevick A et al. (2000) National comprehensive cancer network oncology practice guidelines for cancer related fatigue. *Oncology* **14**: 151–61.

Mok E, Chan F (2002) Perception of empowerment by family caregivers of patients with a terminal illness in Hong Kong. *Int J Palliative Nurs* **8**: 137–45.

Montgomery GH, Weltz CR, Borbjerg DH (2002) Brief pre surgery hypnosis reduces distress and pain in excisional breast biopsy patients. *Int J Clin Expl Hypnosis* **50**(1): 17–32.

Moos RH, Moos BS (2002) The Family Relationships Index (FRI). In: Kissane DW, Block S (eds) *Family Focused Grief Therapy*. Milton Keynes, Bucks: Open University Press, 202–3.

Moorey S, Greer S (2006) *Cognitive Behavior Therapy for People with Cancer*. Oxford: Oxford University Press.

Morgan G (1990) *Images of Organisation*. London: Sage.

Morrison P (1994) *Understanding Patients*. London: Baillière Tindall.

Morrison RS, Siu AL (2000) A comparison of pain and its treatment in advanced dementia and cognitively intact patients with hip fracture. *J Pain Symptom Man* **19**: 240–8.

Moss AH, Oppenheimer EA, Casey P et al. (1996) Patients with amyotrophic lateral sclerosis, receiving long-term mechanical ventilation. Advance care planning and outcomes. *Chest* **110**(1): 249–55.

Moulin DE (1989) Pain in multiple sclerosis. *Neurol Clinics* **7**: 321–31.

Moulin DE, Lessi A, Amireh R, Sharpe WKJ, Boyd D, Merskey H (1996) Randomised trial of oral morphine for chronic non–cancer pain. *Lancet* **347**: 143–7.

Mulkay M (1993) Social death in Britain. In: Clark D (ed.), *The Sociology of Death.* Oxford: Blackwell.

Munroe B (2003) Social work in palliative care. In: Doyle D, Hanks GWC, MacDonald N (eds), *Oxford Textbook of Palliative Medicine*, 2nd edn. Oxford: Oxford University Press, 867–83.

Munroe B, Oliviere D (2003) *Patient Participation in Palliative Care. A voice for the voiceless.* Oxford: Oxford University Press.

Murray S, Kendall M, Worth A et al. (2004) Exploring the spiritual needs of people dying of lung cancer or heart failure: a prospective qualitative interview study of patients and their carers. *Palliative Med* **18**: 39–45.

Murtagh DR, Greenwood KM (1995) Identifying effective psychological treatments for insomnia: a meta analysis. *J Consulting Clin Psychol* **63**(1): 79–89.

Murtagh FM, Preston M, Higginson I (2004) The Liverpool Care Pathway (LCP) influencing the UK national agenda on the care of the dying. *Int J Palliative Nurs* **11**: 132–4.

Muss HB et al. (1979) Written information: consent in patients with breast cancer. *Cancer* **43**: 1549–56.

Muza SR et al. (1990) Comparison of scales used to quantitate the sense of effort to breathe in patients with chronic obstructive pulmonary disease. *Am Rev Respir Dis* **141**: 909–13.

Narayanasamy A (2001) *Spiritual Care: A practical guide for nurses and health care practitioners.* 2nd edn. Wiltshire: Quay Books.

Narayanasamy A (2006) *Spiritual Care and Transcultural Research.* London: Quay Books.

National Bereavement Consortium (2001) Bereavement Care Standards UK project. *Standards for Bereavement Care.* Available at: www.bereavement.org.uk/standards/index.Asp.

National Cancer Action Team (2007) *Advanced Communications Skills Handout.* The National Cancer Action Team: tel 020 7188 9027.

National Cancer Alliance (1996) *'Patient Centred Services'? What Patients Say.* Oxford: NCA.

National Council for Hospice and Specialist Palliative Care Services (1993) *Key Ethical Issues in Palliative Care. Evidence to the House of Lords Select Committee on Medical Ethics.* London: NCHSPCS.

National Council for Hospice and Specialist Palliative Care Services (1995) *Specialist Palliative Care: A statement of definitions.* London: NCHSPCS.

National Council for Hospice and Specialist Palliative Care Services (1997) *Feeling Better: Psychosocial care in specialist palliative care.* London: NCHSPCS.

National Council for Hospice and Specialist Palliative Care Services (2000) *'Our Lives Not Our Illness' – User involvement in palliative care now.* London: National Council for Palliative Care.

National Council for Hospice and Specialist Palliative Care Services (2002) *Vital Judgements.* London: National Council for Palliative Care.

National Council for Palliative Care (2003) *Priorities and Preferences for End of Life Care.* London: NCPC. Available at: www.ncpc.org.uk (accessed 18 August 2006).

National Council for Palliative Care (2005a) *Our Mission Directive.* Available at: www.ncpc.org.uk/mission/index.html (accessed 17 August 2006).

National Council for Palliative Care (2005b) *Palliative Care Explained.* Available at: www.ncpc.org.uk/mission/index.html (accessed 17 August 2006).

National Council for Palliative Care (2005c) *Guidance on the Mental Capacity Act.* London: NCPC.

National Institute for Clinical Excellence (2001) *Effective Health Care – Acupuncture.* The University of York NHS Centre for Reviews 7(2). London: Royal Society of Medicine Press and NICE.

National Institute for Clinical Excellence (2004a) *Supportive and Palliative Care: The research evidence.* London: NICE. Available at: www.nice.org.uk (accessed 24 March 2008).

National Institute for Clinical Excellence (2004b) *Improving Supportive and Palliative Care for Adults with Cancer – The Manual.* London: NICE. Available at: www.nice.org.uk (accessed 24 March 2008).

National Institute for Clinical Excellence (2004c) *Chronic Obstructive Pulmonary Disease. Management of COPD in Adults in Primary and Secondary Care.* London: NICE. Available at: www.nice.org.uk (accessed July 2007).

National Institute for Clinical Excellence (2006) *Guidelines for Dementia Care.* London: NICE. Available at: www.nice.org.uk (accessed August 2007).

National Occupation Standards for Aromatherapy (2002) *New Skills for Health.* London: Health UK.

Neuberger J (1999) *Dying Well.* Hale, Cheshire: Hochland & Hochland Ltd.

Neuberger J (2003) A healthy view of dying. *BMJ* **327**: 207–8.

New Skills for Health (2002) *National Occupational Standards for Aromatherapy.* London: Health UK (New Skills for Health).

Newshan G, Lefkowitz M (2001) Transdermal fentanyl for chronic pain in AIDS: a pilot study. *J Pain Symptom Man* **21**: 69–77.

NHS Confederation (2005) *Leading Edge: Improving End-of-Life Care*: Issue 12. London: NHS Confederation.

O'Brien T (2001) Neurodegenerative disease. In: Addington-Hall JM, Higginson IJ (eds), *Palliative Care for Non Cancer Patients.* Oxford: Oxford University Press, 44–53.

O'Brien T, Kelly M, Saunders C (1992) Motor neurone disease: a hospice perspective. *BMJ* **304**: 471–3.

O'Connor AM, Stacey D, Entwhistle V et al. (2003) Decision aids for people facing health treatment or screening decisions. *Cochrane Database of Systematic Reviews*, Issue 1.

Ohno-Machado L, Resnic FS, Matheny ME et al. (2006) Prognosis in critical care. *Annu Rev Biomed Eng* **8**: 567–99.

Ojoo JC et al. (2002) Patients' and carers' preferences in two models of care for acute exacerbations of COPD: results of a randomised controlled trial. *Thorax* **55**: 167–9.

Olin J, Masand P (1996) Psychostimulants for depression in hospitalised cancer patients. *Psychosomatics* **37**: 57–62.

Oliver D (1998) Opioid medication in the palliative care of motor neurone disease. *Palliative Med* **12**: 113–15.

Ouslander JG, Osterweil D, Morley J, eds (1997) *Medical Care in the Nursing Home.* New York: McGraw-Hill.

Palenicek J, Graham NM, Tie YD (1995) Weight loss prior to clinical AIDS as a predictor of survival. *J AIDS* **10**: 366–73.

Parker M (2004) Medicalizing meaning: demoralization syndrome and the desire to die. *Aust NZ J Psychiatry* **38**: 765–73.

Parkes CM (1972) *Bereavement: Studies of grief in adult life.* London: Penguin Books.

Parkes CM (1985) Cited in *Birth to Old Age in Transition.* London: Open University Press.

Parkes CM (1991) *Bereavement: Studies of grief in adult life.* London: Penguin Books.

Parkes CM (1994) Bereavement as a psychosocial transition: process of adaptation to change. In: Stroebe M, Stroebe W, Hansson RO (eds), *Handbook of Bereavement.* Cambridge: Cambridge University Press, 91–101.

Parkes CM (2005) Bereavement as a psychosocial transition, process of adaptation to change. In: Dickenson D et al. (eds), *Death, Dying and Bereavement.* London: Sage Publications, 325–31.

Parkes CM, Weiss RS (1983) *Recovery from Bereavement.* New York: Basic Books.

Parkes CM, Benjamin B, Fitzgerald RG (1969) Broken heart: a statistical study of increased mortality among widowers. *BMJ* **i**: 740–3.

Parsons T (1951) *The Social System.* London: Routledge & Kegan-Paul.

Passik SD, Breitbart WS (1996) Depression in patients with pancreatic carcinoma: diagnostic and treatment issues. *Cancer* **78**(suppl 3): 615–26.

Passik SD, Kirsh K (2006) Anxiety and adjustment disorders. In: Lloyd-Williams M (ed.), *Psychosocial issues in Palliative Care*. Oxford: Oxford University Press, 66–79.

Payne R, Gonzales G (1996) Pathophysiology of pain in cancer and other terminal diseases. In: Doyle D, Hanks G, Macdonald N (eds), *Oxford Textbook of Palliative Medicine*. Oxford: Oxford University Press, 140–8.

Payne S, Smith P, Dean S et al. (1999) Identifying the concerns of informal carers in palliative care. *Palliative Med* **13**: 37–44.

Payne A, Barry S, Creedon B, Stone C, Sweeney C, O'Brien T (2007) Sensitivity and specificity of a two-question screening tool for depression in a specialist palliative care unit. *Palliative Med* **21**: 193–8.

Pemberton C, Storey L, Havard A (2003) The preferred place of care document: an opportunity for communication. *Int J Palliative Nurs* **19**: 439–41.

Penson J (1990) *Bereavement: A guide for nurses*. London: Harper & Rowe.

Pert C (1997) *Molecules of Emotion*. London: Simon & Schuster.

Pessin H, Potash M, Breitbart W (2006) Diagnosis, assessment and treatment of depression in palliative care. In: Lloyd-Williams M (ed.), *Psychosocial Issues in Palliative Care*. Oxford: Oxford University Press, 81–104.

Pickard S, Glendinning C (2001) Caring for a relative with dementia: the perceptions of carers and CPNs. *Quality in Ageing – Policy, Practice and Research* **2**(4): 3–11.

Piscitelli SC, Gallicano KD (2001) Interactions among drugs for HIV and opportunistic infections. *N Engl J Med* **344**: 984–96.

Pitceathly P, Maguire P (2000) Preventing affective disorders in partners of cancer patients: an intervention story. In: Baider L, Cooper LL, Kaplan De-Nour AD (eds), *Cancer and the Family*, 2nd edn. Chichester: Wiley, 137–54.

Plain English Campaign (2006) www.plainenglish.co.uk (accessed 6 November 2006).

Pomeranz B (2000) Acupuncture analgesia. In: Stux G, Hammerchlag R (eds), *Clinical Acupuncture: Scientific basis*. Berlin: Springer.

Poole K, Froggart K (2002) Loss of weight and loss of appetite in advanced cancer; a problem for the patient, the carer or the health professional. *Palliative Med* **16**: 499–506.

Portenoy RK (1994) Management of common opioid side effects during long-term cancer pain. *Annu Acad Med Singapore* **23**: 160–70.

Portenoy RK, Itri L (1999) Cancer-related fatigue: guidelines for evaluation and management. *Oncologist* **4**: 1–10.

Portenoy RK, Forbes K, Lussier D, Hanks G (2005) Difficult pain problems: an integrated approach. In: Doyle D, Hanks G, Cherny N, Calman K (eds), *Oxford Textbook of Palliative Medicine*, 3rd edn. Oxford: Oxford University Press, 438–58.

Post-White J, Ceronsky C, Kreitzer MJ et al. (1996) Hope, spirituality, sense of coherence and quality of life in patients with cancer. *Oncol Nurse Forum* **23**: 1571–9.

Power R, Tate HL, McGills, Taylor C (2003) A qualitative study of the psychosocial implications of lipodystrophy syndrome on HIV positive individuals. *Sex Transm Infect* **79**: 137–41.

Praill D (2000) Who are we here for? *Palliative Med* **14**: 91–2.

Preece J (2002) Introducing abdominal massage in palliative care for the relief of constipation. *Complem Therapies Nurs Midwifery* **8**: 101–5.

Prince of Wales's Foundation of Integrated Health (2003) *National Guidelines for the use of Complementary Therapies in Supportive and Palliative Care*. London: Prince of Wales's Foundation of Integrated Health. Available at: www.fihealth.org.uk (accessed 14 March 2008).

Quest P (1999) *An Introduction to Reiki. A step-by step guide to reiki practice*. London: Piatkus.

Quinn JF, Strelkaukas A (1993) Psychoimmunologic effects of therapeutic touch on practitioners and recently bereaved recipients: a pilot study. *Adv Nursing Sci* **15**: 13–16.

Radbruch L, Sabatowski R, Loick G et al. (2000) Cognitive impairment and its influence on pain and symptom assessment in palliative care unit: development of a minimal documentation system. *Palliative Med* **14**: 266–76.

Rahe RH (1979) Life events, mental illness: an overview. *J Human Stress* **5**(3): 2–10.

Ram FSF, Picot J, Lightowler J, Wedzicha J (2004) Non-invasive positive pressure ventilation for treatment of respiratory failure due to exacerbation of COPD. *Cochrane Database of Systematic Reviews*, Issue 3.

Ramirez AJ, Graham J, Richards MA, Cull A, Gregory WM, Leaning MS (1995) Burnout and psychiatric disorder among cancer clinicians. *Br J Cancer* **71**: 1263–9.

Randall F, Downie RS (2006) *The Philosophy of Palliative Care: Critique and reconstruction.* Oxford: Oxford University Press.

Randall-Curtis J, Rocker CT (2006) Chronic obstructive pulmonary disease. In: Bruera E, Higginson IJ, Rapamonti C, Von Gunten C (eds), *Textbook of Palliative Medicine.* London: Hodder Arnold, 935–43.

Razavi D, Delvaux N, Marchal S, De Cock M, Farvacques C, Slachmuylder JL (2000) Testing health care professionals' communication skills: the usefulness of highly emotional standardised role playing sessions with simulators. *Psycho-Oncology* **9**: 293–302.

Rees D (1971) The hallucinations of widowhood. *BMJ* **4**: 37–41.

Registered Nurses Association of Ontario (2005) *Nursing Care of Dyspnoea: The 6th vital sign in individuals with chronic obstructive pulmonary disease (COPD).* Available at: www.rnao.org/bestpractices (accessed 24 March 2008).

Regnard C, Hockley J (2004) *A Guide to Symptom Relief in Palliative Care*, 5th edn. Oxford: Radcliffe Medical Press.

Reid D, Field D, Payne S et al. (2006a) Adult bereavement in five English hospices: types of support. *Int J Palliative Nurs* **12**: 430–7.

Reid D, Field D, Paynee S, Relf M (2006b) Adult bereavement in five English hospices: participants, organisations and pre-bereavement support. *Int J Palliative Nurs* **12**: 320–7.

Renfroe K (1988) Effect of progressive relaxation on dyspnoea and anxiety state in patients with COPD. *Heart Lung* **17**: 408–13.

Research Unit in Health and Behaviour Change (RUHBC) (2006a) *Health and Resilience: What does a resilience approach offer health research and policy?* Available at: www.chs.med.ed.ac.uk/ruhbc (accessed February 2007).

Research Unit in Health and Behaviour Change (2006b) *Support Groups and Coronary Heart Disease: Members' and facilitators' views.* Available at: www.chs.med.ed.ac.uk/ruhbc (assessed February 2007).

Resuscitation Council (2001) *Decisions Relating to Cardiopulmonary Resuscitation.* A Joint Statement from the British Medical Association, the Resuscitation Council (UK) and the Royal College of Nursing. Available at: www.resus.org.uk/pages/dnar.htm (accessed 15 March 2006).

Revans R (1964) *Action Learning in Hospitals.* London: McGraw Hill.

Reynolds MW, Nabors L, Quinlan A (2000) The effectiveness of art therapy: does it work? Art therapy. *J Am Art Therapy Assn* **17**: 207–13.

Richardson A, Sitzia J, Cottrell P (2005) 'Working the system'. Achieving change through partnership working: an evaluation of cancer partnership groups. *Health Expectations* **8**: 210–20.

Richardson V (2006) A dual process of grief counselling. Findings from the changing lives of older couples (CLOC). *Study J Gerontol Social Work* **48**: 311–29.

Ridley S (1994) Scoring systems and prognosis for critical illness. *Care of the Critically Ill* **10**(2): 70–2.

Robinson LA, Nuamah IF, Lev E, McCorkle R (1995) A prospective longitudinal investigation of spousal bereavement examining Parkes and Weiss' Bereavement Risk Index. *J Palliative Care* **11**(4): 5–13.

Rogers C (1967) *On Becoming a Person*. London: Constable.

Roper N, Logan W, Tierney AJ (1980) *The Elements of Nursing*. Edinburgh: Churchill Livingstone.

Roscoe JA, Morrow GR, Buchunow P, Tian L, Mattleson S (2002) Acustimulation wristbands for the relief of chemotherapy-induced nausea. *Altern Therap* 8(4): 56–63.

Rothenbacher D, Lutz M, Porzsolt F (1997) Treatment decisions in palliative cancer care: patients' preferences for involvement and doctor's knowledge about it. *Eur J Cancer* 33: 1184–9.

Royal College of Nursing (2003) *Digital Rectal Examination and Manual Removal of Faeces: Guidance for nurses*. London: Royal College of Nursing.

Royal College of Physicians (1986) Physical disability in 1986 and beyond. *J R Coll Physns* 3: 160–94.

Sahler OJ, Hunter BC, Liesveld JL (2003) The effect of using music therapy with relaxation imagery in the management of patients undergoing bone marrow transplantation: a pilot feasibility study. *Alternative Therapies Health Med* 9: 70–4.

Sampson EL, Gould V, Lee D, Blanchard MR (2006) Differences in care received by patients with and without dementia who died during acute hospital admission: a retrospective case note study. *Age Aging* 35: 190–3.

Sanchia A (2000) Changing paradigms in research: do we need to rethink the future? *Progr Palliative Care* 8: 193–202.

Sattman U, Ockenga J, Selbery O et al. (1995) Incidence and prognostic value of malnutrition and wasting in human immunodeficiency virus-infected outpatients. *J AIDS* 8: 239–46.

Saunders C (1963) Cited in Munroe and Oliviere (2003).

Saunders C (2000) Cited in Clark (2006).

Saunders C (2006a) The treatment of intractable pain in terminal cancer. In: Clark D (ed.), *Cicely Saunders Selected Writings 1958–2004*. Oxford: Oxford University Press, 61–4.

Saunders C (2006b) The last frontier. In: Clark D (ed.), *Cicely Saunders Selected Writings 1958–2004*. Oxford: Oxford University Press, 87–91.

Saunders C (2006c) The Templeton Prize speech. In: Clark D (ed.), *Cicely Saunders Selected Writings 1958–2004*. Oxford: Oxford University Press, 157–62.

Saunders C (2006d) Spiritual pain. In: Clark D (ed.), *Cicely Saunders Selected Writings 1958–2004*. Oxford: Oxford University Press, 217.

Schut H, Stroebe MS, van den Bout J et al. (2004) The efficacy bereavement interventions: determining who benefits. In: Stroebe MS, Hansson RO, Stroebe W, Schut H (eds), *Handbook of Bereavement: Consequences, coping and care*. Washington DC: American Psychological Association, 705–37.

Scott G, Whyler N, Grant G et al. (2001) A study of family carers of people with a life threatening illness 1: the carers' needs analysis. *Int J Palliative Nurs* 7: 290–7.

Sengstaken EA, King SA (1993) The problem of pain and its detection among geriatric nursing home residents. *J Am Geriatr Soc* 41: 541–4.

Seo M, Tamura K, Shijo H, Marioka E, Ikegame C, Hirasako K (2000) Telling the diagnosis to cancer patients in Japan: attitude and perceptions of patients, physicians and nurses. *Palliative Med* 14: 105–10.

Serline RC, Mendoza TR, Nakamura Y et al. (1995) When is cancer pain mild, moderate or severe? Grading severity by its interference with function. *Pain* 61: 277–84.

Seymour J, Ingelton C, Payne S, Beddow V (2003) Specialist palliative care: patients' experiences. *J Adv Nurs* 44(1): 24–33.

Seymour J, Clark D, Winslow M (2005) Pain and palliative care: the emergence of new specialties. *J Pain Symptom Man* 29: 2–13.

Shah S, Blanchard M, Tookman A, Jones L, Blizard R, King M (2006) Estimating needs in life-threatening illness: a feasibility study to assess the views of patients and doctors. *Palliative Med* 20: 205–10.

Shealy CN (1974) Six years' experience with electrical stimulation for control of pain. *Adv Neurol* **4**: 775–82.

Sheldon F (1997) *Psychosocial Palliative Care*. Cheltenham: Stanley Thornes.

Sheldon S (2003) Social impact of advanced metastatic cancer. In Lloyd-Williams M (ed.), *Psychosocial Issues in Palliative Care*. Oxford: Oxford University Press, 35–48.

Shen J, Wenger N, Glaspy J et al. (2000) Electroacupuncture for the control of myeloablative chemotherapy-induced emesis: A randomised controlled trial. *JAMA* **284**: 2755–61.

Shepperd S, Harwood D, Gray A et al. (1998) Randomised controlled trial comparing hospital at home care with inpatient hospital care 1: three month follow up of health outcomes. *BMJ* **316**: 1786–91.

Sherwood GD (2000) The power of nurse–client encounters. *J Holistic Nurs* **18**: 159–75.

Shuchter S, Zisook S (1993) The course of normal grief. In: Stroebe M, Stroebe W, Hansson RO (eds), *Handbook of Bereavement: Theory, research and intervention*. Cambridge: Cambridge University Press, 23–44.

Singh KD (1998) *The Grace in Dying: How we are transformed spiritually as we die*. San Francisco, CA: Harper.

Skwarska E et al. (2000) Randomised control trial of supported discharge in patients with exacerbations of chronic obstructive pulmonary disease. *Thorax* **55**: 907–12.

Smart F (2005) The whole truth? *Nursing Man* **11**: 17–19.

Smith C (2000) The role of health professionals in informing cancer patients: findings from The Teamwork Project (Phase one). *Health Expectations* **3**: 217–19.

Snaith et al. (1976) The Leeds scales for the self-assessment of anxiety and depression. *Br J Psychiatry* **128**: 156–65.

Sobin LH, Wittekin C (1997) *UICC TNM Classification of Malignant Tumours*, 5th edn. New York: Wiley-Liss, 74–7.

Solano JP, Gomes B, Higginson IJ (2006) Prevalence of symptoms in advanced disease, based on a systematic review of 64 studies. *J Pain Symptom Man* **31**(1): 58–69.

Souhami R, Tobias J (1998) *Cancer and Its Management*, 3rd edn. Oxford: Blackwell Science.

Speck P (1998) Power and autonomy in palliative care: a matter of balance. *Palliative Med* **12**: 145–6.

Spiegel D (1985) The use of hypnosis in controlling cancer pain. *CA-A Cancer J Clinicians* **4**: 221–31.

Spiegel D, Bloom JR (1983) Group therapy and hypnosis reduce metastatic breast carcinoma pain. *Psychosom Med* **4**: 333–9.

Spiegel D, Spira J (1991) *Supportive/Expressive Group Therapy. A treatment manual of psychosocial intervention for women with recurrent breast cancer*. Stanford, CA: Stanford University of Medicine.

Spiegel D, Bloom J, Yalom I (1981) Group support with patients with metastatic cancer: a randomised prospective outcome study. *Arch Gen Psychiatry* **28**: 527–33.

Spiegel D, Bloom JR, Kraemer HC, Gottheil F (1989) Effect of psychosocial treatment on survival of patients with metastatic breast cancer. *Lancet* **ii**: 888–91.

Spiegel D, Stein SL, Earhart TZ, Diamond S (2000) Group psychotherapy and the terminally ill. In: Chochinor H, Breitbart W (eds), *Handbook of Psychiatry in Palliative Medicine*. Oxford: Oxford University Press, 241–52.

Spielberger CD, Gorsch RI, Lushene RE, Vagg PR, Jacobs GA (1983) *Manual for State–Trait Anxiety Inventory Counselling*. Palo Alto: Psychologist Press.

Spira JL (2000) Existential psychotherapy in palliative care. In: Chochinov HM, Breitbart W (eds), *Handbook of Psychiatry in Palliative Medicine*. Oxford: Oxford University Press, 197–214.

Stannard D (1989) Pressure prevents nausea. *Nursing Times* **85**(4): 33–4.

Stedeford A (1985) *Facing Death: Patients, families and professionals.* London: William Heinemann.

Stedeford A (1994) *Facing Death: Patients, families and professionals*, 2nd edn. Oxford: Sobell Publications.

Stephenson C (1996) Complementary therapies in cancer care: an NHS approach. *Int J Palliative Nurs* 2(1): 15–18.

Stevens S (2006) Assessment of language and communication difficulties in the dementias. In: Bryan K, Maxim J (eds), *Communication Disability in the Dementias.* Chichester: Wiley, 147–83.

Stewart A, Greenfield S, Hays BD et al. (1989) Functional status and well–being of patients with chronic conditions: results from the Medical Outcomes Study. *JAMA* **262**: 907–13.

Stewart MA (1995) Effective physician–patient communication and health outcomes: a review. *Can Med Assn J* **152**: 1423–33.

Stewart M (2001) Towards a global definition of patient centre care. *BMJ* **322**: 444–5.

Stewart M, Belle Brown J, Wayne Weston W et al. (2003) *Patient-centred Medicine: Transforming the clinical method*, 2nd edn. Abingdon: Radcliffe Medical Press.

Stjernswärd J, Clark D (2005) Palliative medicine – a global perspective. In: Doyle D, Hanks G, Cherny N, Calman KC (eds), *Oxford Textbook of Palliative Medicine*, 3rd edn. Oxford: Oxford University Press, 1119–224.

Stockwell F (1972) *The Unpopular Patient.* London: RCN Study of Nursing Care Series.

Storey L (2003) Place of death: Hobson's choice or patient choice? *Cancer Nurs Pract* 3(4): 33–8.

Stroebe M (1992) Coping with bereavement. A review of the grief work hypothesis. *Omega: J Death Dying* **26**: 19–42.

Stroebe M (1998) New direction in bereavement research exploration of gender differences. *Palliative Med* **12**: 5–12.

Stroebe M, Schut H (1996) Bereavement: sex differences in bereavement. *Progr Palliative Care* **4**: 85–7.

Stroebe M, Schut H (1999) The dual process of coping with bereavement: rationale and description. *Death Studies* **23**: 197–224.

Stroebe M, Stroebe W (1994) The mortality of bereavement. In: Stroebe M, Stroebe W, Hansson RO (eds), *Handbook of Bereavement.* Cambridge: Cambridge University Press, 175–95.

Stroebe M et al. (1992) Coping with bereavement: a review of the grief work hypothes *Omega* **26**: 19–4.

SUPPORT (Study to Understand Prognoses and Preferences for Outcome and Risks of Treatment) (1996) A controlled trial to improve care for seriously ill hospitalised patients: The study to understand prognoses and preferences for outcome and risks of treatments (SUPPORT). *JAMA* **274**: 1591–8.

Suttman U, Ockenga J, Selberg O et al. (1995) Incidence and prognostic value of malnutrition and wasting in human immunodeficiency virus-infected outpatients. *J AIDS* **8**: 239–46.

Swarm RA, Karanikolas M, Cousins J (2005) Anaesthetic techniques for pain control. In: Doyle D, Hanks G, Cherny NI, Calman K (eds), *Oxford Textbook of Palliative Medicine*, 3rd edn. Oxford: Oxford University Press, 378–96.

Sweeney C, Neuenschwander H, Bruera E (2005) In: Doyle D, Hanks G, Cherny N, Calman K (eds), *Oxford Textbook of Palliative Medicine*, 3rd edn. Oxford: Oxford University Press, 560–8.

Sweeting H, Gilhooly M (1997) Dementia and the phenomenon of social death. *Sociol Health Illness* **19**(10): 93–117.

Swinton J (2001) *Spirituality and Mental Health Care.* London: Jessica Kingsley.

Sykes N (2005) Constipation and diarrhoea. In: Doyle D, Hanks G, Cherny N, Calman K (eds), *Oxford Textbook of Palliative Medicine*, 3rd edn. Oxford: Oxford University Press, 483–96.

Tanaka K, Akechi T, Okuyama T, Nishiwaki Y, Uchitomi Y (2000) Development and validation of the Cancer Dyspnoea Scale: a multidimensional, brief, self rating scale. *Br J Cancer* **82**: 800–5.

Tate H, George R (2001) The effect of weight loss on body image in HIV positive gay men. *AIDS Care* **13**(2): 163–9.

Telford K, Kralik D, Koch T (2006) *Acceptance and Denial: Implications for people adapting to chronic illness: literature review*. Oxford: Blackwell Publishing Ltd, 457–64.

Thomas K (2003) *Caring for the Dying at Home*. Oxford: Radcliffe Medical Press.

Thomas K (2005) Background to GSF. Available at: www.goldstandardsframework.nhs.uk (accessed 24 March 2008).

Thomas KJ, Fall M, Nicholl J (2001) Access to complementary medicine via general practice. *Br J Gen Pract* **51**: 25–30.

Tiran D (2002) Reviewing theories and origins. In: Mackereth P, Tiran D (eds), *Clinical Reflexology: A guide for health professionals*. London: Churchill Livingstone, 5–15.

Tomer A, Eliason G (1996) Toward a comprehensive model of death anxiety. *Death Studies* **20**: 343–65.

Trijsburg RW, van Knippenberg FC, Rijpma SE (1992) Effects of psychological treatment on cancer patients: a critical review. *Psychosom Med* **54**: 489–517.

Turk D, Feldman DC (2000) A cognitive–behavioural approach to symptom management in palliative care. In: Chochinor H, Breitbart W (eds), *Handbook of Psychiatry in Palliative Medicine*. Oxford: Oxford University Press, 223–39.

Twycross R (1995) *Pain Relief in Advanced Cancer*. London: Churchill Livingstone.

Twycross RG (1997) *Symptom Management in Advanced Cancer*, 2nd edn. Oxford: Radcliffe Medical Press.

Twycross RG (1999) Oral history interview March 3rd 1999 with Faull C. Collection of Dr Faull.

Twycross R, Wilcock A (2001) *Symptom Management in Advanced Cancer,* 3rd edn. Oxford: Radcliffe Medical Press.

Twycross R, Wilcock A (2007) *Palliative Care Formulary*, 3rd edn. Nottingham. Available at: palliativedrugs.com.

Twycross R, Wilcock A, Charlesworth S, Dickman A (2002) *Palliative Care Formulary*, 2nd edn Oxford: Radcliffe Medical Press.

UN AIDS (2001) AIDS epidemic update. December 2001. Available at: www.unaids.

UN AIDS (2006) Report on the global AIDS epidemic. Available at: www.unaids.org (accessed August 2007).

Uretsky BF, Sheahan RG (1997) Primary prevention of sudden cardiac death in heart failure: will the solution be shocking? *J Am Coll Cardiol* **30**: 1589–97.

Urquhart P (1999) Issue of suffering in palliative care. *Int J Palliative Nurs* **5**(1): 35–9.

Vachon M (2003) The emotional problems of the patient. In: Doyle D, Hanks G, Macdonald N (eds), *Oxford Textbook of Palliative Medicine*, 2nd edn. Oxford: Oxford University Press, 883–907.

Vachon M (2005) The emotional problems of the patient in palliative medicine. In: Doyle D, Hanks G, Cherny N, Calman K (eds), *Oxford Textbook of Palliative Medicine*, 3rd edn. Oxford: Oxford University Press, 961–84.

Vachon MLS, Lancee WJ, Ghadirian P, Adair WK (1991) *Final Report on the Needs of Persons Living with Cancer in Quebec*. Toronto: Canadian Cancer Society.

Vachon MLS, Fitch M, Greenberg M, Franssen E (1995) *The Needs of Cancer Patients and Their Families Attending Toronto-Sunnybrook Regional Cancer Center*. Toronto: Canadian Cancer Society.

Vickers AJ (1996) Can acupuncture have specific effects on health? A systematic review of acupuncture antiemesis trials. *J R Soc Med* **89**: 303–11.

Wakefield A (2000) Nurses' response to death and dying: a need for relentless self-care. *Int J Palliative Nurs* **6**: 245–58.

Walker AE, Robins M, Weinfield FD (1985) Epidemiology of brain tumours: the national survey of intracranial neoplasms. *Neurology* **35**: 219–26.

Walker LG (1992) Hypnosis with cancer patients. *Am J Prev Psychiatry Neurol Fall* **3**: 3.

Walker LG, Walker MB, Simpson F et al. (1997) Guided imagery and relaxation therapy can modify host defences in women receiving treatment for locally advanced breast cancer. *Br J Surg* **84**(15 suppl 1): 31.

Walker LG, Walker MB, Ogston K et al. (1999) Psychological clinical and pathological effects of relaxation training and guided imagery during primary chemotherapy. *Br J Cancer* **80**: 262–8.

Wall PD, Sweet WH (1967) Temporary abolition of pain in man. *Science* **155**: 108–9.

Walsh D, Donnelly S, Rybickil (2000) The symptoms of advanced cancer: relationship to age, gender and performance status in 1000 patients. *Support Cancer Care* **8**: 175–9.

Walter T (1994) *The Revival of Death*. London: Routledge.

Walter T (1996) A new model of grief: bereavement and biography. *Mortality* **1**(1): 7–25.

Walter T (1999) *On Bereavement: The culture of grief*. Milton Keynes, Bucks: Open University Press.

Wang X, Kavanagh J (2006) Cancer chemotherapy. In: Bruera E, Higginson IJ, Ripamonti C, Von Gunten C (eds), *Textbook of Palliative Medicine*. London: Hodder Arnold, 880–9.

Ward H, Cavanagh J (1997) A descriptive study of self perceived needs of carers with a range of long term problems. *J Public Health* **19**: 281–7.

Wardell DW, Engebretson J (2001) Biological correlates of Reiki touch. *J Adv Nurs* **33**: 439–45.

Warden V, Hurley AC, Volicer L (2003) Development and psychometric evaluation of the pain assessment in advanced dementia (PAINAD) scale. *JAMA* **4**(9): 9–15.

Warren J, Holloway I, Smith P (2000) Fitting in: maintaining a sense of self during hospitalisation. *Int J Nurs Studies* **37**: 229–35.

Wary B, Pandolfo J, Farnetti S (1993) Ce vieillard a t-il mal? Douleur et antalgie. *Ann Soins Palliatifs* 89–98.

Watson M, Greer S (1983) Development of a questionnaire measure of emotional control. *J Psychosomat Res* **27**: 299–305.

Watson M, Greer S, Young J, Inayat Q, Burgess C, Robertson B (1988) Development of a questionnaire measure of adjustment to cancer: the MAC scale. *Psychol Med* **18**: 203–9.

Watson M, Lucas C, Hoy A (2006) *Adult Palliative Care Guidance*, 2nd edn. South West London, Surrey, West Sussex and Hampshire, Mount Vernon and Sussex Cancer Networks and Northern Ireland Palliative Medicine Group.

Wessex Specialist Palliative Care Units (2007) *The Palliative Care Handbook: Advice on Clinical Management*, 6th edn. Hierographics Ltd, Designer House, Sandford Lane Industrial Estate, Wareham, Dorset BH20 4DY.

Wheeler D, Gilbert CL, Launer CA et al. (1998) Weight loss as a predictor of survival and disease progression in HIV infection. *J AIDS* **18**: 80–5.

White A (1998) Electroacupuncture and acupuncture analgesia. In: Filshie J, White A (eds), *Medical Acupuncture: A Western Scientific Approach*. Edinburgh: Churchill Livingstone. 153–75.

White JC (1950) Neurosurgical treatment of persistent pain. *Lancet* **ii**: 161–4.

Wijkstra J, Lacasse Y, Guyatt GH, Goldstein RS (2002) Nocturnal non-invasive positive pressure ventilation for stable chronic obstructive pulmonary disease. *Cochrane Database Syst Rev* **2**: CD002878.

Wilkinson SM (1991) Factors which influence how nurses communicate with cancer patients. *J Adv Nurs* **16**: 677–88.

Wilkinson SM (1994) Stress in cancer nursing – does it really exist? *J Adv Nurs* **20**: 1079–84.

Wilkinson S (1995) Aromatherapy and massage in palliative care. *Int J Palliative Nursing* **1**(1): 21–30.

Wilkinson S, Mula C (2004) Communication in care of the dying. In: Ellershaw J, Wilkinson S (eds), *Care of the Dying – A pathway to excellence.* Oxford: Oxford University Press, 74–90.

Wilkinson S, Aldridge J, Salmon I, Cain E, Wilson B (1999a) An evaluation of aromatherapy massage in palliative care. *Palliative Med* **13**: 409–17.

Wilkinson S, Bailey K, Aldridge J, Roberts A (1999b) A longitudinal evaluation of a communication skills programme. *Palliative Med* **13**: 341–8.

Wilkinson SM, Fellowes D, Leliopoulou C (2005) Does truth-telling influence patients' psychological distress? *European Journal of Palliative Care* **12**(3): 124–6.

Wilson B (1977) *Stress in Hospital.* Edinburgh: Churchill Livingstone Press.

Wilson KG, Chochinov HM, de Faye MA, Breitbart MD (2000) Diagnosis and management of depression in palliative care. In: Chochinov HM, Breitbart W (eds), *Handbook of Psychiatry in Palliative Medicine.* Oxford: Oxford University Press, 25–43.

Winslow M, Seymour J, Clark D (2005) Stories of cancer pain: a historical perspective. *J Pain Symptom Man* **29**: 22–31.

Wood M (2005) The contribution of art therapy to palliative medicine. In: Doyle D, Hanks G, Cherny N, Calman K (eds), *Oxford Textbook of Palliative Medicine*, 3rd edn. Oxford: Oxford University Press, 1063–8.

Woodruff R, Glare P (2005) AIDS in adults. In: Doyle D, Hanks G, Cherny N, Calman K (eds), *Oxford Textbook of Palliative Medicine*, 3rd edn. Oxford: Oxford University Press, 847–880.

Wool MS (1988) Understanding denial in cancer patients. *Adv Psychosom Med* **18**: 37–53.

Woollam CH, Jackson A (1998) Acupuncture in the management of chronic pain. *Anaesthesia* **53**: 593–5.

Worcester A (1935) *The Care of the Aged, the Dying and the Dead.* (Reprint of the original.) New York: Arno Press, 1977: 48.

Worden W (1997) *Grief Counselling and Grief Therapy*, 2nd edn. London: Tavistock Publications.

World Health Organization (1992) *International Classification of Mental and Behavioural Disorders*, 10th revision. Geneva: WHO.

Wright B (1999) Responding to autonomy and disempowerment at the time of sudden death. *Accident Emerg Nurs* **7**: 154–7.

Wright B (2004) Compassion fatigue and how to avoid it. *Palliative Med* **18**: 3–4.

Yennurajalingam S, Bruera E (2006) Haemorrhage. In: Bruera E, Higginson I, Ripamonti C, Von Gunten C (eds), *Textbook of Palliative Medicine.* London: Hodder Arnold, 808–16.

Young-McCaughan S, Dramig SA, Yoder LH et al. (2002) Physical and psychological health outcomes in patients with cancer participating in a structured exercise programme. *Oncol Nurs Forum* **29**: 334.

Zabalegui A, Sanchez S, Sanchez P (2005) Nursing and cancer support groups. *J Adv Nurs* **51**: 369–81.

Zigmond AS, Snaith R (1983) The Hospital Anxiety and Depression Scale. *Acta Psychiatr Scand* **67**: 361–70.

Zisook S, Shuchter SR (1986) The first four years of widowhood. *Psychiatr Ann* **15**: 288–94.

Zorza R, Zorza V (1980) *A Way to Die.* London: Andre Deutsch.

Index